GERALD SHKLAR, D.D.S., M.S.

Charles A. Brackett Professor of Oral Pathology and Head of the Department of Oral Medicine and Oral Pathology; Director, Oral Cancer Diagnostic Service, Harvard School of Dental Medicine; Lecturer in Oral Pathology, Tufts University School of Dental Medicine; Consultant in Oral Pathology, Massachusetts General Hospital, Children's Hospital Medical Center, Brigham and Women's Hospital; Visiting Oral Pathologist, Boston City Hospital; Diplomate of American Board of Oral Pathology and Diplomate of American Board of Periodontology

Oral Cancer
THE DIAGNOSIS, THERAPY, MANAGEMENT AND REHABILITATION OF THE ORAL CANCER PATIENT

with 26 Contributors

W. B. Saunders Company / 1984

Philadelphia   London   Toronto   Mexico City   Rio de Janeiro   Sydney   Tokyo

W. B. Saunders Company: West Washington Square
Philadelphia, PA 19105

1 St. Anne's Road
Eastbourne, East Sussex BN21 3UN, England

1 Goldthorne Avenue
Toronto, Ontario M8Z 5T9, Canada

Apartado 26370—Cedro 512
Mexico 4, D.F., Mexico

Rua Coronel Cabrita, 8
Sao Cristovao Caixa Postal 21176
Rio de Janeiro, Brazil

9 Waltham Street
Artarmon, N.S.W. 2064, Australia

Ichibancho, Central Bldg., 22-1 Ichibancho
Chiyoda-Ku, Tokyo 102, Japan

Library of Congress Cataloging in Publication Data

Main entry under title:

Oral cancer.

1. Mouth—Cancer.   I. Shklar, Gerald. [DNLM: 1. Mouth
   neoplasms. WU 280 0645]

RC280.M6073 1984   616.99′431   83–20382

ISBN 0–7216–1271–7

Oral Cancer: The Diagnosis, Therapy, Management and
Rehabilitation of the Oral Cancer Patient   ISBN   0-7216-1271-7

Last digit is the print number: 9   8   7   6   5   4   3   2   1

Contributors

JOSEPH B. BARRON, D.M.D.
Lecturer on Prosthetic Dentistry, Co-Director, Maxillofacial Prosthetic Division, Harvard School of Dental Medicine.

R. BRUCE DONOFF, D.M.D., M.D.
Professor and Head, Department of Oral and Maxillofacial Surgery, Harvard School of Dental Medicine; Chief of Service, Department of Oral and Maxillofacial Surgery, Massachusetts General Hospital.

CHESTER W. DOUGLASS, D.D.S., Ph.D.
Associate Professor and Chairman, Department of Dental Care Administration, Harvard School of Dental Medicine.

ELLEN EISENBERG, D.M.D.
Assistant Professor of Oral Pathology, University of Connecticut School of Dentistry.

THOMAS J. ERVIN, M.D.
Assistant Professor of Medicine, Harvard Medical School; Assistant Professor of Medicine, Dana-Farber Cancer Institute.

EMIL FREI, III, M.D.
Professor of Oncologic Medicine, Harvard Medical School; Director and Physician in Chief, Dana-Farber Cancer Institute.

SUMNER P. FRIM, D.M.D.
Assistant Clinical Professor of Oral Pathology, Tufts University School of Dental Medicine; Assistant Clinical Professor of Pathology, Tufts University School of Medicine; Instructor in Oral Medicine and Oral Pathology, Harvard School of Dental Medicine.

MARILIE D. GAMMON, M.S.P.H.
Research Epidemiologist, Department of Dental Care Administration, Harvard School of Dental Medicine.

JOHN L. GIUNTA, D.M.D., M.S.
Professor of Oral Pathology, Tufts University School of Dental Medicine; Lecturer in Oral Pathology, Harvard School of Dental Medicine.

WALTER C. GURALNICK, D.M.D.
Professor of Oral and Maxillofacial Surgery, Harvard School of Dental Medicine; Chief of Ambulatory Services, Massachusetts General Hospital.

WILLIAM J. HORGAN, D.D.S., M.P.H.
Research Fellow in Dental Care Administration, Harvard School of Dental Medicine.

DANIEL D. KARP, M.D.
Assistant Professor of Medicine, Boston University School of Medicine; Director of Clinical Hematology, Boston VA Hospital.

DEBORAH GEORGIAN KOCH, M.A., CCC-SP
Speech-Language Pathologist, Massachusetts General Hospital.

PETER B. LOCKHART, D.D.S.
Assistant Professor of Oral Medicine and Oral Pathology, Harvard School of Dental Medicine; Surgeon, Brigham and Women's Hospital; Consultant in Surgical Oncology, Dana-Farber Cancer Institute.

DEBORAH LUCKS, D.D.S.
Research Fellow in Oral Pathology (Oral Oncology), Harvard School of Dental Medicine.

EDWARD C. MALOOF, D.D.S., M.P.H.
Lecturer in Oral Pathology, Harvard School of Dental Medicine.

PHILIP L. McCARTHY, M.D.
Associate Professor of Oral Pathology and Head, Division of Oral Medicine, Tufts University School of Dental Medicine; Instructor in Dermatology, Harvard Medical School; Assistant Dermatologist, Massachusetts General Hospital; Chief of Dermatology, Carney and Quincy City Hospitals.

ADEYEMI MOSADOMI, D.M.D., M.S.
Professor of Oral Pathology and Dean, School of Dental Sciences, College of Medicine of the University of Lagos, Lagos, Nigeria.

JOSEPH E. MURRAY, M.D.
Professor of Surgery, Harvard Medical School; Chief of Plastic Surgery, Brigham and Women's Hospital; Chief of Plastic Surgery, Children's Hospital Medical Center.

JOEL L. SCHWARTZ, D.M.D., D.M.Sc.
Assistant Professor of Oral Pathology, Harvard School of Dental Medicine.

DAVID SHERMAN, M.D.
Assistant Professor of Radiation Therapy, University of Massachusetts Medical School; Associate Director of Radiotherapy, St. Vincent's Hospital, Worcester, Massachusetts.

GERALD SHKLAR, D.D.S., M.S.
Charles A. Brackett Professor of Oral Pathology and Head, Department of Oral Medicine and Oral Pathology, Harvard School of Dental Medicine; Director of Oral Cancer Diagnostic Service, Harvard School of Dental Medicine.

DENNIS B. SOLT, D.M.D., Ph.D.
Associate Professor of Pathology, Northwestern University Medical and Dental Schools.

STEPHEN T. SONIS, D.M.D., D.M.Sc.
Associate Professor of Oral Medicine and Oral Pathology, Harvard School of Dental Medicine; Chief of Dental Services, Brigham and Women's Hospital; Consultant in Surgical Oncology, Dana-Farber Cancer Institute.

C. C. WANG, M.D.
Professor of Radiation Therapy, Harvard Medical School; Head, Division of Clinical Services, Department of Radiation Medicine, Massachusetts General Hospital.

RALPH R. WEICHSELBAUM, M.D.
Associate Professor of Radiation Therapy, Harvard Medical School; Head of Brigham and Women's Division, Joint Center for Radiation Therapy.

RICHARD E. WILSON, M.D.
Professor of Surgery, Harvard Medical School; Chief, Surgical Oncology, Brigham and Women's Hospital and Dana-Farber Cancer Institute.

Preface

Oral oncology is essentially that branch of oncology that is concerned with the oral cavity. Primarily, it deals with oral cancer and its management. Secondarily, it involves the oral problems of all cancer patients who receive therapy—either radiation therapy or chemotherapy or a combination of these and other modalities. In oral oncology, a close cooperation between the dentist and the physician, and among the various specialists of both professions, is required. Dentists now receive training in the specialized area of oral oncology, and they will be able to guide both professions toward improved care for the patient who has oral cancer and improved oral care for the patient with non-oral cancer who develops oral problems resulting from cancer therapy. The oral oncologist currently plays a significant role in three types of environment: in cancer centers, in university-based dental and medical schools with teaching and research programs that deal with oral cancer, and in community health programs.

Regrettably, the mortality rate from oral cancer is still high. Almost half the patients who have oral cancer die. This amounts to 11,000 deaths per year, while some 28,000 new cases of oral cancer are diagnosed annually in the United States. Incidence and mortality rates vary in other parts of the world, ranging from Hong Kong, Singapore, and France, where the incidence rate is high, to Japan, Mexico, and Israel, where the incidence rate is low. Figures for the United States fall somewhere in the middle of various worldwide surveys of oral cancer.

The major reason for the high mortality rate of oral cancer is late diagnosis, with lesions that are large, deeply invasive, and often metastatic to regional lymph nodes. It is not a tribute to the professions nor to public health authorities that an area of the body that is so easily accessible for examination and a lesion that is so easily diagnosed can still result in so many deaths. In addition to resulting in many deaths, oral cancer results in much morbidity. Late diagnosis and treatment of large invasive lesions often results in extensive mutilation of oral and facial structures, with poor appearance and function following therapy.

Education must be a major thrust if oral cancer is to be found and diagnosed in its early stages, when therapy is simple and highly successful. Such education must be brought to the high-risk population in our society, adequately identified as cigarette smoking, alcohol drinking males with poor oral hygiene and poor nutrition. Public education must be aimed in two directions: the necessity of routine oral examinations by qualified personnel, and the removal or diminution of factors known to be significant in the etiology of oral cancer. Thus, prevention of oral cancer is a reasonable goal, just as is early diagnosis. Prevention of oral cancer also includes the recognition of oral precancerous lesions such as leukoplakia, erythroplasia, and papilloma.

Therapy for oral cancer has improved significantly within the past 25 years. Chemotherapy has now been added to surgical approaches and megavoltage radiation. A combined therapeutic approach is now the rule rather than the exception, with authoritative voices in all specialties joining their talents and experiences for the benefit of the patient.

This book has emerged from a program in oral oncology developed at the Harvard School of Dental Medicine and its affiliated hospitals; the Brigham and Women's Hospital, the Massachusetts General Hospital, the Children's Hospital Medical Center, and the Dana-Farber Cancer Institute. The various authoritative chapters have been prepared by specialists who have been involved in various aspects of the program. It is hoped that this introductory text will serve as a guide to the further development of oral oncology programs throughout the United States and elsewhere. Many clinical cancer education programs have been supported in dental schools by the National Cancer Institute of the National Institutes of Health. The programs were of great value in the development of improved oral cancer teaching and in the development of improved facilities for the early diagnosis of oral cancer. Expanded support will be necessary if oral cancer, a major health problem, is to be brought under proper control and if the high mortality and morbidity figures are to take their place in the history of medicine and stomatology rather than serving as an unpleasant reminder of our inadequacy in solving a relatively simple and straightforward medical and social problem.

Contents

1

Clinical manifestations of oral cancer

WALTER C. GURALNICK, D.M.D.

Oral cancer constitutes 3 to 5 percent of all cancers and accounts for approximately 8000 deaths each year. Because it is among the most obvious of all tumors, its early detection is possible and significantly reduces mortality. The following are suggested as guidelines to early detection: a high index of suspicion; systematic, careful examination of the oral cavity; and awareness of the presenting symptoms of oral carcinoma. The advantage of early detection, before lymph node involvement, is shown by the 70 percent survival rate of patients who do not have nodal involvement. This is in marked contrast to the 30 percent 5-year survival rate of patients whose diagnosis is established after nodal disease exists. It is, therefore, apparent that familiarity with oral cancer is particularly important for dentists, because they, as the primary oral health caretakers, are in the most favorable position to detect the disease in its early stages.

A high index of suspicion of oral lesions is stimulated by knowledge of the epidemiology of oral cancer. There is compelling, statistical evidence that drinking and smoking are major etiologic agents. Knowing this, dentists should be particularly careful to view patients who are known to drink and smoke heavily as being at high risk. These patients should be examined frequently to detect mucosal changes and potential malignancy.

As important as careful history taking and knowledge of the patient are in early detection, examination of the mouth and the neck is critical. Such an examination is easily carried out by the simple skills that are currently taught to all dental students and one's skills are further sharpened by clinical application. Of utmost importance is systematic examination of all the tissues of the oral cavity, including areas that are less readily visualized, such as the retromolar trigone, tonsillar fossa, pos-

terior third of the tongue, floor of the mouth, palate, and oropharynx. A thorough examination of all these areas may disclose suspicious lesions that require diagnosis.

Most neoplasms of the oral cavity are squamous cell carcinoma and are found, in order of frequency, in the lower lip, alveolar ridge (the mandibular far more frequently than the maxillary), floor of the mouth, lateral margin of the tongue, retromolar trigone, and buccal mucosa. The lesions may be quite innocuous in appearance if discovered in the early stage or invasive and destructive if found in the advanced stage. An early lesion may appear as a round, small granular excrescence, arousing suspicion because of the subtle difference from normal mucosa or because it was not noticed at a previous examination. By contrast, an advanced oral carcinoma will appear as an ulcer with friable tissue that bleeds readily when touched. It will also be attached to deeper tissues when examined and, if close to underlying bone, may be found, by x-ray examination, to have caused bone resorption by invasion of the tumor.

Another lesion that commonly causes suspicion is the oral ulcer. It is frequently related to trauma such as that caused by an ill-fitting denture, biting of one's cheek, or laceration of the mucosa by sharp objects. Of utmost importance in cancer screening is the fact that a traumatic ulcer is expected to heal within a week after the causative irritant has been eliminated. If a denture is suspected of causing irritation, it can be either corrected or not worn. The patient should be examined within a week to determine whether the suspected lesion has improved. However, if appreciable healing has not occurred, a definitive diagnosis must be established. This is done by performing a biopsy.

Generally, oral carcinoma appears as a pap-

1

illary configuration, as an ulcer, or as a deeply invasive lesion with minimal surface manifestation. Fortunately, the latter type of lesion is rare. The papillary or verrucous type may have a narrow or broad base and tends to be characterized by slower growth and being less invasive than the other forms. The ulcerative variety grows more rapidly and tends to form an indurated raised margin. As lesions become larger, a combination of papillary and ulcerative areas often arises, as well as considerable induration at the margin of the lesion.

Buccal mucosal lesions often occur in areas of keratosis. The appearance of an early carcinoma may be no different from a desquamated area, often associated with benign, keratotic lesions. Early detection is dependent upon keen and frequent observation and appropriate pathological examination of the tissue. The size of a primary lesion and the extension to regional lymph nodes and other tissues are important criteria for cancer therapy.

In order to clarify the existing knowledge about lesions, nodal disease, and metastasis, the American Joint Committee for Cancer Staging and End Results Reporting developed a TNM staging system in 1977. T represents the size of the lesion on a centimeter scale. N represents nodal disease, and its subgroups refer to the number, size, and location—either unilateral or bilateral—of cervical nodes. M represents distant metastasis, and the numbers indicate its presence or absence.

T categories:
T1—a lesion up to 2 cm in size.
T2—a lesion greater than 2 cm but less than 4 cm.
T3—a lesion greater than 4 cm.
T4—a lesion greater than 4 cm and deeply invasive of underlying tissues.

N categories:
Nx—nodes cannot be assessed.
N0—no clinically positive node.
N1—single clinically positive homolateral node less than 3 cm in diameter.
N2a—single clinically positive homolateral node 3 to 6 cm in diameter.
N2b—multiple clinically positive homolateral nodes, none greater than 6 cm in diameter.
N3a—clinically positive homolateral nodes, one greater than 6 cm in diameter.
N3b—bilateral clinically positive nodes.
N3c—contralateral clinically positive nodes only.

M categories:
M0—no distant metastasis.
M1—distant metastasis.

Cervical metastases should always be suspected, and examination for them should be an integral part of every oral cancer investigation. Statistically, the incidence of cervical metastases for early lesions, T1, is only 10 to 20 percent. By contrast, the incidence of lymph node involvement for T2 lesions is 25 to 30 percent and for T3 and T4 lesions, it is 50 to 70 percent. Again, the prognostic benefits of early detection are apparent.

Oral cancer other than epidermoid or squamous cell carcinoma is rare. Malignant tumors of glandular origin may be found on the palate, an area that contains numerous mucous glands beneath the mucosa.

Although squamous cell carcinoma occurs on the palate, the more common tumors in this site are the mucoepidermoid and adenoid cystic carcinomas of salivary gland origin. They are deceptively benign in appearance, usually manifesting as painless unilateral lumps in the posterior palate adjacent to the molar region. The overlying mucosa is ordinarily intact, and differentiating such tumors from an abcess or benign growth is impossible by observation alone.

The clinical features of oral cancer may resemble those of a variety of benign oral conditions. In Figures 1–1 through 1–8, the appearance of oral cancer is shown, and the unreliability of *tumor appearance alone* as a definitive diagnostic tool is indicated.

CLINICAL FEATURES OF ORAL CANCER IN DIFFERENT AREAS OF THE MOUTH

Lower Lip

The mucous membrane surface of the lower lip is a common site for the development of oral carcinoma. Both smoking and actinic radiation predispose the lower lip to malignant transformation, often resulting in actinic cheilitis and leukoplakia in patients who have a labial carcinoma. The labial mucosa may also show changes in aging, with a thin and wrinkled surface, a red color, and relative dryness. The carcinoma is usually localized, with a raised, indurated margin and a central area of surface necrosis or ulceration. At the skin margin of the lip, invariably there is crusting. Some induration is usually present adjacent to the visible margins of the tumor. In chronic pipesmokers, the pipe stem is often related to

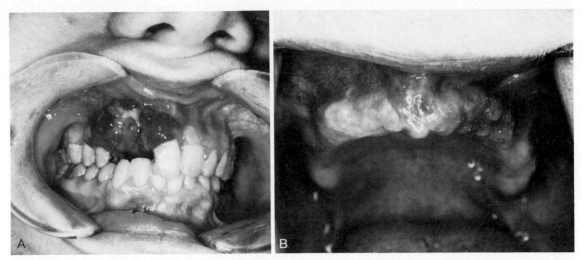

Figure 1–1. *A,* Very suspicious appearing lesion of the alveolar ridge. Tissue diagnosis: pyogenic granuloma. *B,* A relatively innocuous appearing alveolar ridge lesion. Tissue diagnosis: squamous cell carcinoma.

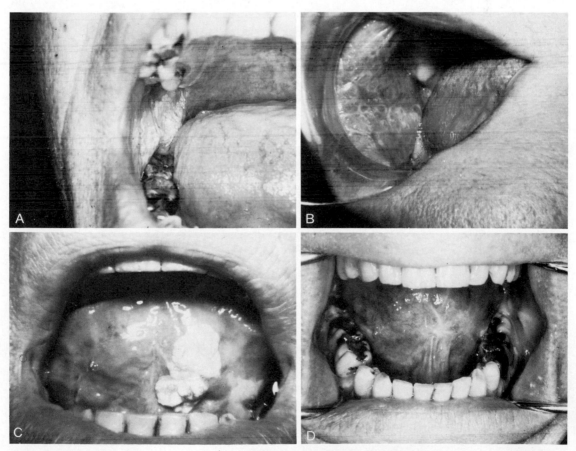

Figure 1–2. *A,* "White" lesion: leukoplakia. (Ten years later, squamous cell carcinoma developed in this area.) *B,* "White" lesion: lichen planus. *C,* "White" lesion of the floor of the mouth in a heavy smoker. Tissue diagnosis: squamous cell carcinoma. *D,* Same patient as in *C* after radiation therapy.

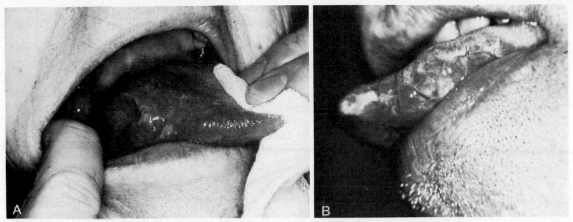

Figure 1–3. *A,* Carcinoma of the tongue, with a very characteristic appearance; craterlike lesion with rolled edges. *B,* Luetic tongue, at high risk for carcinoma.

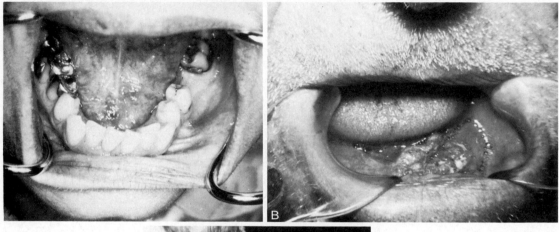

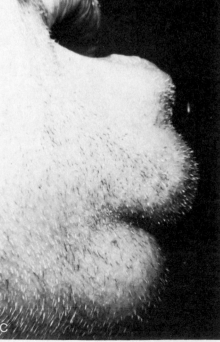

Figure 1–4. *A,* Early detection of a small, erythroplastic lesion of the floor of the mouth. Tissue diagnosis: squamous cell carcinoma—T1NOMO. *B,* Advanced, squamous cell carcinoma of the floor of the mouth. *C,* Direct extension of the tumor into the neck.

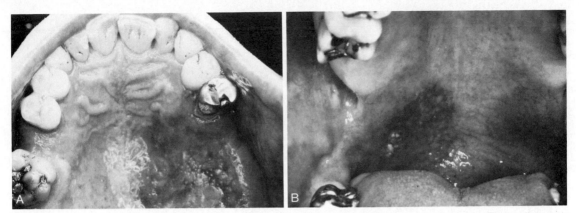

Figure 1–5. *A,* "Red" lesion: erythroplasia of the palate. *B,* A similar appearing "red" lesion. Tissue diagnosis: squamous cell carcinoma.

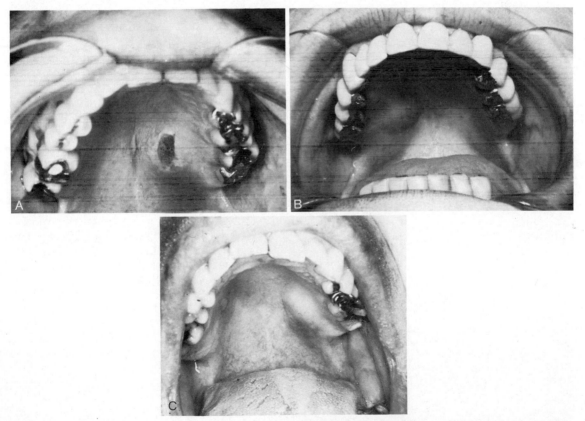

Figure 1–6. *A,* Painless, firm mass on the palate. Histologic diagnosis (from obvious biopsy site): benign, pleomorphic adenoma. *B,* A similar appearing, asymptomatic lump on the palate. Tissue diagnosis: mucoepidermoid carcinoma. *C,* Another similar-looking palatal lump. Tissue diagnosis: squamous cell carcinoma.

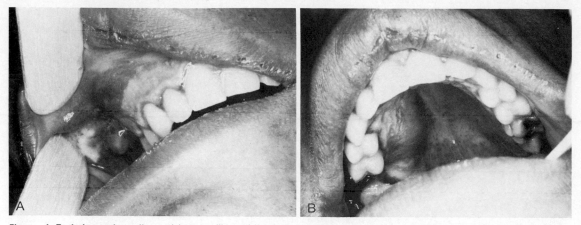

Figure 1–7. *A,* Asymptomatic, sudden swelling of the buccal sulcus. Tissue diagnosis: osteogenic sarcoma of the maxilla. *B,* Rapid extension of the tumor.

the position of the tumor. Carcinoma of the lower lip is relatively painless, grows slowly, and rarely invades deeply. Patients often wait until the lesion is large and extensive before presenting for diagnosis and treatment. Cancer of the lower lip rarely metastasizes. In those few cases that do spread to regional nodes, submental or submandibular (submaxillary) nodes may be involved.

Upper Lip

The mucosa of the upper lip is an uncommon site of oral cancer. Lesions usually originate on the skin and spread to the mucous membrane surface of the upper lip. They tend to be indurated and ulcerated lesions. Basal cell tumors involve the upper lip more often than do epidermoid carcinomas. Metastatic spread to submental or submandibular nodes is possible but rare.

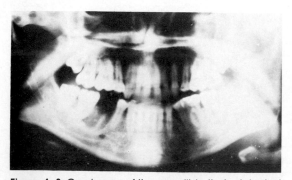

Figure 1–8. Carcinoma of the mandible that originated in the socket of the first molar. Failure of the extraction site to heal normally aroused suspicion. Repeated biopsies proved the lesion to be carcinoma.

Tongue

The tongue is frequently a site of oral carcinoma, and this site always signifies a serious prognosis. Cancer of the tongue usually starts as a small ulcer and gradually infiltrates deeply and extensively, resulting in the tongue losing its normal motility. The patient becomes aware that there is some difficulty or abnormality relating to speaking or swallowing. These symptoms become very marked when a lingual carcinoma spreads to the floor of the mouth, which results in the ventral surface of the tongue becoming attached to the adjacent tissue. Cancer of the tongue, even in its early stage, is painful, and in later stages may be exceedingly painful, with the patient complaining of radiating pain to the neck and ear. The lateral borders of the tongue are more frequently involved than is the dorsal surface. However, if the filiform and fungiform papillae undergo atrophy, leaving a smooth, denuded surface on the dorsal surface of the tongue, this region becomes highly susceptible to leukoplakia and results in a greater risk of the development of carcinoma. The smooth atrophic tongue occurs in cases of severe iron deficiency, vitamin B deficiency, Plummer-Vinson syndrome, tertiary syphilis, and lichen planus.

The tragic aspect of carcinoma of the tongue is that it metastasizes early in its course of development. Both submandibular and jugular nodes become involved.

Floor of the Mouth

The small area beneath and anterior to the tongue may occasionally be the site of an oral cancer lesion. It is usually a small papillary, erosive or an ulcerative lesion. It may be hidden beneath the tongue and may be related to the attachment region of the lingual frenum, which is easily traumatized. Malignancies of the floor of the mouth may be painful, but symptoms are often expressed as an irritation or a feeling of dryness. If the lesion is indurated or papillary, it may be felt by the patient's tongue as being something unusual. Both submandibular and jugular nodes may become involved if the tumor metastasizes.

Buccal Mucosa

The inner surfaces of the cheeks are frequent sites of oral cancer. It may be papillary or erosive in appearance and is often traumatized by the teeth if it is near the occlusal line. Leukoplakic lesions often precede the development of buccal mucosal cancer. There may be pain, but it is not a striking feature of buccal mucosal cancer. Patients may describe a "burning" sensation or may feel a roughened area with their tongue. Submandibular nodes are involved if the lesion metastasizes.

Gingiva

Cancer of the gingiva is not common but does occur and must be suspected in a chronic destructive lesion that results in loss of gingival tissue and exposure of the alveolar bone. The localized appearance of this type of lesion should alert the clinician to the probability that it is not chronic destructive periodontal disease (periodontitis). The latter condition rarely results in ulceration or surface necrosis. Gingival cancer may be painful and often causes bleeding during toothbrushing, alerting the patient to something unusual. Gingival carcinomas tend to be ulcerated lesions on the attached gingiva and usually invade into the underlying alveolar bone. The lower jaw is involved more often than the upper jaw. Metastatic spread from gingival lesions is variable. Lesions of the upper gingiva may involve submandibular and jugular nodes. Lesions of the lower gingiva may involve submental, submandibular, and jugular nodes.

Edentulous Alveolar Mucosa

When the teeth have been lost, the alveolar bone is covered with a thick, well-keratinized mucosa. Cancer often occurs on alveolar mucosa, particularly in patients who have poorly fitting dentures. If the dental appliances produce constant low-grade trauma or irritation, the malignancy may arise in that particular site. The borders of dentures may also traumatize tissues, irritating the floor of the mouth, mucobuccal fold, or palate. Lesions of edentulous alveolar mucosa tend to be erosive or ulcerative with raised margins. They may invade into underlying alveolar bone. Metastatic spread is similar to that of gingival lesions.

Mucobuccal Fold (Vestibule)

This is an unusual site for the development of oral cancer; however, it is occasionally seen here. It may be a papillary or ulcerative lesion and may be close to the labial frenum.

Hard Palate

This is a common site of oral cancer, particularly in smokers. Leukoplakia manifests in the hard palate in heavy smokers, and carcinoma usually develops in an area of leukoplakia in these high-risk patients. The tumor is often papillary or exophytic, rather than flat or ulcerated. Metastatic spread to jugular nodes may occur.

Soft Palate and Uvula

The soft palate and uvula may be involved in oral cancer but are not common sites. Lesions may be ulcers with raised margins or fungating masses with central areas of necrosis or ulceration. Cancer in this region tends to invade early and to produce severe symptoms of pain, particularly when swallowing. Pain from this region may radiate widely and be expressed by the patient as pain in the ear, neck, jaws, or forehead. Metastatic spread to jugular nodes may occur.

The rewards of early detection of oral cancer are measurable and gratifying. The patient whose oral cancer is detected at the T1 stage with no cervical node involvement has a high potential of being cured. By contrast, later discovery markedly alters the patient's prognosis. Diagnostic potential is dependent upon a few simple skills: careful observation and systematic examination of the oral cavity and appropriate use of incisional biopsy procedures.

REFERENCES

1. Keller, A. Z.: Cirrhosis of the liver, alcoholism and heavy smoking associated with cancer of the mouth and pharynx. Cancer, *23*:920, 1969.
2. Krolls, S. O., and Hoffman, S.: Squamous cell carcinoma of the oral soft tissues: a statistical analysis of 14,252 cases by age, sex and race of patients. J.A.D.A., *92*:517, 1976.
3. Ledlie, E. M., and Hammer, M. H.: Cancer of the mouth: a report on 800 cases. Br. J. Cancer, *4*:6, 1950.
4. Lee, E. S., and Wilson, J. S. P.: Carcinoma involving the lower alveolus. Brit. J. Surg., *68*:85, 1973.
5. Lund, C., et al.: Epidermoid carcinoma of the tongue. Acta Radiol. (Stockholm), *14*:513, 1975.
6. Mashberg, A.: Erythroplasia vs. leukoplakia in the diagnosis of early asymptomatic oral squamous cell carcinomas. Cancer, *37*:2149, 1976.
7. Mashberg, A., and Meyers, H.: Anatomical site and size of 222 early asymptomatic oral squamous cell carcinomas: a continuing prospective study of oral cancer. Cancer, *37*:2149, 1976.
8. Shear, M., Hawkins, D. M., and Farr, N. W.: The prediction of lymph node metastases from oral squamous carcinoma. Cancer, *37*:1901, 1976.
9. Shedd, D. P.: Clinical characteristics of early oral cancer. J.A.M.A., *215*:955, 1971.

2

Microscopic pathology of oral cancer

GERALD SHKLAR, D.D.S., M.S.

Most oral malignant tumors (approximately 97 percent) are epidermoid carcinomas. Two to 3 percent of oral malignant neoplasms are adenocarcinomas of various types, and the remaining portion, 1 percent, includes rare primary oral mucosal malignancies such as lymphoma, malignant melanoma, and fibrosarcoma. Essentially, oral cancer signifies epidermoid carcinoma, otherwise termed *squamous cell carcinoma*. Epidermoid carcinoma of the mouth may be well differentiated or may be poorly differentiated or anaplastic. It is not only important that clinicians have a specific diagnosis of epidermoid carcinoma, but the knowledge of the degree of differentiation or grade of tumor will often determine the nature of the overall treatment plan and will aid in the evaluation of prognosis. Apart from other considerations, such as location and size of the lesion, the well-differentiated oral epidermoid carcinoma is treated conservatively and has a good prognosis. The anaplastic oral epidermoid carcinoma, by virtue of its biologic characteristics such as deep invasion and early metastatic spread, must be treated aggressively, often with several therapeutic modalities, and the prognosis should still be guarded. An interesting facet of oral cancer relates to the anatomic site of origin. Carcinomas of the lip are invariably of the well-differentiated variety and have an excellent prognosis. Carcinomas of the tongue, on the other hand, tend to be of the anaplastic variety, and their prognosis is poor, with less than 50 percent of the patients surviving 5 years.

WELL-DIFFERENTIATED EPIDERMOID CARCINOMA

The well-differentiated oral epidermoid carcinoma tends to be papillary or verrucous in overall configuration (Fig. 2–1). Invasion into underlying connective tissue occurs, as in any malignant tumor, but is usually local in nature and rarely involves the underlying bone. Metastasis to regional lymph nodes may occur but is a late phenomenon, and lymph node involvement tends to be absent in most cases.

Histologically, the cells show some pleomorphism, but they are easily discerned as epithelial cells. The nuclei are somewhat larger than normal, and the nuclear-cytoplasmic ratio is altered, but not notably so. The nuclei tend to stain lightly and evenly throughout the lesion (see Figs. 2–1B and C). Mitotic activity is increased, but the mitoses are of the normal variety, with prophase, metaphase, anaphase, and telophase patterns readily discernible. Abnormal or bizarre cell forms are rarely seen. Large amounts of keratin are formed, and this may be the most significant histologic feature that determines the interpretation of a well-differentiated lesion (see Fig. 1A).

Furthermore, the invading cords and nests of epithelium still show differentiation into the stratum germinativum, or basal layer; stratum spinosum, or prickle-cell layer; and stratum corneum, or keratinizing layer. In a well-differentiated carcinoma, keratin can usually be seen with relative ease. However, if there is uncertainty, special stains may be used to

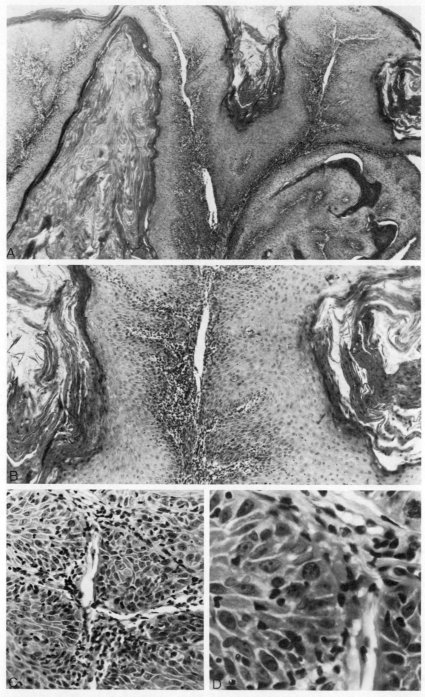

Figure 2–1. *A*, Low-power view (× 50) of papillary, well-differentiated epidermoid carcinoma of the palate. Large amounts of keratin are evident. *B*, High-power view (× 100) of lesion showing both orthokeratin and parakeratin. The epithelial cells appear relatively homogeneous in staining. *C*, High-power view (× 250) showing variability in cell size, shape, and cohesion. *D*, High-power view (× 350) showing large nuclei and altered nuclear-cytoplasmic ratio.

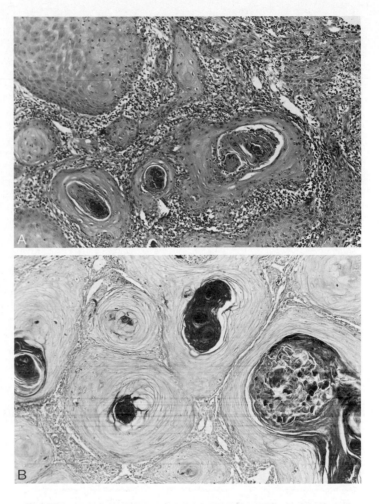

Figure 2–2. A, Well-differentiated epidermoid carcinoma of the buccal mucosa. Note the keratin within the invading projections of the tumor. (Hematoxylin-eosin stain × 100) B, Tumor in A stained to emphasize the presence of keratin. (Ayoub-Shklar modification of the Mallory stain × 100.)

reveal the keratin (Fig. 2–2). The well-differentiated carcinoma also has a relatively well-defined basement membrane, and this can clearly be seen, even in the advancing or invading cords and nests (Fig. 2–3). If desired, the basement membrane can effectively be shown with the periodic acid-Schiff stain for polysaccharides. The basement membrane may be thickened in areas, and there may be some minor discontinuity. The cells of the

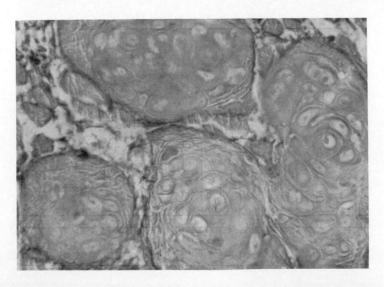

Figure 2–3. Well-differentiated epidermoid carcinoma showing distinct basement membrane. (Periodic acid-Schiff stain × 350.)

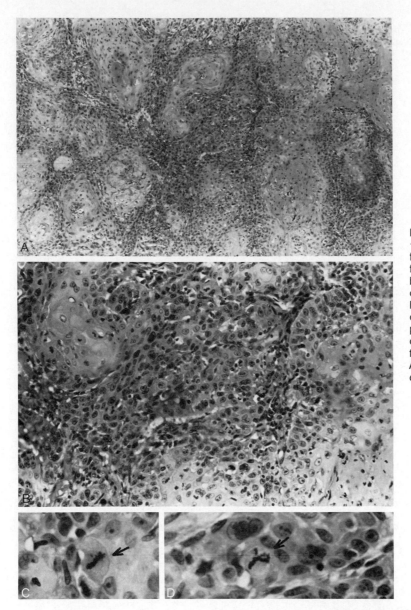

Figure 2–4. *A,* Low-power view (×
100) of moderately well-differentiated epidermoid carcinoma of
the buccal mucosa. Keratin is
being formed but is abnormal and
contains nuclei and entire cells. *B,*
High-power view (× 200) showing
deeply staining nuclei, cellular
pleomorphism, and abnormal keratin formation. *C,* Normal mitotic
figure in metaphase (× 600). *D,*
Abnormal tripolar mitotic figure (×
600).

tumor adhere well to one another, and the
intercellular spaces caused by cell separation
are not obvious.

Chronic inflammatory infiltration is always
present, is primarily lymphocytic in character,
and tends to be localized to the base of the
tumor. Invading cords of tumor are usually
surrounded by lymphocytes (see Figs. 2–1*B*
and 2–2A). Basically, a well-differentiated tumor causes minimal surface necrosis except in
larger lesions. Because the tumor grows
slowly, an adequate blood supply develops,
and the tumor cells remain viable. As the
tumor expands, the surface becomes easily
traumatized and will then undergo ulceration
and necrosis.

In an epidermoid carcinoma that is moderately well differentiated, keratin is formed, but
the tumor is more invasive and the cells are
more variable in size, shape, and chromaticity.
Keratin formation is not as obvious and striking as in the well-differentiated papillary type
of epidermoid carcinoma (Fig. 2–4A and *B*).
There is less keratin, and it appears somewhat
unusual, containing multiple nuclei and entire
cells. In addition to the cellular pleomorphism,
there are numerous normal mitotic figures,
usually in metaphase (Fig. 2–4*C*) and occasional bizarre mitoses, often of the tripolar
variety (Fig. 2–4*D*). Large cells and multinucleated tumor giant cells may be present, but
they are not seen in appreciable numbers. The

demarcation of stratum germinativum, stratum spinosum, and stratum corneum is less distinct than in the very well-differentiated tumor, although there is some semblance of this stratification within the invading cords and nests of epithelium. Nucleoli appear more prominent than in the nuclei of well-differentiated lesions.

ANAPLASTIC EPIDERMOID CARCINOMA

In anaplastic lesions, there is notable cellular pleomorphism (see Figs. 2–5 and 2–6), an absence of keratin (see Figs. 2–5 through 2–8), deep invasion with discontinuity of the basement membrane, separation of cells, and the presence of bizarre cell forms and bizarre mitotic figures. The cells tend to present a rounded rather than a polyhedral shape, and intercellular spaces appear as they lose their normal adherence to one another (Fig. 2–5). Ultrastructural studies show that the cell separation results from the loss of desmosomes and that the discontinuity of the basement membrane results from the loss of basal lamina. Anaplastic carcinomas usually do not have a papillary or verrucous configuration; they tend to invade deeply rather than merely proliferate at the mucosal surface. They are also apt to ulcerate early, because their rapid growth outstrips an effective blood supply. Surface necrosis is a common feature of anaplastic lesions, and cellular degeneration is often apparent. (Fig. 2–6).

Although numerous normal mitoses can be seen, in anaplastic carcinoma, a diagnostic feature of this type of tumor is the presence of abnormal or bizarre mitoses and bizarre cell forms. Bizarre mitoses are large and often tripolar. The cell attempts to divide into three cells instead of two, and the chromosomes appear as three sets in a variety of configurations. Bizarre cell forms include large cells with single large hyperchromatic nuclei or giant cells with multiple nuclei. The nuclei divide, but cytoplasm apparently does not divide synchronously.

As cells separate, they also have a tendency to spindle and resemble connective tissue cells. In a highly anaplastic epidermoid carcinoma, the epithelial origin may not be readily apparent and the lesion may be confused with a sarcoma, because keratin is absent, cellular adherence is uncertain, bizarre cell forms are seen, and pleomorphism is notable. (Fig. 2–7). Findings of ultrastructural studies may occasionally reveal desmosomes and fragments of basal lamina.

Inflammatory infiltration tends to be extensive and diffuse, with numerous polymorphonuclear leukocytes in the infiltrate as well as the lymphocytes, plasma cells, and histiocytes.

SPINDLE CELL CARCINOMA

The term *spindle cell carcinoma* has been used to designate lesions that appear highly anaplastic histologically but may behave less aggressive clinically than their microscopic appearance would suggest. Most of these tumors have been reported to be located on the lip. They are composed of cells that are spindle shaped and that resemble connective tissue cells. Most carcinomas of oral mucosa that appear as spindle-shaped lesions are highly malignant, and their biologic activity does, in fact, conform to their anaplastic appearance (Fig. 2–8). Rarely does a lip lesion appear to be less aggressive than anticipated. Spindle cell carcinomas of the tongue or buccal mucosa are highly aggressive and tend to metastasize early.

MODERATELY DIFFERENTIATED CARCINOMAS

The degree of differentiation of most oral epidermoid carcinomas is somewhere between the well-differentiated and the anaplastic extremes. Nevertheless, the pathologist should attempt to offer an appraisal of the degree of differentiation, because this would be of assistance in the overall clinical management.

HISTOLOGIC GRADING OF ORAL EPIDERMOID CARCINOMA

Many pathologists and most clinicians prefer to use numbers to indicate differentiation or lack of it. Broders[3] originally used Grade 1 to Grade 4 as a means of indicating the percentage of differentiated cells. Grade 1 lesions had 75 percent of cells differentiated, Grade 2 lesions had 50 percent, Grade 3 had 25 percent, and Grade 4 had less than 25 percent. Because many features other than the cells themselves indicate the degree of differentiation, and because the percentages of so-called differentiated cells vary from area to area, the grades today tend to be used loosely in placing a numerical value on the overall degree of differentiation of the tumor. Thus, Grade 1 would indicate a low grade or well-differentiated tumor with significant amounts of keratin being formed and with minimal cellular

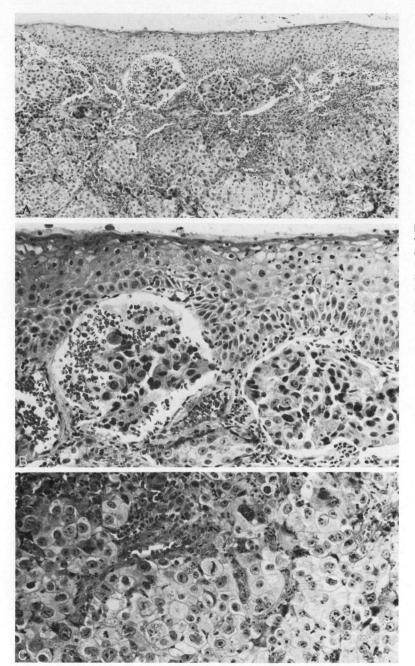

Figure 2–5. *A*, Medium-power view (× 100) of anaplastic carcinoma of the edentulous alveolar ridge, invading deeply and spreading beneath the adjacent surface mucosa. *B*, High-power view (× 200) showing that the epithelium adjacent to the carcinoma is dysplastic and is undermined by rounded tumor cells that are separated from one another. The tumor cells are highly pleomorphic. *C*, Invading tumor cells showing notable pleomorphism and numerous mitoses. There is no evidence of keratinization (× 200).

Illustration continued on opposite page

pleomorphism. Grade 2 would indicate more pleomorphism, less keratin, some bizarre cell forms, and widened intercellular spaces. Grades 3 and 4 would indicate progressively more bizarre patterns and cell separation, spindling, and seeding of underlying connective tissue with small nests of bizarre cells. We prefer to describe the biopsy specimen, and then indicate whether the carcinoma is well differentiated, moderately differentiated, ana-plastic, or highly anaplastic. If the clinician prefers to classify the tumor by grade we would use that system based on our four descriptive terms.

CARCINOMA-IN-SITU

Although the term carcinoma-in-situ is not widely used for oral lesions, it is a reasonable description for a histologically obvious carci-

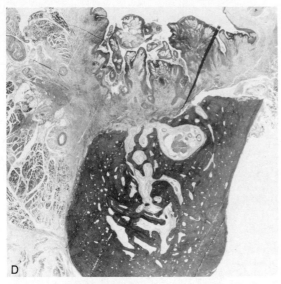

Figure 2–5 *Continued. D,* Carcinoma invading the bone of the mandible (× 50).

noma that is contained within stratified squamous epithelium but that reveals no evidence of invasion or significant extensions into underlying connective tissue. Although this type of lesion is rare in oral mucosa without accompanying hyperkeratosis, occasional cases do occur. This type of lesion has also been called Bowen's disease and erythroplasia of Queyrat as well as other terms. It may remain confined to surface epithelium for extended periods but will eventually become invasive.

DYSPLASTIC LEUKOPLAKIA (PRECANCEROUS LEUKOPLAKIA)

Leukoplakia is a clinical term that signifies a nonspecific white lesion on oral mucosa that is caused primarily by smoking (see Chapter 10).

Microscopically, approximately 90 percent of the cases of oral leukoplakia include varying

Figure 2–6. *A,* Medium-power view (× 100) of epidermoid carcinoma with relative absence of keratin, notable pleomorphism, and cellular degeneration. *B,* High-power view (× 200) showing notable variation in cell size, shape, and chromaticity. Spindling of cells is evident.

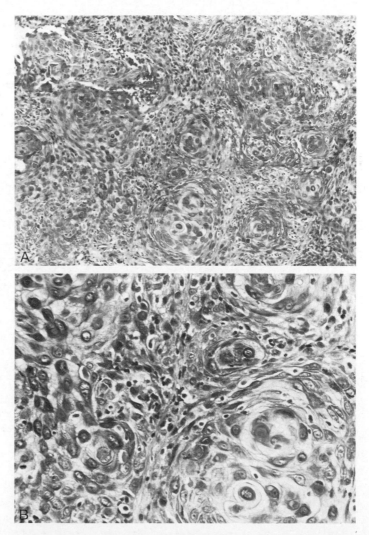

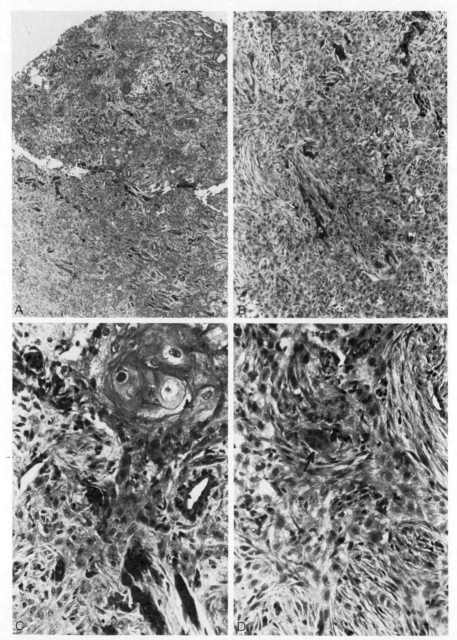

Figure 2–7. *A*, Low-power view (× 50) of anaplastic carcinoma of the tongue. *B*, Medium-power view (× 100) showing absence of keratin and densely packed cells with variation in staining. *C*, High-power view (× 200) showing notable variation in cell shape. *D*, High-power view (× 200) showing spindling of cells and presence of tumor giant cell (arrow).

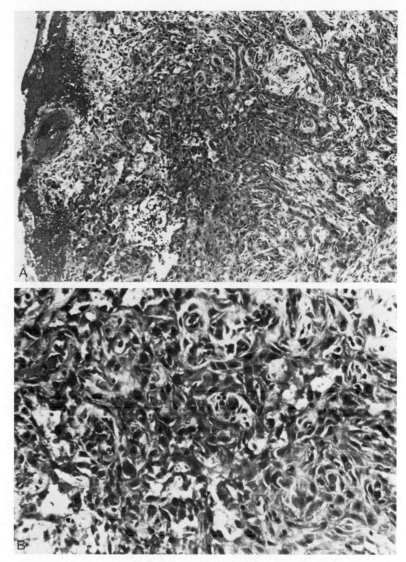

Figure 2–8. *A,* Medium-power view (× 100) of spindle cell carcinoma of the tongue. The surface is necrotic, and the tumor is deeply invasive. No keratin is observed. *B,* High-power view (× 200) showing spindle-shaped cells with minimal adherence to one another.

degrees of hyperkeratosis and chronic inflammation. Ten to 12 percent of the cases present some histologic evidence of dysplasia in addition to keratosis and inflammation. These lesions should be considered precancerous and are essentially in the same general category as carcinoma-in-situ. They should, in fact, be regarded as early preinvasive carcinomas and be treated as such. If untreated, dysplastic leukoplakic lesions will eventually become frank, invasive carcinomas. This may take as long as 10 years, but the eventual development of carcinoma is reasonably certain. Dysplastic leukoplakia is an irreversible lesion and will not regress, even if the patient stops smoking. The mutation from normal to malignant has already occurred. The nondysplastic lesions, on the other hand, will generally regress if the patient stops smoking.

Leukoplakia as a histologic term is to be discouraged. It is a clinical term. However, the possible presence of dysplasia must be diagnosed histologically; thus, a biopsy must be taken of all cases of oral leukoplakia, because it is not possible to determine clinically which cases are precancerous or dysplastic. Microscopically, the term *dysplasia* is used to indicate such features as nuclear hyperchromatism, altered nuclear-cytoplasmic ratio, enlarged nucleoli, loss of normal orientation of cells so that differentiation into strata is obscured, cellular pleomorphism, and abnormalities of keratinization (Figs. 2–9 and 2–10). Separation of cells with widening of intercel-

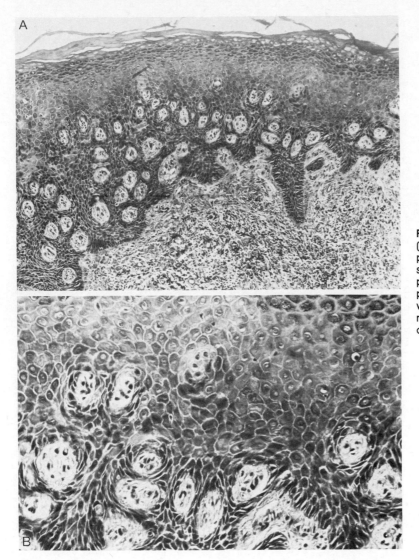

Figure 2–9. A, Low-power view (× 100) of precancerous leukoplakia of the buccal mucosa showing hyperkeratosis, hyperplasia, and dysplasia. B, High-power view (× 200) of dysplasia, with hyperchromaticity, altered nuclear-cytoplasmic ratio, and cellular separation.

lular spaces may also be noted. The term *dyskeratosis* has been used to signify precancerous features. However, the term dysplasia is preferred, because dyskeratosis has also been used to describe certain types of unusual benign diseases.

The relationship between dysplasia and subsequent epidermoid carcinoma has clearly been shown in numerous studies in which oral mucosal carcinoma was experimentally induced.[10] Following applications of carcinogenic chemicals three times per week, dysplasia develops in 6 to 8 weeks and early carcinomas begin to develop in 8 to 10 weeks.

BASAL CELL CARCINOMA

Basal cell carcinoma (basal cell epithelioma) is a common malignant tumor of the skin that occasionally involves the mucosa of the upper lip as an extension from the skin surface. Intraoral or true mucosal basal cell carcinomas have been reported, but these are probably extraosseus ameloblastomas. The basal cell carcinoma and the ameloblastoma are usually indistinguishable microscopically and have a similar derivation. Basal cell carcinomas are well-differentiated tumors, tend to grow slowly, and gradually invade underlying and

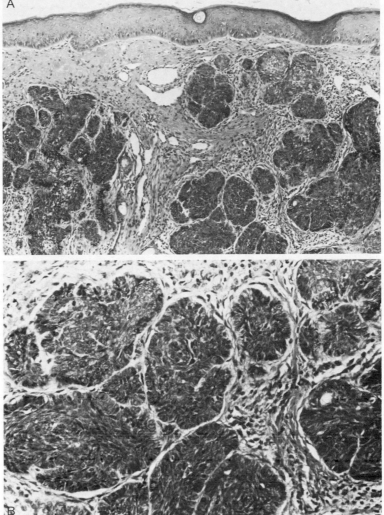

Figure 2–10. *A,* Low-power view (× 100) of basal cell carcinoma of the upper lip, showing proliferating islands of basal cells beneath the surface epithelium. *B,* High-power view (× 200) showing aggregations of deeply staining basal cells.

contiguous tissues but very rarely metastasize. Many different clinical patterns may be seen (see Chapter 26).

Histologically, the basal cell epithelioma is composed of cells that have deeply staining nuclei that resemble the basal layer of stratified squamous epithelium. The cells may be arranged in solid masses (see Fig. 2–10) or may have a reticular or adenoid pattern. Mitoses tend to be few in number, and bizarre mitoses are not observed.

REFERENCES

1. Allen, A. C.: The Skin. A Clinicopathologic Treatise. St. Louis, The C. V. Mosby Co., 1954.
2. Broders, A. C.: Squamous cell epithelioma of the skin. Ann. Surg., *73:*141, 1921.
3. Broders, A. C.: Carcinomas of the mouth; types and degrees of malignancy. Am. J. Roentgenol., *17:*90, 1927.
4. Cataldo, E., Goldman, H., and Shklar, G.: Oral Pathology—An Atlas of Microscopic Pathology, 3rd ed. Boston, Oral Path Press, 1980.
5. Ewing, J.: Neoplastic Diseases, 4th ed. Philadelphia, W. B. Saunders Company, 1940.
6. Hashimoto, K., and Lever, W. F.: Appendage Tumors of the Skin. Springfield, IL, Charles C Thomas, Publishers, 1968.
7. Krompecher, E.: Der Basalzellenkrebs. Jena, G. Fisher, 1903.
8. McCarthy, L.: Histopathology of Skin Diseases. St. Louis, The C. V. Mosby Co., 1931.
9. McCarthy, P. L., and Shklar, G.: Diseases of the Oral Mucosa, 2nd ed., Chapter 34. Philadelphia, Lea and Febiger, 1980.
10. Shklar, G.: Modern studies and concepts of leukoplakia in the mouth. J. Dermatol. Surg. Oncol., *7:*996, 1981.
11. Teloh, H. A., and Wheelock, M. C.: Histogenesis of basal cell carcinoma. Arch. Pathol., *48:*447, 1949.

3

Ultrastructural pathology of oral cancer

GERALD SHKLAR, D.D.S., M.S.

The ultrastructural features of oral squamous cell (epidermoid) carcinoma tend to correlate relatively well with those seen in standard light microscopy. However, the fine details seen by electron microscopy are often a means of explaining some of the characteristic features observed with the light microscope. Thus, the widening of intercellular spaces in the stratum spinosum that is characteristic of anaplastic carcinomas is found to be caused by degeneration or disappearance of desmosomes. Absence of desmosomal attachments permits the cells to separate, and the cell surfaces develop microvillous-like structures that extend into the widened intercellular spaces. Similarly, disruption of the basal lamina explains the deep extension of tumor cells into underlying connective tissue. In general, however, the cellular pleomorphism, altered nuclear-cytoplasmic ratio, nuclear hyperchromatism, and variable nuclear morphology seen in light microscopy are also seen with the electron microscope, although occasionally with superior clarity. The complexity of the preparation of tissues for electron microscopy and the difficulty of locating specific areas of pathology on very small, thin specimens minimizes the usefulness of the electron microscope in diagnostic pathology. There are unusual tumors that may be difficult to diagnose by light microscopy, and in these limited instances, electron microscopy may reveal significant ultrastructural features that lead to a specific diagnosis. Myoblasts may be difficult to distinguish histologically in a rhabdomyosarcoma. Electron microscopy may reveal the characteristic banding more clearly than light microscopy. Oncocytes are characteristically loaded with mitochondria.

In epidermoid carcinoma, the diagnosis is readily made by standard light microscopy; the study of ultrastructural features is primarily done by researchers who are looking into the mechanisms and basic biological characteristics of the tumor and its cellular and subcellular components. The results of ultrastructural studies of oral epidermoid carcinoma have helped to increase our knowledge about these lesions and have provided a clearer understanding of the differences between well-differentiated and anaplastic lesions.

WELL-DIFFERENTIATED EPIDERMOID CARCINOMA

In well-differentiated lesions, the cells are somewhat pleomorphic, the nuclei are large, and the nuclear-cytoplasmic ratio is altered, but the cells are still tightly bound to one another by their desmosomal attachments (see Figs. 3–1 and 3–4), and the basal lamina tends to be relatively intact (Fig. 3–1), with numerous hemidesmosomes that attach the basal lamina to the basal cells of the tumor (Fig. 3–2). Occasional disruption or duplication of the basal lamina occurs, and pseudopodal cytoplasmic projections can be seen extending into the underlying connective tissue.

The nuclear envelope shows irregular indentations. Interchromatin granules are scattered intranuclearly. Heterochromatin may be discerned occasionally. Nucleoli tend to be enlarged, increased in number, marginated, and segregated (Figs. 3–3 and 3–4). Dense clumps of tonofilaments may be found either in perinuclear or peripheral locations within the cytoplasm (Figs. 3–5 and 3–6). Polyribosomes tend to be abundant throughout the cytoplasm.

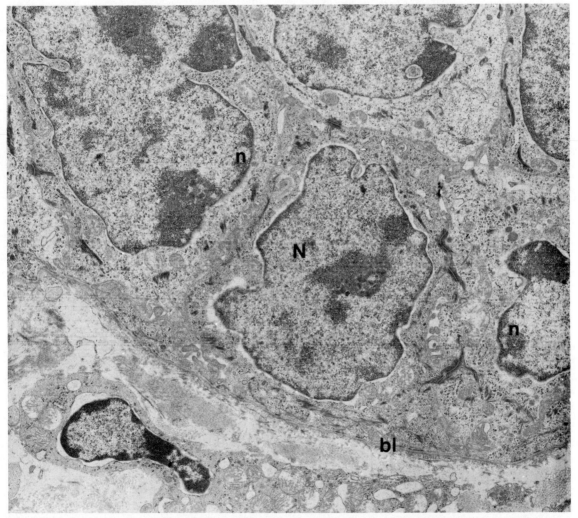

Figure 3–1. Basal cells of well-differentiated epidermoid carcinoma showing basal lamina (bl) at the interface of the epithelium and underlying connective tissue. The nuclei (N) are abnormal in shape, with indentations. There is some segregation and peripheral localization of nucleoli (n) (× 7500).

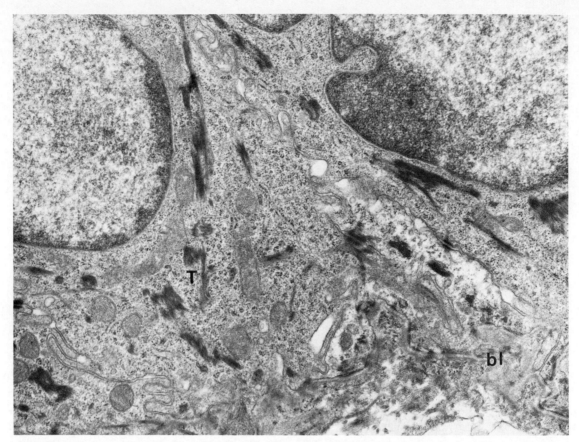

Figure 3–2. High-power view of basal cells in epidermoid carcinoma. The basal lamina (bl) is intact, and hemidesmosomes are apparent at the upper surface of the basal lamina. The view of the nucleus indicates peripheral placement of nucleolar material. Clumping of tonofilaments (T) is noted (× 18,000).

Mitochondria are likely to be swollen and degenerated.

ANAPLASTIC EPIDERMOID CARCINOMA

In less well-differentiated or anaplastic oral epidermoid carcinomas, the abnormal features that are seen in well-differentiated lesions are exaggerated and unusual new structural abnormalities can be observed. The most obvious features are the extremely abnormally shaped nuclei, the relative absence of desmosomes, and the discontinuity of the basal lamina. The nuclei are extremely variable in shape, and the nuclear envelope shows not only indentations but also often deep invaginations (Figs. 3–7 and 3–8). Interchromatin granules extend randomly within the nucleus and perichromatin granules, surrounded by a clear halo, can often be observed at the periphery of the nucleus. Nucleoli are enlarged, increased in number, and scattered. Margination of nucleolar material is commonly observed.

Desmosomes are sparse and the intercellular spaces are widened. Intermediate junctions are rare. Gap junctions and tight junctions are not seen. Plasma membranes of adjacent cells may be straight and parallel, but more often, the membranes form microvillus-like configurations that extend into the large intercellular space. Although few desmosomes may be seen, their structure remains normal. In the cytoplasm, there are notable clumps of tonofilaments. These large, dense bundles may be located perinuclearly or at the periphery of the cell.

Basal lamina is often absent or disrupted in large segments. Cell projections or pseudopodia extend into the connective tissue. Mitochondria may show structural abnormalities such as tubular configurations or they may be large and degenerated, with absence of cristae. Nuclear bodies are an unusual feature that is seen in the more anaplastic carcinomas.

Text continued on page 26

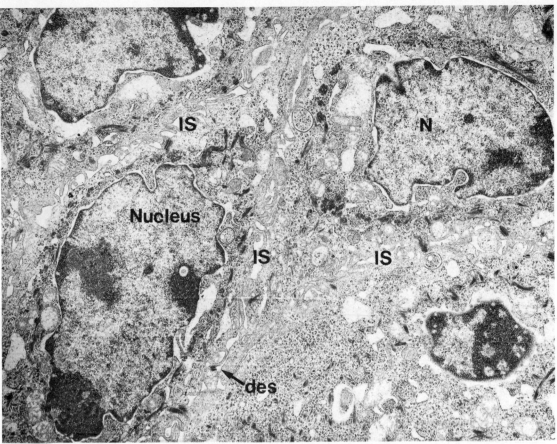

Figure 3–3. Several cells of stratum spinosum in well-differentiated epidermoid carcinoma. Few desmosomes (des) are apparent at the intercellular spaces (IS). Mitochondria appear to be degenerate (× 7500).

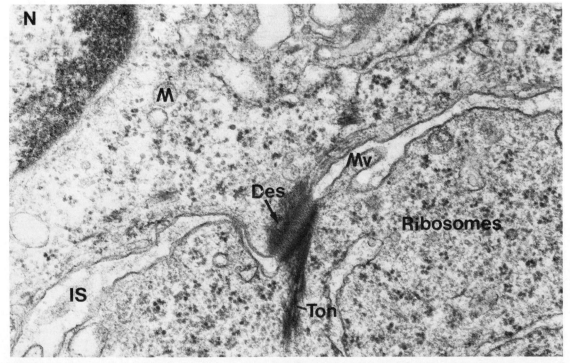

Figure 3–4. High-power view between two cancer cells showing a single desmosome (Des) and tonofilaments (Ton) remaining as an attachment between the cells. The intercellular space (IS) is widened, and the cell surface forms microvillouslike (Mv) structures. Mitochondria (M) appear to be degenerate. Numerous ribosomes are noted in the cytoplasm (× 30,000).

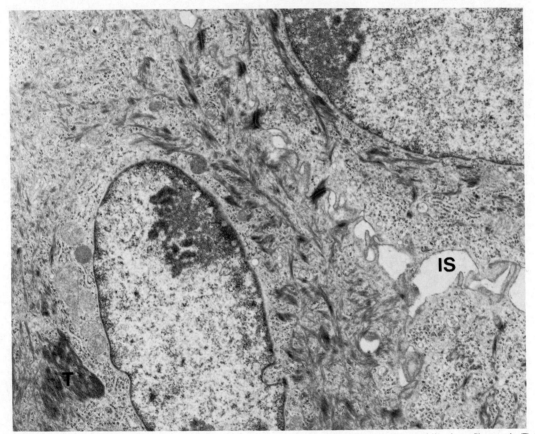

Figure 3–5. Two cancer cells showing a widened intercellular space (IS) and clumping of the tonofilaments (T) (× 12,000).

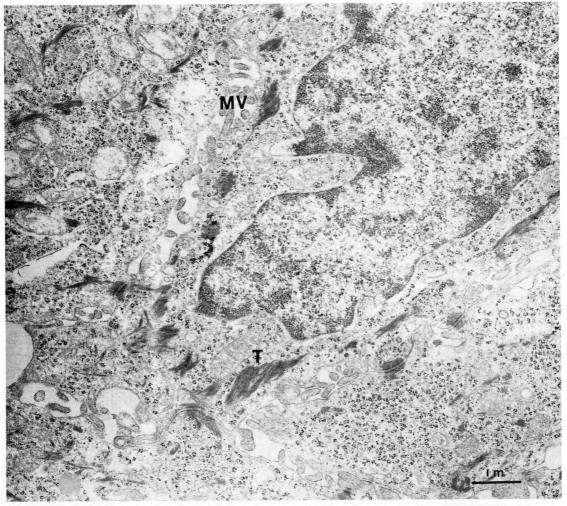

Figure 3–6. Moderately differentiated epidermoid carcinoma cells showing nucleolar segregation and margination, widened intercellular space with microvillous structures (MV), and clumping of the tonofilaments (T) (× 12,000).

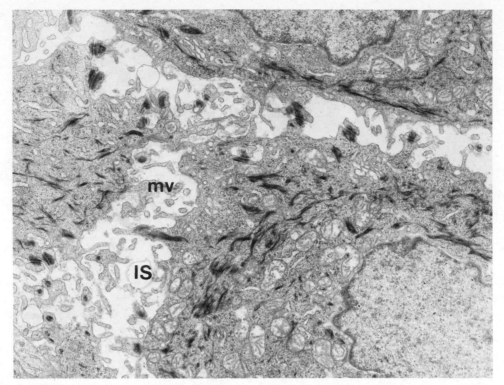

Figure 3–7. Notably widened intercellular spaces (IS) and microvillous structures (mv) in an anaplastic epidermoid carcinoma. Numerous mitochondria are noted in these cells (× 12,000).

The enlargement of nuclei and deep invaginations of nuclear envelopes are familiar features of standard microscopy. The more unusual features of anaplastic carcinoma, such as the presence of both interchromatin and perichromatin granules, probably relate to increased cellular activity, because both are involved in the synthesis of nuclear proteins. Nuclear bodies may also be signs of metabolically active cells, because nuclear proteins have been found in the components of nuclear bodies. Nucleolar margination may represent increased protein synthesis but may also facilitate the exchange of nucleocytoplasmic products. Nucleolar segregation is not unique for malignancy and may result from a variety of drugs, viruses, and radiation.

Movement of anaplastic carcinoma cells is facilitated by loss of cellular attachments and may be mediated in part by contraction of the clumps of tonofilaments and peripherally located microfilaments. Anaplastic cells are rich in polyribosomes, and these may synthesize the proteins required for the locomotion of the cells.

LEUKOPLAKIA

In simple, benign leukoplakia, the major alterations from normal are hyperkeratosis or parakeratosis and varying degrees of chronic inflammatory infiltration. Ultrastructurally, one sees the hyperkeratosis as regular, horizontally oriented layers of flattened lamellae of acellular keratin. Occasionally flattened cells may be present. Keratohyalin granules can be seen in the upper stratum spinosum or in a thin stratum granulosum (Fig. 3–9A). The cells of the stratum spinosum and stratum germinativum appear normal (Fig. 3–9B). Essentially, benign leukoplakia resembles normal skin without skin appendages.

In dysplastic or precancerous leukoplakia, there is often some abnormality in the orientation of the surface keratin, with irregularly shaped and structured lamellae. Some acellular keratin may appear in the stratum spinosum. However, the fundamental pathologic alteration in dysplastic leukoplakia is the abnormal orientation of cells throughout the epithelium and the presence of cells that have altered

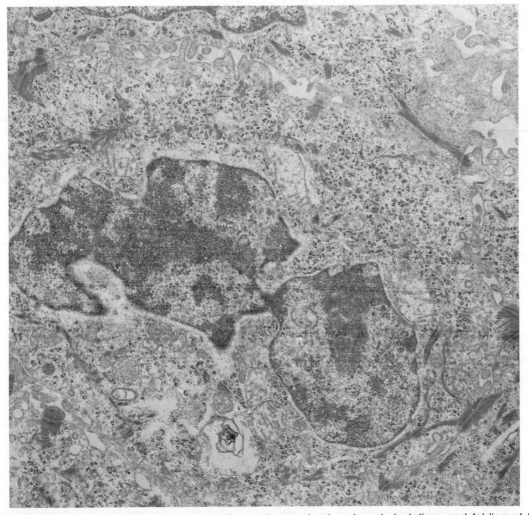

Figure 3–8. Abnormal epithelial cell in anaplastic carcinoma showing deep indentations and folding of the nucleus (× 18,000).

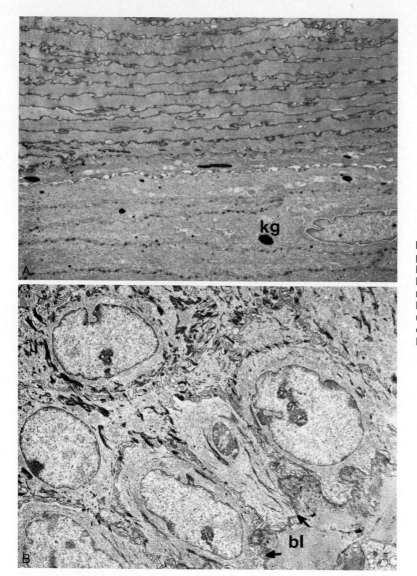

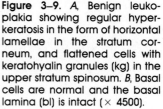

Figure 3–9. *A,* Benign leukoplakia showing regular hyperkeratosis in the form of horizontal lamellae in the stratum corneum, and flattened cells with keratohyalin granules (kg) in the upper stratum spinosum. *B,* Basal cells are normal and the basal lamina (bl) is intact (× 4500).

nuclear-cytoplasmic ratio and irregularly shaped nuclei that contain large amounts of nucleolar material. Deep indentations can often be seen in the nuclei, and nucleolar material may show segregation and margination along the nuclear membrane (Fig. 3–10). Basal lamina usually appears normal, but there may be small areas of discontinuity.

ADENOCARCINOMA

Ultrastructurally, adenocarcinoma, in its various histological classifications, appears as clusters of glandular cells, often in the shape of ductal or acinar structures. The glandular cells have large nuclei with extensive peripheral nucleolar material (Fig. 3–11). The glandular cells may be producing mucin granules or may be relatively free of cytoplasmic granules. A tumor that had more mucin production and excretion would tend to be better differentiated, but in glandular malignancy, the apparent degree of differentiation does not correlate well with clinical behavior, as in epidermoid carcinoma.

REFERENCES

1. Busch, H., and Smetana, K.: The nucleus of the cancer cell. *In* The Molecular Biology of Cancer, Chapter 2. New York, Academic Press, Inc., 1974.
2. Chen, S. Y., and Harwick, R. D.: Ultrastructure of oral squamous cell carcinoma. Oral Surg., *44:*744, 1977.
3. Frithiof, L.: Ultrastructure of the basement membrane

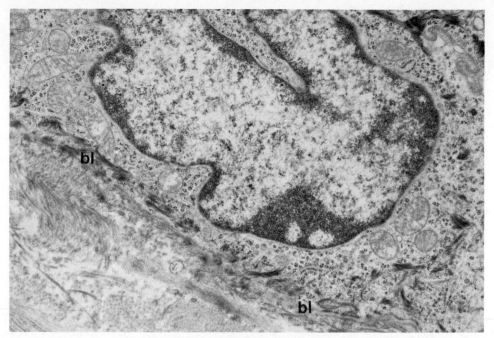

Figure 3–10. Dysplastic leukoplakia showing a basal cell that has large nucleus with indentation and nucleolar segregation and margination. The basal lamina (bl) is intact (× 18,000).

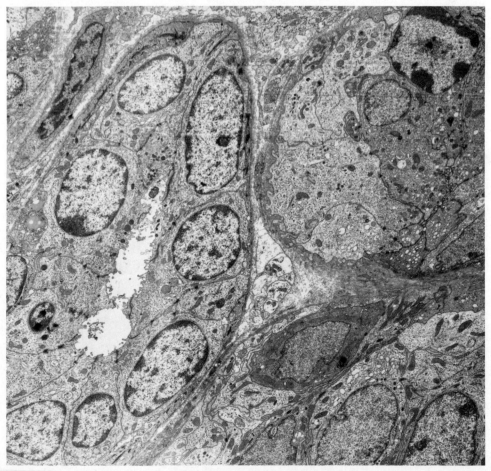

Figure 3–11. Adenocarcinoma showing a group of tumor cells, some of which are producing mucin granules. The cells are arranged in a glandular structure and have large nuclei with peripherally located nucleolar material (× 4500).

in normal and hyperplastic human oral epithelium compared with that in preinvasive and invasive carcinoma. Acta Pathol. Microbiol. Scand. (Suppl.), *200:*3, 1969.

4. Frithiof, L.: Electron microscope observations on structures related to the epithelial basement membrane in squamous cell carcinoma. Acta Otolaryngol., *73:*323, 1972.

5. Ghadially, F. N.: Ultrastructural pathology of the cell. London and Boston, Butterworth Publishers Inc., 1975.

6. Gould, V. E., Memoli, V. A., and Dardi, L. E.: Multidirectional differentiation in human epithelial cancers. J. Submicrosc. Cytol., *13:*97, 1981.

7. Hashimoto, K., DiBella, R. J., and Shklar, G.: Electron microscopic studies of the normal human buccal mucosa. J. Invest. Dermatol., *47:*512, 1966.

8. Malech, H. L., and Lentz, T. L.: Microfilaments in epidermal cancer cells. J. Cell Biol., *60:*473, 1974.

9. Marefat, M. P., Albright, J. T., and Shklar, G.: Ultrastructural alterations in experimental lingual leukoplakia and carcinoma. Oral Surg., *47:*334, 1979.

10. McKinney, R. V., and Singh, B. B.: Basement membrane changes under neoplastic oral mucous membrane. Ultrastructural observations, review of the literature, and a unifying concept. Oral Surg., *44:*875, 1977.

11. Meng, C., Albright, J., and Shklar, G.: Ultrastructural pathology of experimental oral anaplastic carcinoma (in press).

12. Schenk, P.: Microfilaments in human epithelial cancer cells. Z. Krebsforsch. Klin. Onkol., *84:*241, 1975.

13. White, G. H., and Squier, C. A.: A quantitative study of the intercellular and basal attachment apparatus in hamster cheek pouch epithelium during carcinogenesis. J. Dent. Res., *53:*1072, 1974.

14. Woods, D. A., and Smith, C. J.: Ultrastructure of the dermal-epidermal junction in experimentally induced tumors and human oral lesions. J. Invest. Dermatol., *52:*259, 1969.

15. Woods, D. A., and Smith, C. J.: Ultrastructure and development of epithelial cell pseudopodia in chemically induced premalignant lesions of the hamster cheek pouch. Exp. Mol. Pathol., *12:*160, 1970.

4

Oral precancerous lesions

PHILIP L. MCCARTHY, M.D.

A premalignant condition is something that is frequently referred to without any firm commitment as to a generally accepted definition. We feel that the study of oral precancerous lesions is vitally important, because the prevention of oral cancer is most desirable and should take precedence over the diagnosis and therapy of oral cancer.

It is suggested that a premalignant condition be defined as any systemic disorder, specific condition, or environmental factor that renders the oral mucosa more susceptible to the subsequent development of a malignant tumor. These elements may be considered in further detail, concerning the likelihood of cancer without elimination of the offending lesion or condition.

The three major groups of precancerous conditions are:

1. Systemic disorders that predispose oral mucosa to the development of cancer.
2. Specific pathologic conditions of oral mucosa that show a tendency to develop into cancer.
3. Environmental factors or habits that predispose oral mucosa to the development of cancer.

SYSTEMIC DISORDERS

The following systemic disorders must be dealt with in the overall consideration of premalignancy:

1. Immunosuppression.
   Naturally occurring (e.g., lymphoma).
   Artificially induced (e.g., corticosteroids).
2. Syphilis.
3. Iron deficiency anemia (Plummer-Vinson syndrome).
4. Alcoholism, including hepatic cirrhosis.

5. Heredity (genetic predisposition).
6. Oral sepsis.

Immunosuppression

Perhaps the most obvious and significant element related to the ultimate development of cancer is the status of the patient's immune system. It has been shown that when immunosuppression has been present for significant periods of time the likelihood that a malignant tumor will appear is enhanced.[3] This may happen in naturally occurring immunosuppression such as that induced by the lymphomas and also may happen when immunosuppression is artificially induced with immunosuppressive drugs in patients who receive organ transplants.

This significant role of immunity is currently becoming very much appreciated, especially with regard to the management of some forms of widespread or metastatic malignant tumors. Many immunoenhancing agents are being used to enable the patient to control the growth and to limit the spread of the tumor. Much has yet to be learned in this exciting field, but it is obvious that the presence of a normal immune system is important in the prevention and control of malignancies.

Any interference or aberration in the so-called surveillance mechanisms of the host immune system may result in a significant increase in the development of malignant tumors, especially of the lymphoma and reticuloendothelial varieties. This phenomenon has been observed in animals for many years, and the practical application in many has become obvious with the ever-increasing use of organ transplants. It has been shown that a tumor cell represents foreign substance to the host, whether it arises spontaneously, is induced by

31

carcinogenic agents, or is transplanted. The host's responses, namely the immunologic processes, against tumor cells are the same as those that act against any other foreign material.

Immunologic deficiency states such as the Wiskott-Aldrich syndrome or ataxia telangiectasia,[44] are diseases in which the patients not only have an increased susceptibility to infection but also have a faulty surveillance mechanism, which increases their chances of developing a neoplasm. In fact, when the infections that can be life threatening are controlled by antibiotics, a major cause of death is the occurrence and development of a malignant tumor, usually of the reticuloendothelial system and its organs, such as the thymus.

Syphilis

For many years it has been observed that the development of oral cancer is commonly seen in patients who have positive results from serologic tests for syphilis.[20] This phenomenon apparently has proved to be statistically valid, although the relationship, other than epidermoid carcinoma of the tongue, has never been clear. Perhaps patients who develop syphilis may be more prone to poor oral hygiene and have less of a tendency for good health habits, including nutrition.

There is no question as to the effect that spirochetemia has upon the tongue. Spirochetes have a predilection for motile muscular tissue, accounting for the presence of these organisms in large numbers in the tongue during secondary syphilis. As a result, an obliterative endarteritis ensues, which results in a marked atrophy of both the epithelial covering and the musculature of the tongue. The normal protective coating disappears, taking with it the filiform papillae, which are essential in providing a natural protective covering from the many frequent irritative experiences that the tongue normally encounters. As a result, hyperkeratinization develops to replace the normal coating, and eventually, dyskeratosis and subsequent malignant transformation occur in some cases. In our experience, a "bald" syphilitic tongue is one of the susceptible lesions for the development of cancer, especially if the patient continues to be exposed to irritants such as the products of combustion of tobacco, mechanical trauma, and poor oral hygiene.

Iron Deficiency Anemia (Plummer-Vinson Syndrome)

Plummer-Vinson syndrome, which includes dysphagia, glossitis, and koilonychia, occurs most commonly in middle-aged females.[50, 57] Although it has primarily been featured in Scandinavian scientific literature, it has been described in other parts of the world. In addition to the major clinical features, angular cheilitis, achlorhydria, splenomegaly, and abnormal barium swallow have also been attributed to this syndrome. Although iron deficiency is considered to be the most significant element in the etiology, other nutritional factors such as riboflavin deficiency and primary dysphagia have been postulated.

Because of the atrophic mucosa, it has not been surprising that a significant incidence of carcinoma of the oral cavity has been observed in patients who have the Plummer-Vinson syndrome.[1] The early administration of appropriate iron therapy will increase the chances that the mucosa will return to a relatively normal state. Long-standing cases do not respond well to treatment, and malignant transformation may occur despite adequate therapy. Approximately 10 percent or more of the patients who have this condition will eventually develop an epidermoid carcinoma of the mucosa of the mouth, pharyngeal area, or esophagus. In fact, the possibility of multiple primary tumors must be considered because of the extensive atrophic premalignant nature of the mucous membranes.

Alcoholism

It has been established that a relationship exists between heavy intake of alcohol and higher incidence of cancer of the oral cavity.[7] However, it must be noted that most alcoholics also use tobacco, and it is in the combination of the two that the most striking increases in the incidence of mouth cancer have been observed. A heavy drinker who does not smoke has approximately the same increased risk of developing cancer of the mouth as a heavy smoker who does not drink. However, when heavy drinking and heavy smoking are combined, there is an enormous increase in the risk of the development of oral cancer.[15] It has been estimated that people who drink *and* smoke heavily will have a 1500 percent higher incidence of malignancy than those who do not engage in either.

The means by which alcohol may exert a carcinogenic effect are unknown. There are wide geographic and gender variations in the incidence of cancers thought to be linked to alcohol.

Further investigation must be undertaken to determine whether alcoholism acts as an immunosuppressive phenomenon or whether tobacco and alcohol are synergistic in their capacity to induce malignant transformation. However, based on current epidemiologic studies, it is clear that the heavy drinker who smokes is at high risk of developing oral cancer. Many alcoholics suffer from nutritional deficiencies, particularly vitamin B deficiency, and this, too, may play a role in the alcohol-tobacco-cancer predisposition.

Hepatic Cirrhosis

Several studies have linked hepatic cirrhosis to carcinoma of the oral cavity.[48, 49] In addition to a higher incidence of oral cancer, the age of onset was earlier and the survival rates were poorer in the cirrhotic patient. Perhaps, because alcoholism is a frequent cause of cirrhosis, a common denominator exists, which accounts for the higher incidence of oral cancer in both conditions. Statistics have shown a higher relationship between carcinoma of the tongue (44.4 percent), palate, tonsillar region, and floor of the mouth (59 percent) and hepatic cirrhosis. In Trieger's studies, the average age of the patients who had cirrhosis was 57 years, whereas the average age of noncirrhotics with cancer was 70 years. The 5-year survival rate of cancer victims who had cirrhosis was 19 percent, whereas the control group had a 40.3 percent survival rate.

Genetic Factors

Genetic factors are an important consideration with all malignancies. The tendency to develop certain tumors follows a direct hereditary pattern, frequently an autosomal dominant one. In one disorder, dyskeratosis congenita, a sex-linked recessive trait may be present. Other patients have an increased susceptibility to tumors induced by solar irradiation, exemplified by actinic cheilitis. The influence of solar irradiation will largely depend upon the genetic endowment of the individual. Because of their lightly pigmented skin, Caucasians have a high incidence of solar-induced tumors. Other significant inheritable diseases that have significant tendencies to develop into malignancy include xeroderma pigmentosum, ataxia telangiectasia, Wiskott-Aldrich syndrome, and the basal-cell nevus syndrome.

Oral Sepsis

Although it may be difficult to accurately evaluate the influence of infection on the oral mucosa, it seems obvious that chronic intraoral infection has a harmful effect on the well-being of the oral cavity. Products of bacterial proliferation, including bacterial toxins, may have an irritating reaction, which when combined with other elements such as immunosuppression, nutritional deficiencies, and alcoholism, can enhance the risk of ultimately developing a malignant growth.

PATHOLOGIC CONDITIONS

Some specific pathologic conditions of the oral mucosa have a tendency to undergo malignant transformation.

Leukoplakia

Leukoplakia is the most common precancerous lesion, and approximately 10 to 15 percent of all cases eventually develop into epidermoid carcinomas if untreated.[4, 25] It is a relatively common condition in heavy smokers who are older than fifty years of age, and both the association with smoking and the precancerous relationship have been known and understood for many years. Schwimmer first used the term *leukoplakia* in 1877 to describe these white, plaquelike lesions of oral mucous membrane,[8, 9, 38] although the condition had previously been described under a variety of other names. Sturgis and Lund[45] studied 312 cases of leukoplakia and found that 12 percent of the lesions developed into carcinoma. McCarthy studied a series of 316 cases and graded the lesions on the basis of both their clinical and microscopic patterns.[23]

Grade I represented the initial reaction of the mucous membrane to irritation; clinically the lesion was a red, granular area that gradually became slightly gray. Inflammatory infiltration without epithelial proliferation was seen microscopically. Grade II lesions were bluish-white patches or plaques, sharply outlined but without palpable induration. The lesions revealed hyperkeratotic changes and inflammation on microscopic evaluation. Grade III lesions were indurated plaques, white, possibly wrinkled, and sharply outlined. Microscopically, severe hyperkeratosis and inflammation were noted. Grade IV lesions were indurated, leathery plaques with fissures, erosions, and occasional warty proliferations of the surface. Microscopically, early malignant changes were noted. This gradation of lesions in leukoplakia, with the Grade IV lesions representing early malignant changes, was of considerable importance in differentiating leukoplakial lesions into various types based on both clinical and microscopic features.

In a correlated clinical and histopathologic survey of 90 cases, Renstrup found hyperkeratosis and parakeratosis in 71 cases, epithelial hyperplasia in 24 cases, and dyskeratotic alterations in 2 cases.[34] The lesions were found to occur with greatest frequency on the buccal mucosa, followed by the alveolar mucosa, tongue, lip, palate, floor of the mouth, and gingiva. Shafer and Waldron reviewed 332 tissue specimens of clinical oral white lesions and found hyperkeratosis or parakeratosis in 105 cases; hyperkeratosis or parakeratosis with àcanthosis in 190 cases; hyperkeratosis, parakeratosis, and acanthosis with focal atypia in 26 cases; carcinoma-in-situ in 6 cases; and invasive carcinoma in 27 cases.[39]

It is now known that microscopic evidence of dysplasia is the most significant feature that can be used prognostically in determining whether a given case of oral leukoplakia may develop into a malignancy. The results of all recent studies have confirmed this concept and have helped to clarify the histologic features of dysplasia.

In a recent study of 723 patients who had oral leukoplakia in India, Mehta and colleagues found epithelial dysplasia in 10.7 percent.[24] Roed-Peterson found dysplasia in 15 percent of 331 cases of leukoplakia in Denmark.[35]

Banoczy and Csiba, in a histologic study of 500 cases of oral leukoplakia, defined dysplasia and offered criteria for its evaluation.[4, 5] Forty-eight cases (9.6 percent) revealed the presence of epidermoid carcinoma, and 120 cases (24 percent) showed some evidence of epithelial dysplasia. Among the histologic criteria used for determining dysplasia were irregular epithelial stratification, hyperplasia of the basal layer, drop-shaped rete pegs, increased number of mitotic figures, loss of polarity of basal cells, increased nuclear-cytoplasmic ratio, nuclear polymorphism, nuclear hyperchroma-

tism, enlarged nucleoli, keratinization of single cells or cell groups in the prickle-cell layer, and loss of intercellular adherence. Dysplasia was considered mild if only two of the histologic features were present, moderate when two to four of the features were seen, and severe when five or more features were observed. Most cases of dysplasia were moderate. Severe dysplasia occurred most often with the erosive clinical form of leukoplakia rather than the simple or verrucous form. Most carcinomas that were discovered initially in the leukoplakial lesions occurred on the tongue. Nine additional carcinomas (13.2 percent) developed within dysplastic leukoplakial lesions over periods that ranged from 1 to 20 years.

The largest study of oral leukoplakia cases was carried out by Waldron and Shafer in 1975 with 3256 cases.[53] Carcinoma or severe epithelial dysplasia was found in 7.6 percent of the cases, and mild to moderate dysplasia was found in 12.2 percent. In all these studies, the most frequent occurrence of dysplasia occurred in people who were older than 50 years. Various types of histochemical studies have been done, and none have resulted in clearly defining those cases of leukoplakia with dysplastic or dyskeratotic alterations.[41, 42]

Clinical features of oral leukoplakia may be variable and primarily depend upon the degree of surface keratinization. Initial, early lesions may appear as granular red and gray areas. More advanced lesions are raised and appear white, often with erythematous margins (Figs. 4–1 and 4–2). Severe, long-standing involvment may consist of thick, leathery white plaques, often verrucous in areas. Zones of erosion or fissuring may also be noted. Lesions may be localized or diffuse. Symptoms are minimal.

Unfortunately, there is not a good correlation between severity of clinical features and histologic evidence of dysplasia. For this reason, all cases of oral leukoplakia must be biopsied and presence of dysplasia must be noted. These cases should be considered as early preinvasive malignancy and managed as such. Cases without evidence of dysplasia should be followed periodically, and further biopsies should be taken if the lesions appear clinically altered, such as by thickening or fissuring (Figs. 4–3 through 4–5).

The etiology of oral leukoplakia is complex, but smoking is the major exciting cause.[29, 36] Another local exciting cause may be chronic irritation such as that caused by poorly fitting dental appliances or by neurotic cheekbiting.

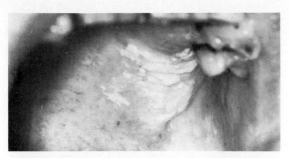

Figure 4–1. Leukoplakia of the palate.

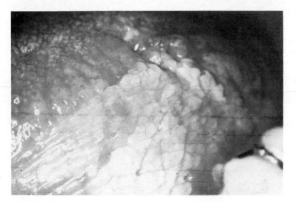

Figure 4–2. Leukoplakia on the lateral border of the tongue.

There also appear to be several predisposing causes, such as hereditary factors; hormonal factors, including estrogen deficiency[27]; nutritional factors; and, rarely, syphilis with its resultant atrophic glossitis.

Some individuals have hereditary resistance to the development of dysplastic leukoplakia, despite the amount of smoking that they engage in and the clinical severity of their lesions. Quigley and associates found neither oral carcinomas nor histologic evidence of dysplasia in a group of "reverse smokers."[32]

Dyskeratosis Congenita (Zinsser-Engman-Cole Syndrome)

This extremely rare syndrome is characterized by keratinization of the oral mucosa, reticular cutaneous hyperpigmentation, nail dystrophy, and pancytopenia.[43] There is a sex-linked recessive inheritance pattern. The initial lesions may be noted as early as the fourth or fifth year as a reticulated hyperpigmentation on the neck, face, and trunk. The nail dystrophy is characterized by poor growth, thinness, and longitudinal ridges and grooves. Palmar and plantar hyperkeratosis with occasional bullae after trauma is a common feature. Purpuric lesions can be seen as the hematologic abnormalities develop.

Involvement of the oral mucous membrane is significant and is characterized by extensive keratinization. The most commonly observed sites are the tongue and buccal mucosa. A primary lesion that consists of a bulla that eventually ruptures apparently leads to the eventual keratinization. The likelihood that a squamous cell carcinoma will develop has been well documented, and all cases should be followed very carefully for such an occurrence. There is no specific treatment for this disorder.

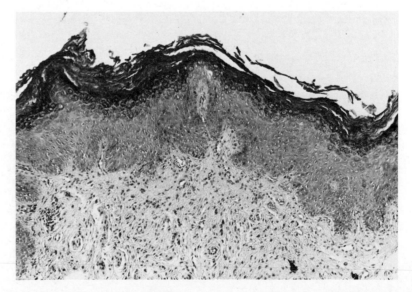

Figure 4–3. Biopsy of buccal mucosal leukoplakia showing notable hyperkeratosis ($\times$ 150).

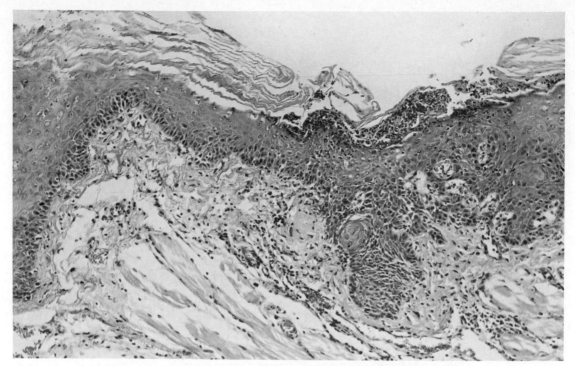

Figure 4–4. Leukoplakia showing hyperkeratosis and dysplasia (× 100).

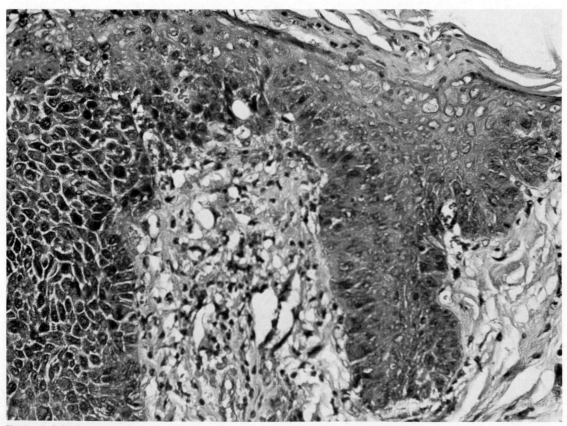

Figure 4–5. High-power view of leukoplakia showing dysplasia (left) with altered nuclear-cytoplasmic ratio, nuclear hyperchromaticity, cell separation, and spindling of cells (× 250).

Oral Florid Papillomatosis

Oral florid papillomatosis is a rare condition of the oral mucosa that is characterized by multiple papillomas, generally clustered in cauliflowerlike lesions that involve extensive areas, and is seen principally in middle-aged and older individuals.[14, 54] The onset may be moderately rapid, although many cases develop over a period of months to years.

Histologically they appear benign, with acanthosis, papillomatosis, vacuolated epithelial cells, and a well-oriented basal cell layer. There may be some lymphocytes, plasma cells, and eosinophils in the underlying connective tissue.

Clinically they can cause a great deal of confusion and concern, because their behavior is more likely to indicate a malignant tumor than can be predicted by studying the lesion histologically. They are invasive and may produce extensive tissue destruction. Therapy consists of approaching this condition with all the modalities used in true malignancy, e.g., surgery, x-ray, cryotherapy, and chemotherapy.

One must understand, however, that although the papillomas appear as a malignant disease, they do not metastasize. The most significant question, perhaps, is whether they eventually become true carcinomas or remain as locally destructive, histologically benign processes.[37] This may only be of academic interest, because the management should be decisive and extensive, as if one were dealing with a truly malignant neoplasm.

Bowen's Disease (Erythroplasia of Queyrat, Carcinoma-in-Situ)

The only controversy that might exist about Bowen's disease is whether it is premalignant or is in reality a very early superficial carcinoma. It is generally agreed that in time, if left untreated, an invasive squamous cell carcinoma will result.[12] Bowen's disease is rare, occurring principally in elderly people. The usual clinical appearance is that of a red, velvety, slightly elevated surface that resembles granulation tissue with patches of keratinization. The floor of the mouth and soft palate and the retromolar regions are the common sites.[56] When the diagnosis has been made, the lesion should be treated as a true carcinoma and appropriate therapeutic measures should be taken, such as surgery or cryosurgery. Mashberg and associates reported that 90 per-

cent of a series of 150 early asymptomatic oral carcinomas had an erythroplastic component, and they have emphasized this feature as an important aid in the diagnosis of early oral cancer.[22]

Lichen Planus

In recent years, there has been considerable confusion about the possibility of lichen planus being considered a premalignant condition.[2, 6, 31, 33, 51] It is the author's feeling that in most instances the appearance of carcinoma in the oral cavity of patients who have pre-existing lichen planus is coincidental. One must realize that lichen planus and oral carcinoma are not rare diseases, and consequently, the two conditions will appear together occasionally following the law of averages.[10, 18] The only possible exception is in patients, especially the elderly, who have experienced long-standing lichen planus of the bullous, erosive, or atrophic variety.[13] Eventually, a profound atrophy may develop, which renders the tissues more susceptible to irritants, and subsequent dysplastic leukoplakia and carcinoma may follow.

Krutchkoff and coworkers reviewed the statistical evidence regarding the potential malignant transformation of lichen planus and found it unconvincing.[19] In their study, they also found poor documentation in many of the published reports of carcinoma developing in lesions of lichen planus.

In general, however, we do not believe that lichen planus should be included in the group of premalignant conditions.

ENVIRONMENTAL FACTORS AND HABITS

Some environmental factors and habits are injurious to the oral mucosa and increase the risk of oral malignancy.

Smoking

There is well-established evidence that the incidence of oral cancer in increased by the smoking of tobacco.[26, 50, 58] Smoking is undoubtedly the most significant and widespread carcinogenic habit, and the only variables are determined by the form of smoking and the presence of concomitant practices, such as excessive alcohol intake. In the past, it has been thought that most oral cancer is associated with pipe and cigar smokers and tobacco chewers. However, in our experience, it is the

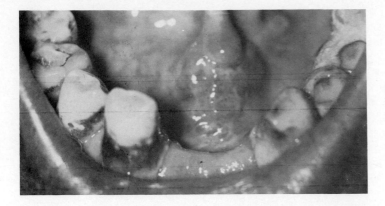

Figure 4–6. Epidermoid carcinoma of the floor of the mouth in a patient who has used betel nut for many years.

cigarette smokers who are developing more premalignant and malignant lesions today. The development of new primary oral cancers in those patients who have been successfully treated for a previous malignancy is alarmingly common in those who continue to smoke. Knowledge of the specific ingredient or product of combustion of tobacco that is carcinogenic is not well understood at this time. Until further investigation incriminates a specific element of tobacco smoke or tobacco, it must be considered a major environmental hazard and all use of tobacco should be discouraged.

It is also probable that mucous membrane changes brought about by the effects of tobacco are reversible and that when one discontinues smoking, the mucosa may again be restored to reasonably normal condition. This may depend upon the duration and intensity of the use of tobacco and other factors such as age and inherent susceptibility. In any event, the discontinuance of the habit is obviously preferable to its continued use until an understanding of the problem may make it possible to remove the hazardous substances from tobacco or to develop measures to inhibit their activity.

Betel Nut Chewing

Betel nut chewing, which is considered a cause of cancer, has been extensively studied in India, Ceylon, the Malaysian peninsula, and the Phillipines.[47] The betel nut is wrapped in a leaf of the betel plant. Calcium hydroxide, tobacco, and coconut are usually added. This habit is associated with a high incidence of oral malignancy (Fig. 4–6).

Actinic Cheilitis

Long-term exposure to the rays of the sun results in damage to the lips, especially the lower lip. The result of the actinic radiation is atrophy, crusting, scaling, and telangiectasia. These changes make the lip more vulnerable to further damage from other sources, and the possibility of the development of carcinoma increases.[28] Gradually, indurated areas develop, and one should suspect a developing carcinoma (Fig. 4–7).

Treatment consists of destruction of the damaged tissue by chemical or surgical means, allowing a fresh new epithelium to replace the premalignant tissue.

Figure 4–7. Atrophy and crusting of the lip in actinic cheilitis.

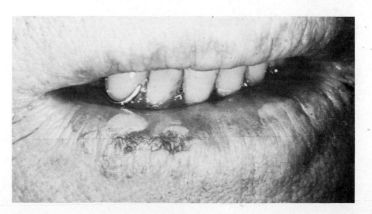

Radiation Stomatitis

After ionizing radiation has been delivered to the oral mucosa, irreversible degenerative and progressive damage ensues. The degree of damage and the likelihood of malignant degeneration will depend upon the total amount of irradiation and the manner in which it was delivered. Every effort should be made to protect this mucosa from insults related to trauma in any form.

Trauma

Trauma to the tissues of the oral cavity is a constant occurrence and takes place in a variety of ways. Mechanical trauma is probably the most common form of oral mucosal trauma, because the mucous membranes are in constant direct contact with hard material (teeth, prosthetic appliances, and food). Added to this are innumerable habits such as biting and thrusting that are carried on consciously or subconsciously. In addition, objects composed of varied hard materials are frequently thrust into the mouth in many neurotic habits.

Thermal irritation of the oral mucosa is also universal, because most people consume food and drink that is heated to temperatures that would not be tolerated against the skin surface. Frequently, erosions from the effects of excessively hot substances such as melted cheese and fried foods are noted on the oral mucosa.

Various kinds of chemicals are introduced into the oral cavity and may result in inflammatory reactions, ranging from erythema to necrotic slough. Unfortunately, many such irritants, particularly aspirin and phenol, have been recommended as topical remedies for several oral conditions.

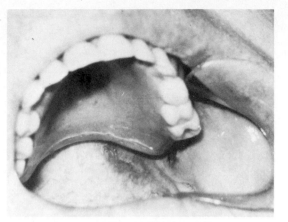

Figure 4–9. The denture in position.

It is obvious, therefore, that trauma to the oral cavity is both common and frequently severe, occurring in many different ways for a variety of reasons. However, the role it plays per se in the development of malignant disease is obscure at the present time. Obviously, in most instances of oral cancer, a variety of factors, such as immunity, heredity, and chemical nature of the irritant, are probably operating. However, until the role of trauma is properly clarified, there should be an awareness of its possible influences, and every effort should be made to eliminate them (Figs. 4–8 and 4–9).

REFERENCES

1. Ahlbom, H. E.: Simple achlorhydric anemia, Plummer-Vinson syndrome and carcinoma of the mouth, pharynx and esophagus in women. Br. Med. J., 2:331, 1936.
2. Andreason, J. O., and Pindborg, J. J.: Cancerudirkling i oral lichen planus. Nord. Med., 70:861, 1963.
3. Baldwin, R. W.: Immunology of maligancy. Summation. Br. J. Cancer, 27:309, 1973.
4. Banoczy, J., and Csiba, A.: Comparative study of the clinical picture and histopathologic structure of oral leukoplakia. Cancer, 29:1230, 1972.
5. Banoczy, J., and Csiba, A.: Occurrence of epithelial dysplasia in oral leukoplakia. Analysis and follow-up study of 12 cases. Oral Surg., 42:766, 1976.
6. Cernea, P., Kuffer, R., and Brocheriou, C.: L'epithelioma sur lichen plan buccal. Actual. Odontostomatol., 25:473, 1971.
7. Chafetz, M. E.: Heavy drinking adds to the rise of cancers of the mouth and throat. J.A.M.A., 229:1023, 1974.
8. Cooke, B. E. D.: Leukoplakia buccalis and oral epithelial naevi: a clinical and histological study. Br. J. Dermatol., 68:151, 1956.
9. Eichenlaub, F. J.: Leukoplakia buccalis. Arch. Dermatol., 37:590, 1938.
10. Fulling, H. J.: Cancer development in oral lichen planus. A follow-up study of 327 patients. Arch. Dermatol., 108:667, 1975.

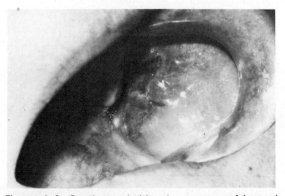

Figure 4–8. Carcinoma arising in an area of buccal mucosa that was traumatized by a poorly fitting denture.

11. Hobaek, A.: Leukoplakia oris. Acta. Odontol. Scand., 7:61, 1946.

12. Hugo, E., and Conway, H.: Bowen's disease: its malignant potential and relationship to systemic cancer. Plast. Reconstr. Surg., 39:190, 1967.

13. Janner, M., von Muissus, E., and Rohde, B.: Lichen planus als fukultative Prakanzerose. Dermatol. Wchnschr., 153:513, 1967.

14. Kaulen-Becker, L.: Orale floride papillomatose. Z. Haut Geschlechtskr., 48:1, 1973.

15. Kissin, B., Kaley, M. M., Wen, H. S., et al.: Head and neck cancer in alcoholics. J.A.M.A., 224:1174, 1973.

16. Klein, G., and Klein, E.: Immune surveillance against virus-induced tumors and nonrejectability of spontaneous tumors: contrasting consequences of host versus tumor evolution. Proc. Natl. Acad. Sci., 74:2121, 1977.

17. Kramer, I. R.: Oral leukoplakia. Proc. Roy. Soc. Med., 73:765, 1980.

18. Kronenberg, K., Fretzin, D., and Potter, B.: Malignant degeneration of lichen planus. Arch. Dermatol., 104:304, 1971.

19. Krutchkoff, D. J., Cutler, L., and Laskowski, S.: Oral lichen planus: the evidence regarding potential malignant transformation. J. Oral Pathol., 7:1, 1978.

20. Levin, M., Kress, L., and Goldstein, H.: Syphilis and cancer: reported syphilis prevalance among 7761 cancer patients. NY State J. Med., 42:1737, 1942.

21. Lynch, H. T., (ed.): Cancer Genetics. Springfield, IL., Charles C. Thomas, Publisher, 1976.

22. Mashberg, A., Morrissey, J. B., and Garfinkel, L.: A study of the appearance of early asymptomatic oral squamous cell carcinoma. Cancer, 32:1436, 1973.

23. McCarthy, F. P.: Etiology, pathology, and treatment of leukoplakia buccalis. Arch. Dermatol., 34:612, 1936.

24. Mehta, F. S., et al.: Epidemiologic and histologic study of oral cancer and leukoplakia among 50,915 villagers in India. Cancer, 24:844, 1969.

25. Mincer, H. H., Coleman, S. A., and Hopkins, K. P.: Observations on the clinical characteristics of oral lesions showing histologic epithelial dysplasia. Oral Surg., 33:389, 1972.

26. Moore, C.: Cigarette smoking and cancer of the mouth, pharynx, and larynx. J.A.M.A., 218:553, 1971.

27. Nathanson, I. T., and Weisberger, D. B.: The treatment of leukoplakia buccalis and related lesions with estrogenic hormone. N. Engl. J. Med., 221:556, 1939.

28. Nicolau, S. G., and Bolus, L.: Chronic actinic cheilitis and cancer of the lower lip. Br. J. Dermatol., 76:278, 1964.

29. Pindborg, J. J., et al.: Studies on oral leukoplakias V. Clinical and histologic signs of malignancy. Acta Odontol. Scand., 21:407, 1963.

30. Pindborg, J. J., Roed-Peterson, B., and Renstrup, G.: Role of smoking in floor of mouth leukoplakias. J. Oral Pathol., 1:22, 1972.

31. Potter, B., and Fretzin, D.: Well-differentiated epidermoid carcinoma arising in hypertrophic lichen planus. Arch Dermatol., 94:805, 1966.

32. Quigley, L., Shklar, G., and Cobb, C. M.: Reverse cigarette smoking in Caribbeans. Clinical, histologic, and cytologic observations. J. Am. Dent. Assoc., 72:867, 1966.

33. Reisman, R. J., et al.: The malignant potential of oral lichen planus—diagnostic pitfalls. Oral Surg., 38:227, 1974.

34. Renstrup, C.: Leukoplakia of the oral cavity. Acta Odontol. Scand., 16:99, 1958.

35. Roed-Peterson, B.: Cancer development in oral leukoplakia: follow-up of 331 patients. J. Dent. Res., 50:711, 1971.

36. Roed-Peterson, B., Banoczy, J., and Pindborg, J. J.: Smoking habits and histologic characteristics of oral leukoplakias in Denmark and Hungary. Br. J. Cancer, 28:575, 1973.

37. Samitz, M. H., Ackerman, A. B., and Lantis, L. R.: Squamous cell carcinoma arising at the site of oral florid papillomatosis. Arch. Dermatol., 96:286, 1967.

38. Schwimmer, E.: Leukoplakia buccalis. Vierteljahrsschr. Derm. Syph., 1:511, 1877.

39. Shafer, W. G., and Waldron, C. A.: A clinical and histopathologic study of leukoplakia. Surg. Gynecol. Obstet., 112:411, 1961.

40. Shklar, G.: The precancerous oral lesion. Oral Surg., 20:58, 1965.

41. Shklar, G.: Oral leukoplakia. Studies in enzyme histochemistry. J. Invest. Dermatol., 48:153, 1967.

42. Shklar, G.: Patterns of keratinization in oral leukoplakia. Arch. Otolaryngol., 87:400, 1968.

43. Sorrow, J. M., and Hitch, J. M.: Dyskeratosis congenita: first report of its occurrence in a female and a review of the literature. Arch. Dermatol., 88:340, 1963.

44. Stiehm, E. R., and McIntosh, R. M.: Wiskott-Aldrich syndrome: review and report of a large family. Clin. Exp. Immunol. 2:179, 1967.

45. Sturgis, S. N., and Lund, C. C.: Leukoplakia buccalis and keratosis labialis. N. Engl. J. Med., 210:996, 1934.

46. Tappeiner, J., and Wolff, K.: Floride oral papillomatose (oral florid papillomatosis). Wien. Klin. Wochenschr., 83:795, 1971.

47. Tennekoon, G. E., Bartlett, G. E., and Bartlett, G. C.: Effect of betel chewing on the oral mucosa. Br. J. Cancer, 23:39, 1969.

48. Trieger, N., et al: Cirrhosis and other predisposing factors in carcinoma of the tongue. Cancer, 11:357, 1958.

49. Trieger, N., et al: Significance of liver dysfunction in mouth cancer. Surg. Gynecol. Obstet., 108:230, 1959.

50. Vogler, W. R., et al.: A retrospective study of etiological factors in cancer of the mouth, pharynx, and larynx. Cancer, 15:246, 1962.

51. von Schettler, D., and Koberg, W.: Interessante Einzelbeobachtungen. Lichen ruber planus der Mundschleimhaut mot maligner Entartung. Zentralbl. Chir., 37:1101, 1970.

52. Waldron, C. A., and Shafer, W. G.: Current concepts of leukoplakia. Int. Dent. J., 10:350, 1960.

53. Waldron, C. A., and Shafer, W. G.: Leukoplakia revisited. A clinicopathologic study of 3256 oral leukoplakias. Cancer, 36:1386, 1975.

54. Wechsler, H. L., and Fisher, E. R.: Oral florid papillomatosis. Arch. Dermatol., 86:480, 1962.

55. Weisberger, D.: Precancerous lesions. J. Am. Dent. Assoc., 54:507, 1957.

56. Williamson, J. J.: Erythroplasia of Queyrat of the buccal mucous membrane. Oral Surg., 17:308, 1964.

57. Wynder, E. L., and Fryer, J. H.: Etiologic consideration of the Plummer-Vinson (Paterson-Kelly) syndrome. Ann. Intern. Med., 49:1106, 1958.

58. Wynder, E. L., Bross, I., and Feldman, R.: A study of the etiologic factors in cancer of the mouth. Cancer, 10:1300, 1957.

5

Experimental pathology of oral cancer

GERALD SHKLAR, D.D.S., M.S.

The aim of experimental pathology has been to develop reasonable experimental models for the different forms of oral cancer and to use these model systems in a variety of studies that involve the major clinical problems in oral oncology—those related to diagnosis, prognosis, and therapy. Several well-defined and extensively studied models have been developed for oral mucosal carcinoma as well as for salivary gland malignancies.

The most widely studied oral mucous membrane tumor model has been the experimental epidermoid carcinoma of hamster buccal pouch. First developed by Salley[40] in 1954, it was more extensively studied by Morris[30] and others and has since proved to be an ideal example of well-differentiated epidermoid carcinoma. It is induced by triweekly topical application by brush of a 0.5 per cent solution of 7,12-dimethylbenz(a)anthracene (9,10-dimethyl-1,2-benzanthracene)(DMBA) in mineral oil. There is a consistent sequence of histologic changes that occur in the affected pouch mucosa, with hyperkeratosis and chronic inflammation occurring at 4 to 6 weeks, hyperkeratosis and dysplasia occurring at 6 to 8 weeks, carcinoma-in-situ at 8 to 10 weeks, papillary and frankly invasive carcinoma at 10 to 12 weeks, and extensive tumors with invasion and surface necrosis at 12 to 14 weeks (Figs. 5–1 and 5–2). Information gained from recent studies of hamster buccal pouch tumors include the following:

1. The development of epidermoid carcinoma is invariably preceded by a hyperkeratotic and dysplastic lesion comparable to human oral leukoplakia of the dysplastic or precancerous variety, as shown by Santis and associates.[42]

2. Chronic irritation to the buccal pouch mucosa with topical application of carcinogen was found to augment carcinogenesis, with the irritation induced by croton oil[57] or mechanical stimulation[36] acting as a cocarcinogenic influence.[2, 3] Even the buccal pouch irritation induced by topically applied vitamin A was found to enhance buccal pouch carcinogenesis.[18, 31] Chronic irritation to the human oral mucosa is generally considered to be a factor in determining the site of tumor development in a susceptible host.

3. Manipulation and incision of the developing carcinomas do not result in alteration of tumor growth, deeper invasion of the lesions, or metastasis.[48] The results of these studies indicate evidence that repudiates the outdated clinical concept concerning the so-called danger of biopsy in spreading tumor cells and in facilitating invasion and metastasis.

4. As in human cancer, the hamster buccal pouch carcinoma is affected by the organism's immune response and immunologic capability generally. Following the discovery that immunosuppressive drugs such as cortisone[45, 46] and methotrexate[49] serve to enhance or augment carcinogenesis, it was found that specific antilymphocyte serum had a similar effect and enhanced the rapidity of tumor development by depressing the animal's cell-mediated immune response.[13, 66] Whereas cortisone merely speeded up tumor development, antilymphocyte serum and antimetabolite drugs such as methotrexate resulted in the development of more anaplastic carcinomas, with deeper invasiveness into underlying tissues. After the tumors had developed, the systemic use of certain types of antimetabolite drugs could cause regression of the tumors by effecting a

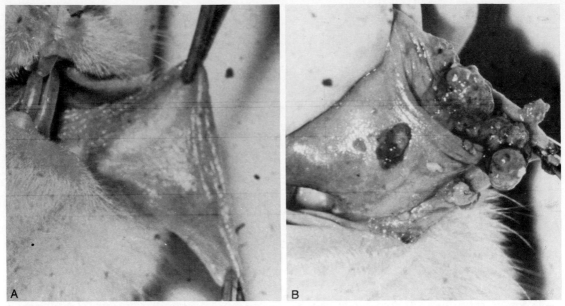

Figure 5–1. *A,* White leukoplakic lesions developing in the buccal pouch of a hamster after 6 weeks of DMBA applications. *B,* Numerous large tumors after 14 weeks of DMBA applications.

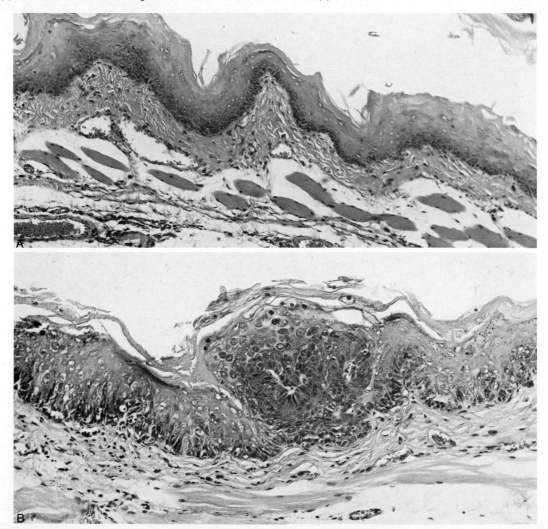

Figure 5–2. *A,* Microscopic features of hamster buccal pouch showing hyperkeratosis. *B,* Buccal pouch epithelium showing hyperkeratosis, dysplasia, and early carcinoma (× 150).

Illustration continued on opposite page

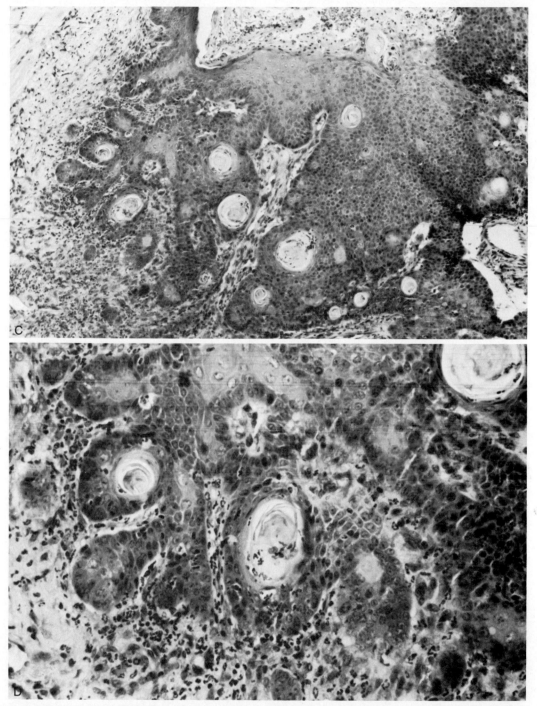

Figure 5–2 *Continued. C,* Well-differentiated, invasive carcinoma of buccal pouch (× 150). *D,* High-power view showing invasion of underlying connective tissue and cellular pleomorphism (× 300).

destruction of the epithelial cells within the tumor. The antitumor effect of different drugs resulted in considerable variation, with azathioprine appearing to be more effective on hamster buccal pouch carcinomas than many other chemotherapeutic drugs that are currently used for the treatment of cancer.[43]

5. Immunoenhancing agents such as Bacillus Calmette-Guérin (BCG)[14] and levamisole[8, 50] have been found to inhibit the development of buccal pouch tumors and may be useful in the future for immunotherapy in the overall management of human oral cancer.

6. Alcohol consumption is known to be a predisposing factor in human oral cancer, and the use of both alcohol and tobacco is so significant in epidemiologic studies of oral cancer that this disease can be considered an environmental malignancy.[37] Alcohol-drinking hamsters develop tumors more rapidly in the buccal pouch model[10] and the mechanism may relate to the chronic liver damage seen in these animals (Fig. 5–3). Protzel and associates found that oral tumors that were induced by carcinogenic chemicals in mice developed more readily in those animals whose livers had been damaged by alcohol or carbon tetrachloride.[35] Condensates of tobacco smoke have been used to induce buccal pouch tumors,[17, 29] but tobacco itself, in a finely ground form (snuff), appeared to have a relatively minimal effect upon the oral mucous membrane.[16] The ingredients of betel quid also failed to induce hamster buccal pouch lesions.[7] The carcinogen benzo(a)pyrene (3,4-benzpyrene), which is found in tobacco smoke condensate, does not induce hamster buccal pouch tumors when used in techniques similar to those for DMBA or methylcholanthrene. It is a much weaker carcinogen and may require some cocarcinogenic influence for the expression of its carcinogenic potential in the oral mucosa of experimental animals.

7. The hamster buccal pouch model is being

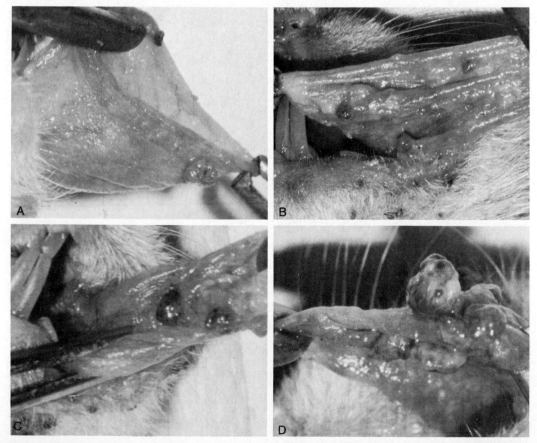

Figure 5–3. Effect of alcohol on chemical carcinogenesis of the oral mucosa of the hamster. *A,* Normal pouch with two small tumors painted with DMBA for 12 weeks. *B,* Pouch painted with DMBA for 12 weeks, and the animal drank alcohol. Extensive involvement of the entire pouch. *C,* The control animal was painted with DMBA for 14 weeks. Several tumors are noted. *D,* DMBA and alcohol animal after 14 weeks. The entire pouch has developed large tumors.

used to explore newer concepts in chemoprevention of cancer. Retinoids have been found to significantly delay the development of buccal pouch leukoplakia and carcinoma,[54] as they have been shown to delay tumor development in other experimental carcinoma models such as lung,[39] skin,[4] and bladder.[61] Retinoids studied in relation to hamster buccal pouch carcinogenesis have been 13-*cis*-retinoic acid and retinyl acetate. It had previously been shown that vitamin A deficiency had acted to augment oral carcinogenesis.[38] The mechanism of the retinoid action in tumor inhibition has not yet been established, but a stimulation of cell-mediated immunity has been postulated.[22, 54] Vitamin E has also been found to significantly delay the development of experimental hamster pouch carcinomas.[48a, 64a] Dietary supple-

ments of zinc were also found to inhibit the development of hamster buccal pouch tumors.[33] Chloropromazine was another substance found to be antineoplastic in the hamster buccal pouch model, but the mechanism of action has not been clarified, although it was suggested that the chloropromazine acted by its membrane- and lysosome-stabilizing properties so that less carcinogen would penetrate past the cell membrane.[32] Inhibition of experimental oral carcinogenesis has recently been demonstrated by the systemic administration of prostaglandin inhibitors such as aspirin and indomethacin (Fig. 5–4).[30c] If a low dosage of chemical carcinogen were used experimentally rather than the very potent 0.5 percent solution of DMBA, the tumor development could actually be prevented

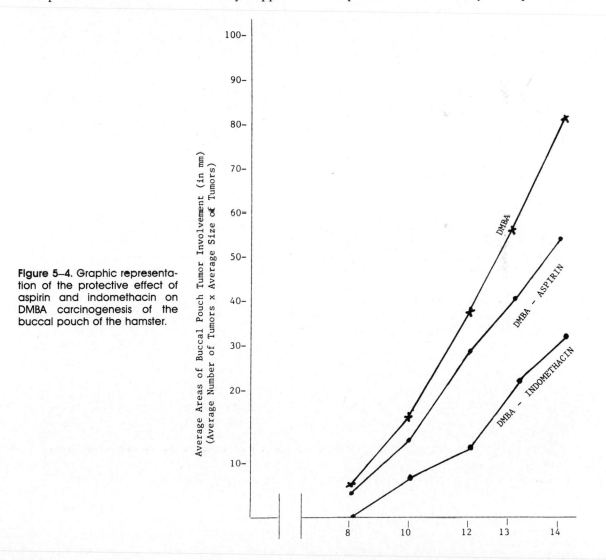

Figure 5–4. Graphic representation of the protective effect of aspirin and indomethacin on DMBA carcinogenesis of the buccal pouch of the hamster.

Number of Weeks After Start of Experiment

rather than merely retarded. This was shown with ibuprofen and a 0.1 percent solution of DMBA as the carcinogen.[6a]

8. Buccal pouch mucosa is an excellent tissue for the study of potential carcinogenicity of various medicaments and substances to be used in the mouth. Potential oral mucosal carcinogens can be applied three times per week to pouch mucosa for periods up to 6 months or even 1 year. If there is no histologic evidence of dysplasia, it is unlikely that the material will be carcinogenic for human oral mucosa.

9. Carcinogenesis of oral mucosa apparently requires activity of a carcinogen at the epithelial surface. When DMBA was combined with dimethyl sulfoxide to penetrate mucosa more readily, epithelial carcinogenesis was retarded and sarcomas developed within the underlying connective tissue.[55] The retardation of the development of epithelial malignancies may also be caused by the degeneration of the epithelium following the subepithelial activity of the carcinogen. It has been shown that radiation-damaged buccal pouch epithelium is less susceptible to hydrocarbon-stimulated malignancy than is normal or relatively undamaged buccal pouch epithelium.[53] Kinetics of pouch carcinogenesis have been studied.[35a]

10. Both precancerous leukoplakia and buccal pouch carcinoma were found to have an altered metabolism, as shown by the findings of enzyme histochemistry (Fig. 5–5).[44, 60] Human oral cancer and leukoplakia had a similar increase in lactic dehydrogenase activity. Because of these findings, it has been suggested that histochemistry be used for early diagnosis of oral cancer. Unfortunately, the cytologic and histologic tests that were devised were unwieldy and did not yield results superior to those in standard cytologic and biopsy techniques.

11. Recent studies in hamster buccal pouch carcinogenesis have shown that carcinogenesis may be a two-phase phenomenon, with initiation occurring at a very early stage and promotion occurring somewhat later.[30b, 42a] Solt and Shklar have shown that clones of transformed cells, positive for γ-glutamyl transpeptidase activity, can be found after only three applications of carcinogen.[60a] These "initiated" cells could be promoted by further DMBA applications or by some noncarcinogen promoter. The transformed or initiated cells may continue to proliferate despite the inhibitory effect that DMBA is known to exert on normal cell replication.

The hamster buccal pouch carcinoma can be transplanted to the abdominal cavity of inbred or neonatal hamsters.[26] The transplanted tumor grows more rapidly than the primary, chemically induced tumor and is more undifferentiated histologically. It can be serially transplanted abdominally and becomes stabilized and anaplastic after three generations of transplantation. It can then be transplanted to the buccal pouch and will serve as a model of anaplastic epidermoid carcinoma, more closely simulating human oral carcinoma than the original, primary, well-differentiated hamster buccal pouch tumors (Fig. 5–6).[25] The hamster buccal pouch carcinoma can be grown in tissue culture. Recently, a cell line has been developed by Odukoya and associates from culture of an experimentally induced epidermoid carcinoma of the buccal pouch.[30a] The cell line can be used to produce a series of similar tumors by inoculation of cells into buccal pouches. The cell line can be useful in a variety of immunologic studies involving the host's response to oral cancer.

Although the hamster buccal pouch carcinoma model has proved extremely useful in a variety of studies, it has certain deficiencies when related to human oral cancer. The carcinomas tend to be well differentiated and papillary, whereas human oral cancer, with the exception of labial malignancies, tends to be anaplastic histologically and more aggressive clinically. Human oral cancer often metastasizes to regional nodes and occasionally to major organs, whereas the hamster model does not metastasize, and all techniques to induce metastasis have failed. Initial attitudes that the hamster buccal pouch is an "immunologically privileged site" and contains no lymphatic supply have been disproved by both immunologic and histologic investigations. However, the buccal pouch is a unique tissue configuration that is absent in humans; thus, a more natural site was sought.

Experimental cancer of the tongue was developed as a tumor model in an attempt to answer some of the critique. As initially reported by Fujita and colleagues, the technique employed trauma to the tissue, followed by topical application of carcinogen in acetone.[11] Marefat and Shklar found the trauma to be unnecessary and have used the technique of painting DMBA in acetone on the lateral border of the tongue three times per week.[23, 24] Leukoplakia and epidermoid carcinoma develop more slowly on the tongue than on pouch mucosa, but the lesions develop in a consistent

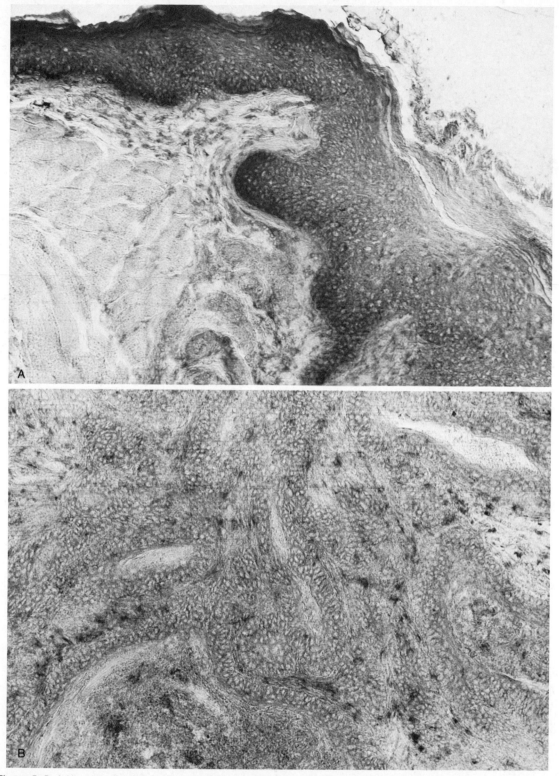

Figure 5–5. *A,* Normal and dysplastic hamster buccal pouch epithelium stained for esterase activity. The dysplastic leukoplakic area at right shows diminution of enzyme (× 200). *B,* Epidermoid carcinoma showing relative absence of esterase activity (× 200).

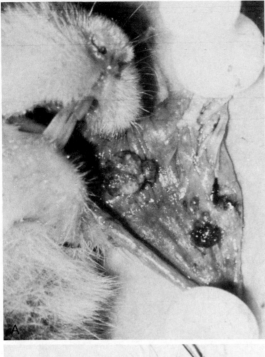

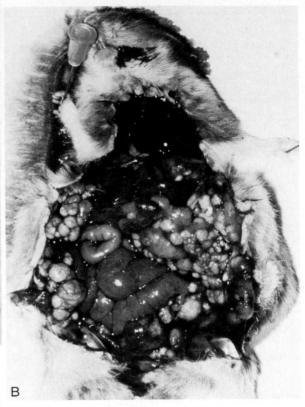

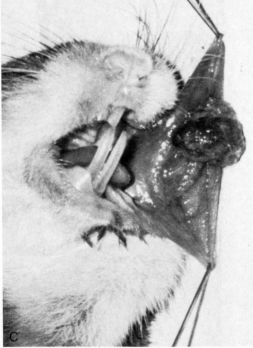

Figure 5–6. *A,* Carcinomas induced by DMBA in hamster buccal pouch. *B,* Multiple carcinomas growing in abdominal cavity after serial transplantation to newborn hamsters. *C,* Anaplastic carcinoma growing in buccal pouch after transplantation from abdomen.

Illustration continued on opposite page

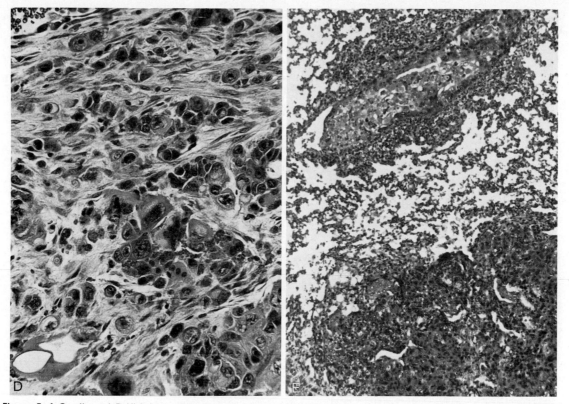

Figure 5–6 *Continued.* *D,* Histology of anaplastic carcinoma. Note the grossly abnormal cells (× 300). *E,* Anaplastic carcinoma metastatic to lung (× 100).

sequence, and the carcinomas tend to be more anaplastic than those in the pouch model. Hyperkeratosis and chronic inflammation occur at 6 to 8 weeks, hyperkeratosis and dysplasia at 8 to 10 weeks, carcinoma-in-situ at 10 to 12 weeks, papillary and invasive carcinoma at 12 to 14 weeks, and extensive lesions with necrosis at 14 to 16 weeks. Metastatic spread is not found consistently in this system but does occur occasionally.

The chemically induced lingual carcinomas tend to be more anaplastic and more invasive than the buccal pouch tumors and thus more closely resemble human oral mucosal epidermoid carcinoma (Fig. 5–7). The anaplastic pattern of experimental lingual carcinoma can be studied ultrastructurally.[51] The basal lamina is more disorganized than that seen in well-differentiated experimental epidermoid carcinomas; cellular pleomorphism is more pronounced; fewer desmosomal attachments are observed; and there is prominent clumping of tonofilaments. The lingual carcinoma model can also be used for the same types of studies that have been applied to the hamster buccal pouch system. A retinoid, 13-*cis*-retinoic acid, has been shown to significantly delay the in-

duction and development of lingual tumors and also to result in more well-differentiated lesions histologically.[51, 52]

Epidermoid carcinomas can be produced in other oral sites by application of carcinogens, but the yield is less consistent.[1, 18] The carcinogen in oil tends to be washed away by saliva. A technique was developed to induce oral carcinoma in any site by applying pure DMBA powder, which was covered and held in position against the mucosa by cyanoacrylate, a true mucous membrane adherent.[21]

Malignant tumors of salivary gland origin can be studied in a rat submandibular gland model by implantation of a small pellet of pure DMBA. After initial necrosis of the tissue that is adjacent to the pellet of carcinogen, adenocarcinomas and epidermoid carcinomas develop, with the latter type of malignancy developing from a cyst wall that often forms around the area of glandular necrosis.[6] Species specificity has been shown to be highly significant in salivary gland carcinogenesis, with the same technique resulting in fibrosarcomas rather than carcinomas in the hamster.[5] The salivary gland model can be used for the study of cocarcinogenic influences and for the effects

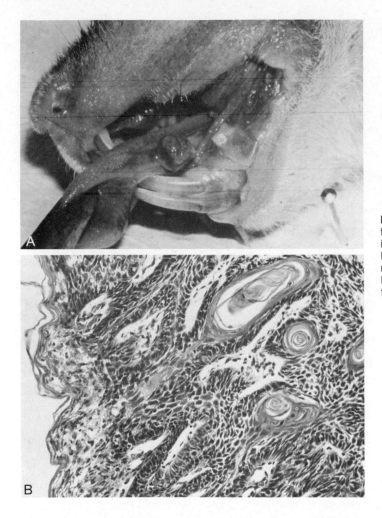

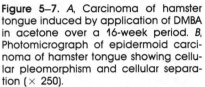

Figure 5–7. *A,* Carcinoma of hamster tongue induced by application of DMBA in acetone over a 16-week period. *B,* Photomicrograph of epidermoid carcinoma of hamster tongue showing cellular pleomorphism and cellular separation (× 250).

of antimetabolite drugs, stress, and other systemic influences upon carcinogenesis (Fig. 5–8).

Salivary gland carcinogenesis is also sensitive to genetic differences within a species. Variations in experimental carcinogenesis of the submandibular gland were shown in three strains of rat: Wistar, Sprague-Dawley, and Long-Evans.[64]

Experimental salivary gland adenocarcinomas can also be induced by injecting mice with polyoma virus (Fig. 5–9), as originally shown by Gross in 1953.[15] However, the virus induces leukemia and many other tumors in experimental animals, including a variety of odontogenic tumors of the jaws.[62]

The rat and hamster have also been used in studies related to the therapy of oral cancer. The skin-sparing and bone-sparing attributes of megavoltage radiation were originally shown by Meyer and associates who compared cobalt 60 radiation with standard 200 KV ra-

diation upon the oral mucosa, teeth, and jaws of rats. They also showed that oral trauma was less likely to lead to severe tissue damage and osteoradionecrosis in oral tissue irradiated with cobalt 60 than in oral tissues irradiated with 200 KV radiation of comparable doses, such as 1500 rads.[28] Hamster buccal pouch cancer has been used in the study of surgical therapeutic techniques such as cryosurgery and electrosurgery.[34] It has also been used to study diagnostic techniques such as oral cytology.[9]

Methotrexate, the first widely used chemotherapeutic drug, was originally shown to be highly toxic to oral mucosa in hamsters, causing atrophy of oral mucosal epithelium as well as collagen degeneration in the underlying connective tissue.[47] These findings subsequently became well known in humans who receive various potent chemotherapeutic agents. A severe stomatitis that has large areas of mucosal necrosis is often a limiting factor in the dosage of the chemotherapeutic drug

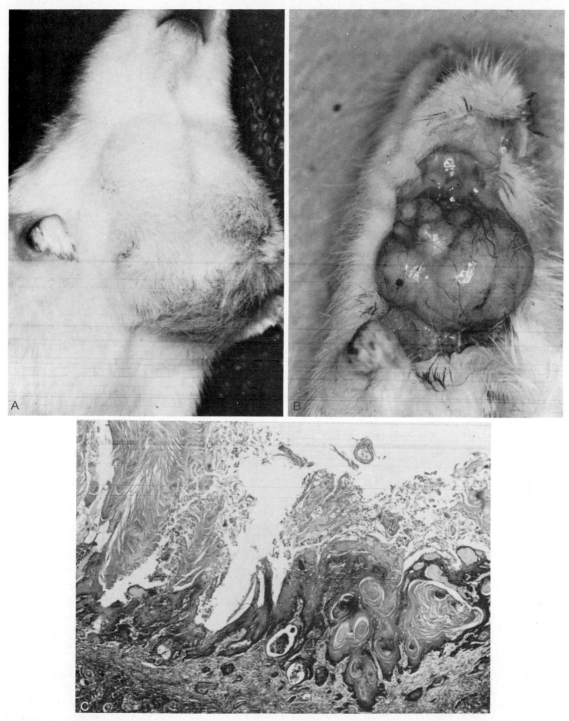

Figure 5–8. *A,* Salivary gland tumor induced by implantation of pellet of DMBA in rat. *B,* Dissection to show nodular carcinoma induced in the salivary gland of a rat. *C,* Microscopic view of an experimental rat salivary gland carcinoma arising as a cystic lesion (× 100).

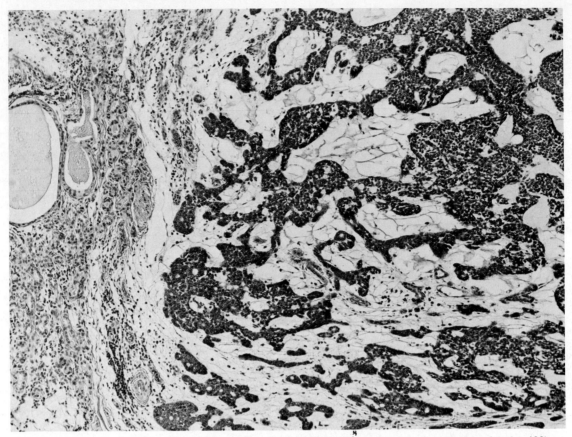

Figure 5–9. Adenocarcinoma arising in parotid gland *(left)* of mouse infected with polyoma virus (× 100).

that is used. Protective substances would be very welcome to chemotherapists, and the hamster could serve as an appropriate experimental animal for their development, because its oral mucosa is highly reactive to antimetabolite drugs.

Essentially, results of studies in the experimental pathology of oral cancer have provided information about its development and clinical course as well as its fundamental biologic characteristics. Findings have suggested the importance of immune phenomena that determine the growth of oral cancer and its spread and have indicated immunotherapy as a possible therapeutic modality. They have also suggested the possibility of chemoprevention, using appropriate nutritional supplements. The role of environmental etiologic agents in oral cancer has also been shown experimentally, particularly that of alcohol acting as a cocarcinogenic influence with known carcinogenic chemicals. The results of studies using animals

have also provided information about therapeutic modalities and may, in the future, be used to develop better diagnostic tests for early detection of cancer. The hamster buccal pouch model may also be the most appropriate testing site for the possible carcinogenicity of various new oral medicaments, dentifrices, and dental materials.

The hamster buccal pouch mucosa undergoing malignant transformation may also be used for many fundamental studies that involve fine structural alterations.[21, 67]

Studies are currently being carried out to identify the mechanisms by which chemical carcinogens act upon the oral mucosa to induce cellular alterations and mutations. Shuler and Latt found that topical application of carcinogen to buccal pouch mucosa resulted in induction of sister chromatid exchange.[56] Slaga and associates[58, 59] and others[63, 65] have recently shown that chemical carcinogens such as 7,12-dimethylbenz(a)anthracene are metabolized to

dihydrodiols and diol-epoxides, which are more effective in tumor initiation and mutagenesis.

REFERENCES

1. Al-Ani, S., and Shklar, G.: Effects of a chemical carcinogen applied to hamster gingiva. J. Periodontol., 37:36, 1966.
2. Berenblum, I.: The mechanism of carcinogenesis: a study of the significance of cocarcinogenic action and related phenomena. Cancer Res., 1:807, 1941.
3. Berenblum, I.: Irritation and carcinogenesis. Arch. Pathol., 38:233, 1944.
4. Bollag, W.: Prophylaxis of chemically induced benign and malignant epithelial tumors by vitamin A acid (retinoic acid). Eur. J. Cancer, 8:689, 1972.
5. Cataldo, E., and Shklar, G.: Chemical carcinogenesis in the hamster submaxillary gland. J. Dent. Res., 33:253, 1964.
6. Cataldo, E., Shklar, G., and Chauncey, H. H.: Experimental submaxillary gland tumors in rats. Histology and histochemistry. Arch. Pathol., 77:305, 1964.
6a. Cornwall, H., Odukoya, O., and Shklar, G.: Oral mucosal tumor inhibition by ibuprofen. J. Oral Maxillofac. Surg., 41:795, 1983.
7. Dunham, L. J., and Herrold, K. M.: Failure to produce tumors in hamster cheek pouch by exposure to ingredients of betel quid: histopathologic changes in the pouch and other organs by exposure to known carcinogens. J. Natl. Cancer Instit., 29:1047, 1962.
8. Eisenberg, E., and Shklar, G.: Levamisole and hamster pouch carcinogenesis. Oral Surg., 43:562, 1977.
9. Fischman, S. L., and Greene, G. W.: Cytologic changes during experimental carcinogenesis. Acta Cytol., 10:289, 1966.
10. Freedman, A., and Shklar, G.: Alcohol and hamster buccal pouch carcinogenesis. Oral Surg., 46:794, 1978.
11. Fujita, K., Kaku, T., Sasaki, M., et al.: Experimental production of lingual carcinomas in hamsters by local application of 9,10-dimethyl-1,2 benzanthracene. J. Dent. Res., 52:327, 1973.
12. Giunta, J., and Shklar, G.: Studies on tongue carcinogenesis in rats with and without cyanoacrylate adhesive. Arch. Oral Biol., 17:617, 1972.
13. Giunta, J., and Shklar, G.: The effect of antilymphocyte serum on experimental hamster buccal pouch carcinogenesis. Oral Surg., 31:344, 1971.
14. Giunta, J., Reif, A. E., and Shklar, G.: Bacillus Calmette Guérin and antilymphocyte serum in carcinogenesis. Arch. Pathol., 98:237, 1974.
15. Gross, L.: A filterable agent recovered from AK leukemic extracts causing salivary gland carcinomas in C3H mice. Proc. Soc. Exp. Biol. Med., 83:414, 1953.
16. Homburger, F.: Mechanical irritation, polycyclic hydrocarbons, and snuff. Arch. Pathol., 91:411, 1971.
17. Kendrick, F. J.: Some effects of chemical carcinogen and of cigarette smoke condensate upon hamster cheek pouch mucosa. Health Sci., 24:3698, 1964.
18. Levij, I. S., and Polliack, A.: Lymphoma-like hamster cheek pouch with topical vitamin A palmitate. Pathol. Microbiol., 34:288, 1969.
19. Levij, I. S., Rwomushana, J. W., and Polliack, A.: Effect of topical cyclophosphamide, methotrexate, and vinblastine on 9,10-dimethyl-1,2-benzanthracene (DMBA) carcinogenesis in the hamster cheek pouch. Eur. J. Cancer, 6:187, 1970.
20. Levy, B. M.: Experimental oral carcinogenesis. J. Dent. Res., 42:321, 1963.
21. Listgarten, M. A., Albright, J. T., and Goldhaber, P.: Ultrastructural alteration in hamster cheek pouch epithelium in response to a carcinogen. Arch. Oral Biol., 8:145, 1963.
22. Lotan, R. A., and Dennert, G.: Stimulatory effect of vitamin A analogs on induction of cell-mediated cytotoxicity in vivo. Cancer Res., 39:55, 1979.
23. Marefat, P., and Shklar, G.: Experimental production of lingual leukoplakia and carcinoma. Oral Surg., 44:578, 1977.
24. Marefat, P., and Shklar, G.: Lingual leukoplakia and carcinoma. An experimental model. Prog. Exp. Tumor Res., 24:259, 1979.
25. Meng, C. L., Shklar, G., and Albright, J.: A transplantable anaplastic oral cancer model. Oral Surg., 53:170, 1982.
26. Merk, L., Shklar, G., and Albright, J.: Transplantation of hamster buccal pouch carcinoma to neonatal hamsters. Oral Surg., 47:533, 1979.
27. Mesrobian, A., and Shklar, G.: Gingival carcinogenesis in the hamster, using tissue adhesive for carcinogen fixation. J. Periodontol., 40:603, 1969.
28. Meyer, I., Shklar, G., and Turner, J.: Tissue healing and infection in experimental animals irradiated with cobalt 60 and orthovoltage. Oral Surg., 21:333, 1979.
29. Moore, C., and Miller, A. J.: Effect of cigarette smoke tar on hamster cheek pouch. Arch. Surg., 76:786, 1958.
30. Morris, A. L.: Factors influencing experimental carcinogenesis in the hamster cheek pouch. J. Dent. Res., 40:3, 1961.
30a. Odukoya, O., Schwartz, J., Weichselbaum, R., et al.: An epidermoid carcinoma cell line derived from hamster DMBA-induced buccal pouch tumors. J. Natl. Cancer Inst., 71:850, 1983.
30b. Odukoya, O., and Shklar, G.: Two-phase carcinogenesis in hamster buccal pouch. Oral Surg., 54:547, 1982.
30c. Perkins, T. M., and Shklar, G.: Delay in hamster buccal pouch carcinogenesis by aspirin and indomethacin. Oral Surg., 53:170, 1982.
31. Polliack, A., and Levij, I. S.: The effect of topical vitamin A on papillomas and intraepithelial carcinomas induced in hamster cheek pouches with 9,10-dimethyl 1,2-benzanthracene. Cancer Res., 29:327, 1969.
32. Polliack, A., and Levij, I. S.: Antineoplastic effect of chlorpromazine in chemical carcinogenesis in the hamster cheek pouch. Cancer Res., 32:1912, 1972.
33. Poswillo, D. E., and Cohen, B.: Inhibition of carcinogenesis by dietary zinc. Nature, 231:447, 1971.
34. Poswillo, D. E.: Cryosurgery and electrosurgery compared in the treatment of experimentally induced oral carcinoma. Brit. Dent. J., 131:347, 1971.
35. Protzel, M., Giardina, A. C., and Albano, E. H.: The effect of liver imbalance in the development of oral tumors in mice following the application of benzpyrene or tobacco tar. Oral Surg., 18:622, 1964.
35a. Reiskin, A. P., and Berry, R. J.: Cell proliferation and carcinogenesis in the hamster cheek pouch. Cancer Res., 28:898, 1968.
36. Renstrup, G., Smulow, J., and Glickman, I.: Effect of chronic mechanical irritation on chemically induced carcinogenesis in the hamster cheek pouch. J. Am. Dent., 64:770, 1962.
37. Rothman, K., and Keller, A.: The effect of joint exposure to alcohol and tobacco on risk of cancer of

the mouth and pharynx. J. Chronic Dis., *25*:711, 1972.

38. Rowe, N. H., and Gorlin, R. J.: The effect of vitamin A deficiency upon experimental carcinogenesis. J. Dent. Res., *38*:72, 1959.

39. Saffiotti, U., Montesano, R., Sellakumar, A. R., et al.: Experimental cancer of the lung. Inhibition by vitamin A of the induction of tracheobronchial squamous metaplasia and squamous cell tumors. Cancer, *20*:857, 1967.

40. Salley, J. J.: Experimental carcinogenesis in the cheek pouch of the Syrian hamster. J. Dent. Res., *33*:253, 1954.

41. Salley, J. J.: Histologic changes in the hamster cheek pouch during early hydrocarbon carcinogenesis. J. Dent. Res., *36*:48, 1957.

42. Santis, H., Shklar, G., and Chauncey, H. H.: Histochemistry of experimentally induced leukoplakia and carcinoma of the hamster buccal pouch. Oral Surg., *17*:307, 1964.

42a. Schribner, J. D., and Suss, R.: Tumor initiation and promotion. Int. Rev. Exp. Pathol., *8*:137, 1978.

43. Sheehan, R., Shklar, G., and Tennenbaum, R.: Azathioprine effect on experimental buccal pouch tumors. Arch. Pathol., *21*:264, 1971.

44. Shklar, G.: Metabolic characteristics of experimental hamster pouch carcinomas. Oral Surg., *20*:336, 1965.

45. Shklar, G.: Cortisone and hamster buccal pouch carcinogenesis. Cancer Res., *26*:2461, 1966.

46. Shklar, G.: The effect of cortisone on the induction and development of hamster buccal pouch carcinomas. Oral Surg., *23*:241, 1967.

47. Shklar, G.: The effect of 4-amino-N¹⁰-methyl-pteroylglutamic acid on oral mucosa of experimental animals. J. Oral Ther. and Pharmacol., *4*:374, 1968.

48. Shklar, G.: The effect of manipulation and incision on experimental carcinoma of hamster buccal pouch. Cancer Res., *28*:2180, 1968.

48a. Shklar, G.: Oral mucosal carcinogenesis in hamsters: inhibition by vitamin E. J. Natl. Cancer Inst., *68*:791, 1982.

49. Shklar, G., Cataldo, E., and Fitzgerald, A. L.: The effect of methotrexate on chemical carcinogenesis of hamster buccal pouch. Cancer Res., *26*:2218, 1966.

50. Shklar, G., Eisenberg, E., and Flynn, E.: Immunoenhancing agents and experimental leukoplakia and carcinoma of the hamster buccal pouch. Prog. Exp. Tumor Res., *24*:269, 1979.

51. Shklar, G., Flynn, E., Szabo, G., et al.: Retinoid inhibition of experimental lingual carcinogenesis— ultrastructural observations. J. Natl. Cancer Inst., *65*:1307, 1980.

52. Shklar, G., Marefat, P., Kornhauser, A., et al.: Retinoid inhibition of lingual carcinogenesis. Oral Surg., *49*:325, 1980.

53. Shklar, G., Meyer, I., Stevens, W., et al.: Hamster pouch carcinogenesis in tissue irradiated with orthovoltage and cobalt 60. Oral Surg., *30*:431, 1970.

54. Shklar, G., Schwartz, J., Grau, D., et al.: Inhibition of hamster buccal pouch carcinogenesis by 13-*cis*-retinoic acid, Oral Surg., *50*:45, 1980.

55. Shklar, G., Turbiner, S., and Siegel, W.: Chemical carcinogenesis of hamster mucosa. Reaction to dimethyl sulfoxide. Arch Pathol., *87*:637, 1969.

56. Shuler, C. F., and Latt, S. A.: Sister chromatid exchange induction resulting from systemic, topical, and systemic-topical presentations of carcinogens. Cancer Res., *39*:2510, 1979.

57. Silberman, S., and Shklar, G.: The effect of a carcinogen (DMBA) applied to the hamster's buccal pouch in combination with croton oil. Oral Surg., *16*:1344, 1963.

58. Slaga, T. J., Huberman, E., DiGiovanni, J., et al.: The importance of the "bay region" diol-epoxide in 7,12 dimethylbenz(a)anthracene skin tumor initiation and mutagenesis. Cancer Lett., *6*:213, 1979.

59. Slaga, T. J., Gleason, G. L., DiGiovanni, J., et al.: Potent tumor-initiating activity of the 3,4-dihydrodiol of 7,12-dimethylbenz(a)anthracene in mouse skin. Cancer Res., *39*:1934, 1979.

60. Solt, D. B.: Localization of gamma-glutamyl transpeptidase in hamster buccal pouch epithelium treated with 7,12 dimethylbenz(a)anthracene. J. Natl. Cancer Instit., *67*:193, 1981.

60a. Solt, D. B., and Shklar, G.: Rapid induction of γ-glutamyl transpeptidase-rich intraepithelial clones in 7,12 dimethylbenz(a)-anthracene-treated hamster buccal pouch. Cancer Res., *42*:285, 1982.

61. Sporn, M. B., Dunlop, N. M., Newton, D. L., et al.: Prevention of chemical carcinogenesis by vitamin A and its synthetic analogs (retinoids). Fed. Proc., *35*:1332, 1976.

62. Stanley, H. R., Dawe, C. J., and Law, I. W.: Oral tumors induced by polyoma virus in mice. Oral Surg., *17*:547, 1964.

63. Tierney, B., Hewer, A., MacNicoll, A. D., et al.: The formation of dihydrodiols by the chemical or enzymic oxidation of benz(a)anthracene and 7,12-dimethylbenz(a)anthracene. Chem. Biol. Interact., *23*:243, 1978.

64. Turbiner, S., and Shklar, G.: Variations in experimental carcinogenesis of submandibular gland in three stains of rats. Arch. Oral Biol., *14*:1065, 1969.

64a. Weerapradist, W., and Shklar, G.: Vitamin E inhibition of hamster buccal pouch carcinogenesis. Oral Surg., *54*:304, 1982.

65. Wong, L. K., Wang, A., and Daniel, F. B.: Oxidative metabolites of 7,12-dimethylbenz(a)anthracene. Further investigation of the K-region epoxide. Drug Metab. Dispos., *8*:28, 1980.

66. Woods, D. A.: Influence of antilymphocyte serum on DMBA induction of oral carcinomas. Nature, *224*:276, 1969.

67. Woods, D. A., and Smith, C. J.: Ultrastructure of the dermal-epidermal junction in experimentally induced tumors and human oral lesions. J. Invest. Dermatol., *52*:259, 1969.

6

Biopsy techniques for oral lesions

SUMNER P. FRIM, D.M.D.

The early recognition, diagnosis, and treatment of oral pathologic conditions are important in helping to ensure a favorable prognosis for the patient. It has been shown that the cure rate for oral cancer is higher when an early definitive treatment has been initiated. Lesions of the oral cavity are easily visualized with appropriate lighting, and palpation may offer information about the surface texture of the lesion and surrounding induration. When an oral lesion is discovered, a detailed history, including its duration, pain, and changes in its size and appearance is required. Information should be sought concerning the presence of other lesions, and these lesions should be examined, if possible. A detailed medical history and a thorough clinical examination, hematologic study, urinalysis, and chest x-rays may be indicated. Dental radiographs may be necessary to eliminate the possibility of odontogenic infection. Radiographs of the jaws may also be useful in determining whether an oral lesion also involves the underlying bone. At the present time, the only known way to establish an accurate diagnosis of a lesion is by microscopic examination.

Removal of tissue for histopathologic examination is referred to as a biopsy, and this is the most effective technique for the diagnosis of neoplasms and in distinguishing benign from malignant tumors. Its accuracy in the diagnosis of malignant oral tumors is almost 100 percent.[3] The oral biopsy is also useful in the diagnosis of dermatologic diseases, such as lichen planus, lupus erythematosus, pemphigus, and pemphigoid. It is also of value in the diagnosis of precancerous leukoplakia and in the initial diagnosis of systemic diseases with oral manifestations, such as amyloidosis,[4] Sjögren's syndrome,[6] and cystic fibrosis.[5]

The oral biopsy is a simple procedure that is carried out quickly and safely, and should be performed whenever a suspicious lesion is seen. It is an indispensable procedure in the diagnosis of oral cancer and is valuable in planning proper treatment, in checking the progress of treatment and the extensiveness of the disease, and in evaluating the results.[1, 9–11] Among the benefits of oral biopsy are the relative absence of scarring and the rarity of infection or other complications.

The results of recent experiments involving animals have indicated that a properly performed biopsy does not increase the dangers of metastasis of the neoplastic cells.[7] It is, however, important that an adequate diagnostic sample of tissue be obtained. Most oral biopsies are performed under local anesthesia, although in cases in which access is difficult, general anesthesia may be preferred. Care should be taken to avoid injecting local anesthesia into the lesion. It either may be infiltrated into the lesion's periphery or conduction anesthesia should be used. Squeezing of the lesions should be avoided. Many pathologists prefer to have some adjacent normal tissue with the abnormal tissue, although it is not necessary for diagnosis.

The removal of necrotic tissue, usually in the center of the lesion, should be avoided, because it has no diagnostic value. The biopsy specimen should immediately be placed in the proper fixative solution, which is 10 percent formalin, for routine histopathology. Drugs that alter the staining characteristics of the tissues (i.e., methylene blue, Merthiolate, Betadine) should not be applied to the lesion prior to the biopsy.

A negative biopsy report means only that no malignancy was revealed by the slide or slides reviewed. One should remember that this does not necessarily mean that the patient is free of malignancy (though this usually is the case in a well-performed biopsy). If a

55

malignancy is strongly suspected, based on clinical judgment, and if recuts of the block tissue reveal negative results, a second or even third biopsy should be performed. On the other hand, when there is a high suspicion of malignancy, which may necessitate an immediate surgical procedure, it is advantageous to hospitalize the patient for the biopsy, so that appropriate surgical excision can be performed as soon as possible. Time is of great importance in cancer management.

PURPOSES OF BIOPSY

The purposes of a biopsy include the following:

1. To make a speedy, definitive, accurate diagnosis of the lesion.

2. To aid in determining the prognosis of the lesion.

3. To aid in deciding the best treatment (surgery, cryosurgery, radiation, chemotherapy, or any appropriate combinations).

4. To determine whether the extent of the surgery is adequate and whether all margins of the specimen are free of tumor infiltration when complete excision of the lesion has been attempted.

5. To confirm or negate a clinical diagnosis.

6. To reassure the patient who has cancerphobia that the lesion is innocuous.

Any abnormal tissue discovered in the oral cavity should be biopsied, but it should be emphasized that indiscriminate biopsy without a thorough history and clinical examination of the patient should be discouraged. For example, in patients who have suspicious gingival hyperplasia or lymph node enlargement, a complete blood count may be necessary, because the oral lesion may represent local evidence of systemic disorders. Enlarged gingival tissue may be the first clinical manifestation of leukemia.

LESIONS TO BE BIOPSIED

Lesions to be biopsied include:

1. Hyperkeratotic lesions of the lips and oral mucosa.

2. Chronic ulcers of the lips, tongue, and mucosa that do not heal within 12 to 14 days of discovery.

3. Tissue enlargement that cannot be explained on a traumatic or bacterial basis.

4. All tissues excised in routine procedures from the oral cavity, such as the removal of hyperplastic tissue in ridge correction for dentures.

5. All pigmented lesions should be completely excised, because there is always the possibility that this type of lesion may be a malignant melanoma.

6. When a vascular lesion is suspected, caution should be exercised, and it may be necessary to hospitalize the patient, in anticipation of massive hemorrhage and its control.

7. All periapical dental lesions that show evidence of increasing in size or that have a history of pain or discomfort, including periapical granulomas and radicular cysts. If a radiolucent area is noted on a routine dental radiograph and if it is asymptomatic, the biopsy may be postponed and the clinical course of the lesion may be followed.

8. Primordial, follicular, and fissural cysts. It should be noted that when microscopically examined, a small but significant number of follicular cysts show ameloblastic epithelial proliferation in their walls or true ameloblastomas.

9. Bone lesions that are accompanied by pain, numbness, or other symptomatology, or bone lesions that show expansion on periodic radiographs.

It would be advantageous if the biopsy were performed in the same setting (e.g., hospital) in which the definitive treatment was to be instituted. However, the purpose of biopsy is to establish a diagnosis as early as possible so that curative treatment may be begun with minimal delay. The patient who presents with oral cancer in the office of a general practitioner may not return for a biopsy because of the fear of what may be found. Thus, it is essential that a biopsy be taken that day by the generalist (if the generalist feels adequately trained to undertake this procedure) or that the generalist refer the patient to a person who can perform the biopsy.

BIOPSY METHODS

Excisional Biopsy

Excisional biopsy refers to the total removal of the lesion surgically. It is the method of choice when the size and the location of the lesion permit a wide margin of normal tissue (not less than 0.5 cm in all directions from the periphery of the lesion) to be included in the specimen. The depth of the lesion is also an important factor in its removal (Figs. 6–1 through 6–3).

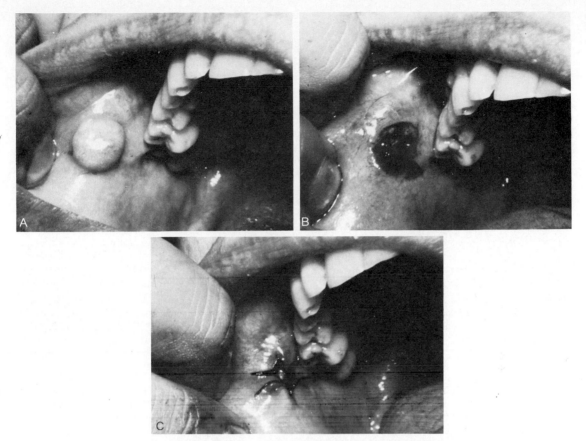

Figure 6–1. Excisional biopsy of a tumor of the right buccal mucosa, diagnosed histologically as a fibroma. *A*, Tumor in situ. *B*, Excision of the tumor. *C*, Closure of the biopsy wound with silk sutures.

Incisional Biopsy

Incisional biopsy is the removal of a representative portion of the lesion with a scalpel. If the lesion is extensive, several representative portions may be removed and should be marked with proper identification to indicate the area from which they were taken. After the section of the tissue has been cut with a sharp knife, dissemination of the malignant cells may be prevented by immediately cauterizing the wound to coagulate the tissue fluid and the blood in the exposed vessels that have been cut (Figs. 6–4 and 6–5).

Electrosurgery

Electrosurgery is not recommended for use in the oral cavity, because the high-frequency cutting knife causes coagulation of tissue with loss of cellular detail along the path of the incision, making it difficult to accurately interpret microscopic findings. In order to obtain well-preserved tissue with this technique, a large biopsy must be taken.

Punch Biopsy

The oral cavity and surrounding area rarely require use of the punch biopsy technique. It is a method that has widely been used in obtaining tissue from organs and areas that are not readily accessible without an extensive surgical procedure. Its disadvantages include lack of visualization of the area to be examined, tissue specimens may not be typical of the lesion, and only a small quantity of tissue may be obtained. On the other hand, a variety of biopsy punches can be used for routine oral biopsy instead of a surgical scalpel. The dermal punch can be used to obtain a small but useful specimen.

Aspiration Biopsy

In the aspiration biopsy technique, a large gauge needle and aspirating syringe are used.[2] This method is widely used in obtaining bone marrow specimens and is favored by orthopedic surgeons for bone lesions that are not easily attainable surgically. Its disadvantages

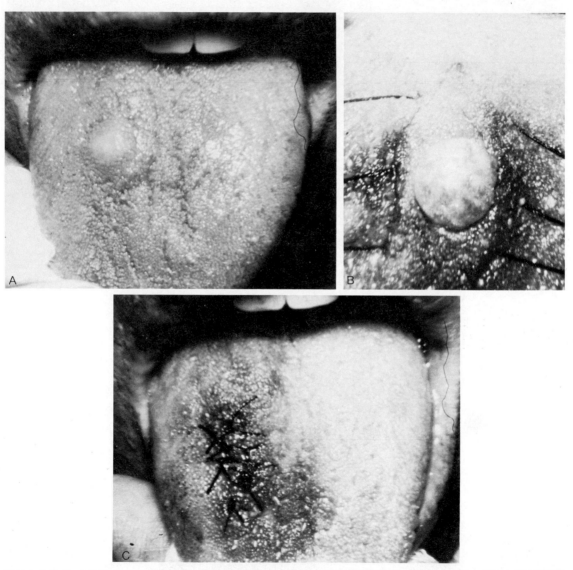

Figure 6–2. Nodular lesion on the dorsum of the tongue, diagnosed histologically as a granular cell myoblastoma. *A,* Tumor in situ. *B,* Sutures have been placed outside the incision line for rapid closure. *C,* Lesion has been excised, and the sutures have been tied.

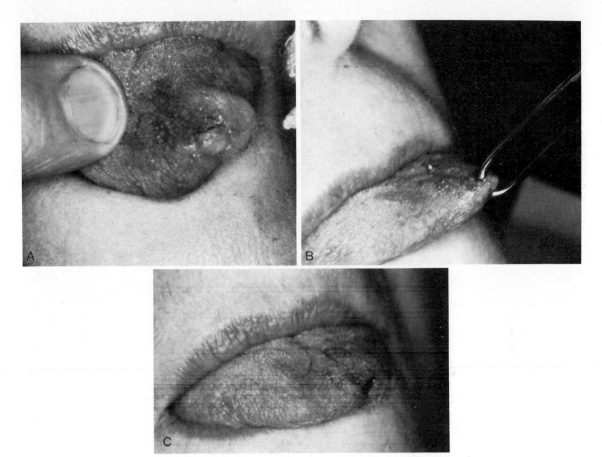

Figure 6–3. Small lesion on the tip of the tongue, diagnosed histologically as a fibroma. *A,* Lesion in situ. *B,* Tongue steadied with forceps prior to excision. *C,* Lesion has been excised. Sutures were not required.

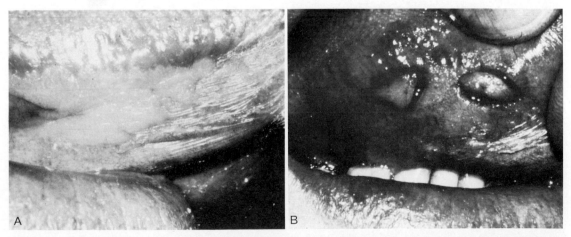

Figure 6–4. *A,* White lesion on the ventral surface of the tongue, diagnosed histologically as parakeratosis and spongiosis, consistent with the diagnosis of white sponge nevus. *B,* Two incisional biopsies, one with a triangular and one with an elliptical outline.

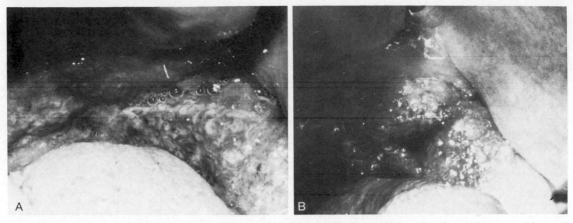

Figure 6–5. *A*, Large epidermoid carcinoma involving the left palate, posterior alveolar mucosa, and buccal mucosa. *B*, Incisional biopsy with a triangular outline. Sutures were not required.

are that limited amounts of material are obtained and that the pathologist must be experienced in the interpretation of the small tissue fragments. Often, it is not possible for the pathologist to make a definitive diagnosis with assurance.

Silverman Needle Biopsy

This procedure is useful in deep-seated lesions (i.e., neoplasms of the salivary glands, neck masses, or soft-tissue tumors of bone). With this needle, one can remove a strip of intact tissue, 1.5-mm wide and about 1.5-cm long, which can be sectioned and studied like an ordinary surgical biopsy. This method is superior to the ordinary aspiration biopsy, which is often unsatisfactory because it furnishes only detached clusters of cells for diagnosis and often does not get any of the tumor cells. It should be emphasized that in all needle biopsies a negative result may be inconclusive.

Cytologic Smears

Smears that use exfoliative cytology, as in the Papanicolaou technique, are commonly used in examining regions such as the uterine cervix. In the mouth, however, exfoliated cells cannot be studied in saliva because of its proteolytic enzymes. Cells must be obtained by curettage or scraping a lesion with a wooden tongue depressor or a metal or plastic instrument. Oral cytologic examination may be carried out as a screening process rather than obtaining a biopsy. However, biopsies are always necessary to confirm a positive or negative diagnosis, because the reliability of the oral cytologic smear in the diagnosis of a malignant tumor is no higher than 85 percent.[8]

INSTRUMENTATION

Instrumentation for surgical excision or incisional biopsy includes:
1. Sterile tray.
2. Local anesthesia and syringe.
3. Scalpel with No. 15 Bard Parker blade.
4. Gauze sponges.
5. Appropriate sutures (000–0000 plain gut for subcutaneous closure, 000–0000 black silk for mucous membrane, and 00000 nylon for skin closure).
6. Tissue forceps.
7. Suture needles.
8. Wide-mouth bottle containing 10 percent formalin.

There are few cases of biopsy in which postoperative complications occur if the proper precautions and attention to sterility are maintained. Primary closure of the wound to obtain proper healing is always desirable. The routine use of antibiotics is not indicated or recommended, because the same care should be taken to maintain sterility as in any surgical procedure. Care should be taken to avoid blood vessels and vascular tumors so that hemorrhage will not be a problem.

DESCRIPTION OF BIOPSY TECHNIQUES

Excisional Biopsy

1. Proper infiltration of a local anesthetic around periphery of the lesion is accomplished.
2. Two elliptical incisions are made around

opposite ends, demarcating the section of tissue to be removed. In order to facilitate a smooth closure of the wound, the length of the specimen should be approximately three times the size of its width.

3. The lesion is held with slight tension with an Allis forceps, and the base of the lesion is undermined with a scalpel.

4. When the specimen is freed from the underlying tissue, it is immediately placed into a bottle that contains a 10-percent formalin solution.

5. Margins of the wound are held with an Adson tissue forceps, and the wound is closed with simple interrupted 000 silk sutures (see Fig. 6–1C).

6. In the rare case of excessive hemorrhage, the bleeding vessels can be clamped with the point of a hemostat and either coagulated or tied off before closure.

7. A wide margin of normal tissue, at least 0.5 cm in all directions from the periphery, should be included in the specimen.

The tongue is extremely vascular, and hemorrhage may occasionally become a problem. The sutures for closure of the wound are placed outside the incision lines, and the incision is made around the lesion. The lesion is then excised, and without any delay, a closure is accomplished, providing early control of hemorrhage.

If the lesion is small enough, insertion of sutures may not be indicated and postoperative pressure on the wound area may create adequate hemostasis (see Fig. 6–3).

Incisional Biopsy

1. A pie-shaped wedge, which includes apparently normal and abnormal tissue and the underlying connective tissue, is removed (see Figs. 6–4 and 6–5).

2. An elliptical incision is made, beginning in the normal tissue, crossing the margin of the lesion at right angles, and extending toward the center of the lesion. The second incision is made in a similar manner, connecting the ends of the first incision.

3. The deepest extent of the lesion must be included.

4. The specimen is removed, and closure is accomplished with interrupted 000 silk sutures, if necessary.

5. Multiple specimens from different areas of a large lesion may be obtained in a similar manner and properly marked with sutures for identification.

Biopsy of Lesions in Bone

1. Proper infiltration of a local anesthetic is accomplished.

2. A proper flap is made, exposing the site of the lesion in the bone and extending over normal bone.

3. Bone that overlies the lesion is carefully removed either by using a No. 15 scalpel blade and curette if it is of parchment consistency from an expanding lesion or by a straight handpiece with a crosscut surgical tissue bur or dental rongeur if the overlying bone is dense.

4. After the window in the bone has been made, the entire lesion, or part of it if it is quite extensive, may be curetted out, removed, and placed in a specimen jar that contains 10 percent formalin (Fig. 6–6).

5. The bone is then smoothed with a dental bone file and irrigated with a sterile normal saline solution, the flap is reapproximated, and multiple interrupted 000 silk sutures are inserted.

6. It should be noted that when parchment bone is present, aspiration of the lesion may be attempted, using a syringe with a No. 21 gauge needle. If the syringe fills with blood, the lesion may be a hemangioma. The needle and syringe are then removed, the flap is reapproximated and sutured in place. Provisions must then be made to hospitalize the patient for a biopsy procedure, which will probably result in total removal of the lesion. The procedure should be performed in the operating room, with close monitoring of the

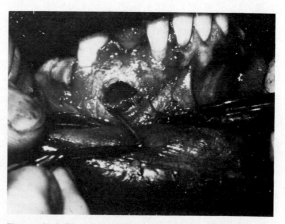

Figure 6–6. Flap is laid back for biopsy of the lesion in the right side of the mandible and appears as a radiolucent area on dental radiographs. Microscopic diagnosis of the cyst wall revealed chronic inflammation.

patient and whole blood available for transfusion, if necessary.

SUMMARY

Biopsy is a simple and safe procedure for the removal of tissue for pathologic diagnosis. Careful diagnosis will hopefully result in appropriate treatment for patients. It is essential that the clinician thoroughly examine the patient so that oral lesions will be found in the early stage and will be diagnosed and treated immediately. Early biopsy is indicated for all lesions after a thorough history has been taken, a clinical examination has been done, and appropriate laboratory tests have been completed. All tissue removed must be submitted for histopathologic examination, regardless of how benign it may appear.

Properly performed biopsies have almost a 99-percent rate of accuracy. Lesions that appear clinically to require extensive treatment for cancer should be referred directly to the proper facility for both diagnosis and treatment, because the faster the treatment, the better the prognosis for the patient.

REFERENCES

1. Burch, R., Jr., and Crouse, V. L.: Biopsy techniques. Dent. Clin. North Am., 3:769, 1959.
2. Frable, W. J., and Frable, M. A.: Thin-needle aspiration biopsy: the diagnosis of head and neck tumors revisited. Cancer, 43:1541, 1979.
3. Giunta, J., Meyer, I., and Shklar, G.: The accuracy of the oral biopsy in the diagnosis of cancer. J. Oral Surg., 28:552, 1969.
4. Lehner, T.: Oral biopsy in the diagnosis of amyloidosis. Isr. J. Med. Sci., 4:1000, 1968.
5. Meskin, L. H., Bernard, B., and Warwick, W. J.: Biopsy of the labial mucous salivary glands in cystic fibrosis. J.A.M.A., 188:82, 1964.
6. Sapiro, S., and Eisenberg, E.: Sjögren's syndrome (sicca complex). Oral Surg., 45:591, 1978.
7. Shklar, G.: The effect of manipulation and incision on experimental carcinoma of hamster buccal pouch. Cancer Res., 28:2180, 1968.
8. Shklar, G., Cataldo, E., and Meyer, I.: Reliability of cytologic smear in the diagnosis of oral cancer. A controlled study. Arch. Otolaryngol., 91:158, 1970.
9. Stern, M.: Oral tumors, including biopsy techniques. Dent. Clin. North Am., 15:423, 1971.
10. Thoma, K. H.: Oral Surgery, 5th ed., Vol. 1. St. Louis, The C. V. Mosby Co., 1969, pp. 120–124.
11. Warren, S.: Biopsy in Relation to Tumor Diagnosis, in Cancer. A Manual for Practitioners, 4th ed. Boston, American Cancer Society, Massachusetts Division, 1968, pp. 34–38.

7

Oral cytology and other diagnostic aids

GERALD SHKLAR, D.D.S., M.S.

Oral Cytology

Following the pioneering efforts of Papanicolaou[8] in the use of cytodiagnostic techniques for early cancer of the uterine cervix and other sites, these techniques were applied to lesions of the oral cavity, with the hope that early malignant tumors could be disclosed while they were small and asymptomatic.[7, 18]

In general, oral cytology is a simple and reasonably effective technique for the rapid initial evaluation of a suspicious oral lesion. The diagnostic accuracy of oral cytology is not as high as that of biopsy, and oral cytology should not be used as a final and definitive diagnostic procedure. However, the simplicity of its use, its high acceptability among patients, and its constant availability make oral cytology an ideal test in many situations.

Oral cytology is useful in screening large numbers of patients for oral cancer when the location of the screening facility (community center, school, neighborhood health center) is far from clinics or hospitals, where surgical and diagnostic facilities are available. It is helpful in corroborating a clinical impression of oral cancer when the patient refuses a biopsy at the initial visit. It is also valuable in following regression or recurrence of oral cancer after radiation therapy, when multiple biopsies could be detrimental to the healing of the tissue.

Oral cytology is an important diagnostic aid in various oral diseases other than cancer. It may be diagnostic for common viral diseases that affect the mouth and oropharynx, such as herpetic stomatitis, herpangina, and herpes zoster. It can be used to reveal the acantholytic cells of pemphigus, and with appropriate staining, the mycelia and spores of mycotic lesions such as candidiasis will also be disclosed.

Oral biopsy is a safe and relatively simple procedure that has virtually no complications, and its diagnostic accuracy is close to 100 percent, with figures of 97 and 98 percent reported.[2] Oral cytology, although a simple technique, has been shown to have a diagnostic accuracy of only 86 percent in carefully controlled studies in which large numbers of oral malignancies were subjected to both cytodiagnostic and histologic techniques.[16, 17] This indicates that oral cytology has a reasonably good diagnostic capability but should not be relied upon for *definitive* diagnosis of oral lesions. It is a very useful test and should be part of the overall diagnostic procedure for many oral disease states. However, it should not be used as the sole test for the diagnosis of an oral lesion, but rather as an adjunct in the overall diagnostic management. Furthermore, there are certain types of oral lesions, particularly hyperkeratotic lesions, in which oral cytology is of limited value and should not be used.

In general, it is always wise and virtually mandatory to correlate the cytology of an oral lesion with its histopathologic features. In oral cytology, a lesion or suspicious area must be found before the procedure can be of value. The suspicious area should be scraped, and the cells that are removed should be placed on a slide, fixed, and submitted for staining and microscopic evaluation. Exfoliative cytology per se is of limited value in the mouth. Cells exfoliated from oral mucosa are usually washed away in saliva and rapidly destroyed by the proteolytic enzymes in saliva and by the indigenous oral microflora of bacteria and fungi. Maintaining reasonable cellular morphology in saliva spit into a container or with a mouthwash technique is not possible, and such techniques have limited value.

A major advantage of the oral cavity over other cancer sites is that the region can be easily examined, and any areas of pathology can be observed and evaluated clinically. If the lesion is suggestive of cancer, it should be biopsied. If the appearance of the lesion makes one suspicious, it can still be biopsied, but a cytologic smear may be taken instead and a follow-up visit scheduled. If the lesion is still present, a biopsy should be taken, even if the cytologic smear were negative.

Fundamentally, careful oral examination is the basis for the detection of oral cancer. A knowledge of the appearance of normal oral structures and tissues is essential for the recognition of a small area of discoloration or altered size or shape that may indicate a suspicious area of disease. The lips of the patient must be retracted to examine the labial mucosa and vestibule. The tongue must be grasped with a piece of surgical gauze and moved to the right and left so that the posterior lateral borders of the tongue can properly be visualized. The floor of the mouth can be examined by raising the tongue. In carrying out an oral examination, an adequate light source is necessary and a mouth mirror is very helpful. If a suspicious lesion is discovered, a smear can be taken immediately. Obviously, the smear becomes a valueless procedure if the oral examination has not been properly carried out and if there is no lesion. It must be understood that small oral lesions are often asymptomatic and the patient may not be aware of the lesion until it reaches a considerable size and produces pain and discomfort.

There are several types of oral lesions in which the cytologic smear is of limited value and should not be used.

1. Hyperkeratotic lesions such as leukoplakia consist of a significantly thickened layer of surface keratin. In the dysplastic or precancerous form of leukoplakia, abnormal cells exist in the tissue but cannot be removed by scraping because of the thick keratin. In fact, few cells are seen in a smear of a hyperkeratinized surface; only fragments of keratin without nuclei are visible. It has been suggested that the keratin be removed with a knife or dental drill, and then the lesion could be smeared. However, this procedure is more traumatic than a biopsy and less effective diagnostically.

2. Lesions beneath the oral mucosal surface may be malignancies, but a surface smear cannot reach these tumor cells. Nodular lesions should be biopsied.

3. Skin is normally covered with a thick keratin layer, and thus, cytologic smears are not feasible. Lip is essentially skin on its dry surface, and suspicious lesions in this area should be biopsied.

TECHNIQUE OF OBTAINING CYTOLOGIC SPECIMEN

In the mouth, smears are obtained by scraping the surface of the oral mucosa. An effective instrument for this purpose is the wooden tongue depressor. The end can be scraped firmly over the lesion to be smeared, and the wooden surface accumulates large numbers of cells from the tissue surface. The wooden blade should be scraped along the mucosal surface several times. If the tissues are dry, the wooden blade should be moistened prior to its use by dipping the end in water or in saliva in the floor of the patient's mouth. When the specimen has been collected, the end of the blade is smeared on a glass slide using a rotatory movement. The specimen of cells must be fixed immediately to retain the cellular morphology. Fixation can be accomplished by immersing the slide in a solution of 70 percent alcohol or in ether-alcohol (50/50) for 15 to 20 minutes. The alcohol may be poured onto a slide and left there for a similar length of time. The slide is then removed from the alcohol and permitted to dry in the air by being positioned somewhat vertically so that the alcohol flows off onto a blotter or paper towel. Rapid and effective fixation can be accomplished by using an aerosol spray that contains alcohols and drying agents. Common hair sprays can be used for this purpose, as well as the more expensive aerosols that are sold as cytologic fixatives. The slide is sprayed from a distance of 10 to 15 cm and dries within several minutes.

When dry, the slide may be stained immediately or set aside for future staining. If the smear is to be sent to a laboratory for diagnosis, it must be fixed prior to mailing. The staining will be carried out in the laboratory. Papanicolaou's technique is still superior to most other differential staining techniques.

Various plastic and metal instruments may be used for collecting cytologic specimens, but they have no advantage over the wooden tongue depressor. The smooth surface of the metal or plastic does not collect large numbers of cells as it glides along the tissues.

The slides are usually evaluated as positive

for tumor cells, suggestive, suspicious, or negative.

CYTOLOGY OF NORMAL ORAL MUCOSA

Oral mucosa consists of three layers: the basal layer, or stratum germinativum; the prickle cell layer of polyhedral cells, or stratum spinosum; and the surface layer of flattened cells, or stratum corneum. There may be no keratin in this surface layer, as in buccal mucosa, or there may be varying degrees of keratinization, with a moderate amount in the hard palate. With Papanicolaou's stain, cells from the stratum corneum are orange-brown in color, with or without nuclei, and oval or flattened (Figs. 7–1 through 7–3). Cells of the stratum spinosum stain blue or red, contain nuclei, and are polyhedral in shape (Fig. 7–2).

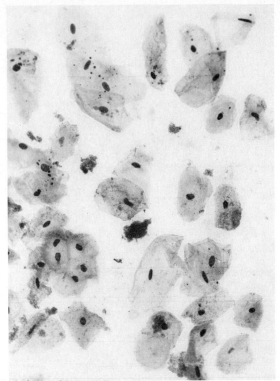

Figure 7–2. Cytologic smear of normal buccal mucosa. Cells stain pink or light blue, and contain small nuclei.

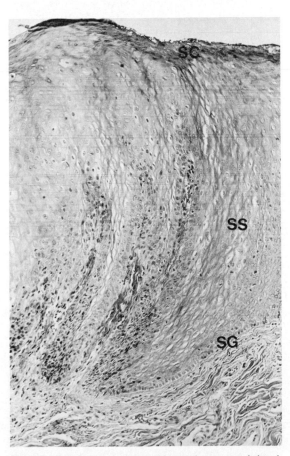

Figure 7–1. Biopsy specimen of buccal mucosa stained with Papanicolaou technique. The stratum corneum (SC) stains orange-red; the stratum spinosum (SS) stains pink in the upper layers and purple-blue in the lower layers. The stratum germinativum (SG) stains blue (× 200).

Cells of the upper stratum spinosum tend to stain red or purple. Cells of the lower stratum spinosum stain purple or blue. The nuclei are small in relation to the overall size of the cell. Occasional basal layer cells may appear in an oral smear and are characterized by somewhat larger nuclei that have a deeper stain, less cytoplasm, and a round or oval rather than a polyhedral outline.

CYTOLOGY OF INFLAMMATORY AND ULCERATIVE LESIONS OF ORAL MUCOSA

In chronic inflammatory lesions of oral mucosa, there is often some degree of epithelial hyperplasia and one may find cells with slightly larger nuclei than those seen in a smear of uninflamed tissue. Inflammatory cells may also be present in the cytologic smear. In ulcerative lesions, there may be many erythrocytes in the smear, as well as polymorphonuclear leukocytes (Fig. 7–4). There is always some degree of hemorrhage when the smear is taken in ulcerative lesions because the surface epithelium is absent. Colonies of bacteria may also be evident.

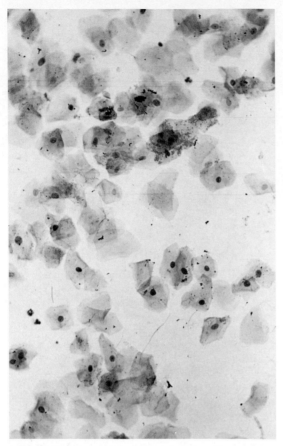

Figure 7–3. Cytologic smear of palate with numerous non-nucleated orange cells that represent the stratum corneum.

CYTOLOGY OF HYPERKERATOTIC LESIONS

In hyperkeratotic lesions, many cell forms are seen that do not have nuclei, representing the upper part of the widened stratum corneum. In hyperkeratotic lesions with dysplasia or early neoplastic transformation (leukoplakia), the major cellular alterations occur in the basal layer and in the lower stratum spinosum. Because the surface of the lesion consists of a dense layer of keratin, it is difficult to rub off a sufficient number of cells from the deeper layers for adequate cytologic interpretation. Thus, cytology should not be used in hyperkeratotic lesions; only biopsy should be used. All lesions interpreted clinically as leukoplakia must be biopsied for evidence of dysplasia or early neoplastic alterations.

CYTOLOGY OF ORAL CARCINOMA

Cytologic investigation of suspicious oral lesions represents the major use of the technique and its major value in the overall early diagnosis of oral cancer. It is only with the increasing discovery of small early lesions that current therapeutic results for oral cancer will improve substantially, and oral cytology can play a significant role in the discovery of small, asymptomatic lesions that may not arouse sufficient suspicion in a busy clinician.

Tumor cells manifest in extremely variable appearances and to a large extent depend upon the degree of differentiation of the oral neoplasm. Oral malignant tumors are epidermoid carcinoma in more than 95 percent of cases. The remaining small percentage includes adenocarcinomas that develop from oral mucous glands and the extremely rare melanomas, fibrosarcomas, and lymphomas. Oral epidermoid carcinomas either may be of the well-differentiated, or "low grade" variety, or may be poorly differentiated or of the "high grade" variety. The term *anaplastic* may also be used for these poorly differentiated lesions (see Chapter 3).

The well-differentiated lesions develop slowly, metastasize late, and tend to grow as papillary configurations rather than invading deeply into the underlying tissues. These tumors develop keratin; the cells resemble normal cells except for an altered nuclear-cytoplasmic ratio; and the different epithelial layers are represented within the papillary folds or within the invading projections. Bizarre mitoses and bizarre cell forms are generally not found.

In a cytologic smear of the well-differentiated type of oral carcinoma, the cells may show less cytoplasm and larger nuclei (Figs. 7–5 and 7–6). However, this altered nuclear-cytoplasmic ratio may not be clearly evident in a well-differentiated epidermoid carcinoma, and the cytologic smear may be difficult to interpret as a carcinoma. This type of carcinoma may occasionally result in a normal-appearing smear and a false-negative interpretation. Even on biopsy, the correct diagnosis may be difficult in some well-differentiated carcinomas. However, in a biopsy there is usually enough cellular material present so that an abnormal orientation of cells may be distinguished.

Anaplastic oral epidermoid carcinoma me-

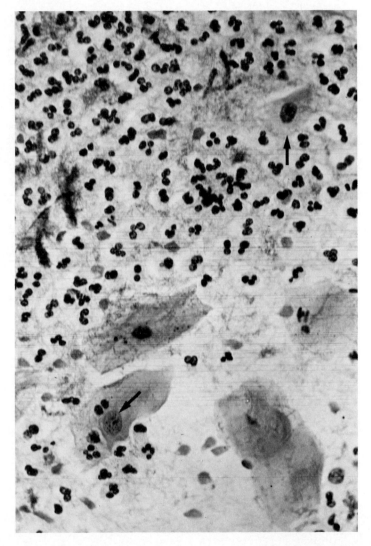

Figure 7–4. Cytologic smear of an ulcerated lesion showing numerous polymorphonuclear leukocytes and several cells that have larger nuclei (arrow) from hyperplastic epithelium.

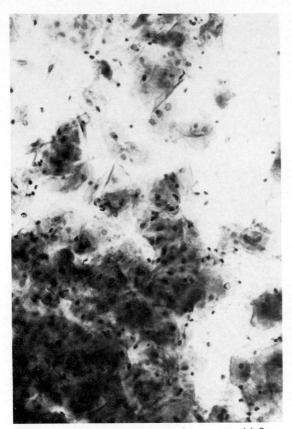

Figure 7–5. Highly cellular smear from an oral inflammatory lesion.

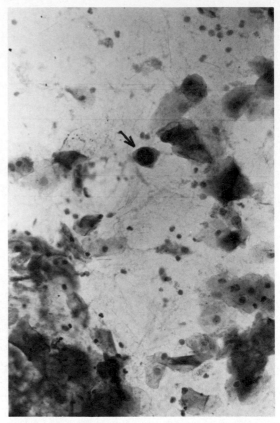

Figure 7–6. Cytologic smear with a suspicious cell (arrow). The nucleus is large and hyperchromatic. The lesion was diagnosed by biopsy as epidermoid carcinoma.

tastasizes early to regional lymph nodes, grows rapidly, and invades deeply into the surrounding and underlying tissue. Histologically, these lesions present a notable proliferation of epithelial cells with abnormal orientation; thus, the different epithelial layers cannot be distinguished. Keratin either does not develop or is present only in small amounts. The cells are notably abnormal, with large, hyperchromatic nuclei and little cytoplasm (Fig. 7–7). Bizarre giant cells and abnormal mitotic figures are usually present. The epithelial cells also lose their junctional adherence and tend to separate from one another.

In a cytologic smear of anaplastic carcinoma, the nuclear-cytoplasmic reversal is obvious and abnormal cell forms can be seen (Fig. 7–8). These may be tumor giant cells with several nuclei, elongate cells with "tails," often referred to as "tadpole cells," and large cell forms with bizarre mitotic figures.

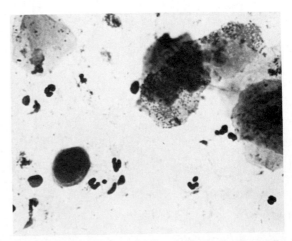

Figure 7–7. A cancer cell with a large hyperchromatic nucleus and several normal epithelial cells colonized by oral bacteria.

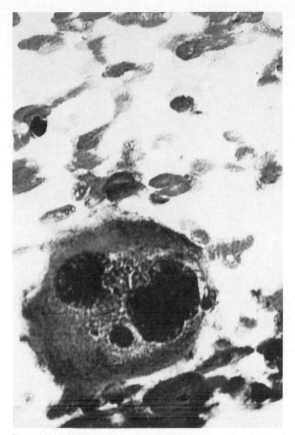

Figure 7-8. High-power view of a bizarre multinucleated cancer cell on a cytologic smear.

CYTOLOGY OF ORAL MALIGNANT TUMORS OTHER THAN EPIDERMOID CARCINOMA

Cytology of oral malignancies other than epidermoid carcinoma reveals bizarre cell forms with deeply staining large nuclei. Biopsy reveals the nature of the malignancy. If the oral malignancy is metastatic rather than a primary tumor, extensive studies may be necessary before the primary cancer can be revealed. The most common tumors that metastasize to the mouth and jaws are carcinoma of the lung, adenocarcinomas of the breast and prostate, gastrointestinal malignancies, and hypernephroma.

FAILURES OR FALSE-NEGATIVE RESULTS

Results of carefully controlled studies have revealed a false-negative rate of approximately 15 percent. The 85-percent rate of reliability

in tumor disclosure still makes oral cytology a valuable screening procedure. The 15-percent rate of error can be ascribed to various problems, including:

1. Smear has not removed a sufficient number of cells from the site involved.

2. Tumor has not been at the surface.

3. Tumor cells are present in cytologic smear, but the carcinoma is well differentiated, so that the cells are misinterpreted as normal cells.

However, this problem must be seen with some perspective. The anaplastic tumors manifest numerous bizarre cells at the surface, and these cells are easily distinguished on a smear. Most anaplastic tumors are found on smears, and these are the dangerous lesions that require immediate therapy. The well-differentiated lesions, which are involved in most of the errors that are made in cytologic evaluation, have a good prognosis, even if they are discovered late and treated as large lesions. Unfortunately, the smear does miss the occasional very early lesion that has notably abnormal cells only in the lower layers of the epithelium. Biopsy would readily aid in the diagnosis of this type of lesion. However, the value of cytology in overall oral cancer diagnosis can be substantial, particularly in the screening process for high-risk populations.

CYTOLOGY OF ORAL LESIONS OTHER THAN TUMORS THAT MANIFEST ABNORMAL CELLS

Cytology is a useful and important technique for the diagnosis of viral diseases of the oral cavity, such as herpetic stomatitis and herpes zoster, as well as dermatologic diseases such as pemphigus, whose initial manifestations may be in the mouth. The application of the technique to these lesions was first described by Tzanck[20] and has been widely used since that time. These diseases reveal abnormal cells that could be confused with tumor cells on cytologic smears. However, the clinical manifestations of these diseases would preclude their confusion with oral cancer.

In viral diseases, the oral lesions tend to be small vesicles that rupture within 24 to 48 hours, leaving ulcers surrounded by enythema. The base of the ulcer must be scraped with a wooden applicator or tongue depressor to obtain the cells with diagnostic features. In these virally modified cells, the nuclei are large, hyperchromatic, and usually lobulated. Giant cells that have multiple nuclei may also be present. The cytologic picture is essentially similar in herpetic stomatitis, herpes zoster, and herpangina.[5]

The oral cytologic smear may reveal enough evidence for a tentative diagnosis of pemphigus, but the disease is sufficiently serious to warrant a diagnosis based on all available information. This must include a biopsy of the oral lesions and possibly immunofluorescent antibody studies, in addition to cytology. The fundamental tissue change in pemphigus in acantholysis, or intraepithelial vesiculation, which develops between the basal layer of the epithelium and the lower layers of the stratum spinosum. This tissue separation is the result of the loss of intercellular bridges between the epithelial cells in this zone.

Cytologic smears of the pemphigus lesion reveal numerous cells with an altered nuclear-cytoplasmic ratio, large hyperchromatic nuclei, and rounded cell outlines with serrated margins.[15]

Vital Staining of Cancer Cells with Toluidine Blue

The application of a vital dye that stains cancer cells and leaves normal tissue relatively unstained was presented by Richard in 1963 as an important clinical test for the delineation of carcinoma-in-situ and areas of dysplasia in mucosal tissue of the uterine cervix.[23] Niebel and Chomet,[22] Shedd and associates,[24] and Strong and colleagues[25] have stressed the value of this simple test in its application to the oral cavity and to the early detection of malignancy. The dye is a basic metachromatic nuclear stain of the thiazine group and stains the nuclear material of malignant cells but has little effect upon the nuclei of normal cells. It is applied topically, using a cotton applicator, in a 1 or 2 percent aqueous solution (toluidine blue) remains in the mouth for a minimum of 30 seconds before being rinsed. The area to be examined should be rinsed with water and dried with a gauze sponge prior to application of the dye. Toluidine blue does not stain normal tissue and will not stain the surface keratin of precancerous leukoplakia. It will stain malignant tumors, as well as a variety of inflammatory lesions that may resemble carcinoma clinically, such as traumatic ulcers, pyogenic granulomas, and erosive lichen planus.

Although there are many false-positive readings, there are relatively few false-negative results. The test could be repeated after waiting 10 to 14 days for the inflammatory lesions to heal, but a biopsy should properly and quickly be obtained in any suspicious-looking lesion that stains positively with toluidine blue.

The staining of carcinoma and dysplastic lesions can be variable, as discussed by Mashberg.[21] In practice, one must consider any type of staining to be positive for the test and either wait for the lesion to heal within 10 to 14 days and perform a biopsy at that time or perform a biopsy earlier if the clinical history suggests that the lesion has been present for more than 10 days.

Toluidine blue can be a valuable adjunct to clinical examination when cancer is suspected. It can be useful in oral cancer screening programs as a simple, rapid, and noninvasive test to indicate a possible malignancy. Any positive lesion should, of course, be subsequently biopsied for definitive diagnosis. The test could also be used during oral examinations by dentists and physicians as an adjunct to clinical evaluation of an oral lesion.

In addition to its use as a cancer detection test, toluidine blue staining can be used by the surgeon to assist in identifying the outer margins of the carcinoma prior to planning the appropriate surgical procedures.

REFERENCES

Oral Cytology

1. Folsom, T. C., White, C. P., Bromer, L., et al.: Oral exfoliative study: review of the literature and report of a three-year study. Oral Surg., *33*:61, 1972.
2. Giunta, J., Meyer, I., and Shklar, G.: The accuracy of the oral biopsy in the diagnosis of cancer. Oral Surg., *28*:552, 1969.

3. Ingram, R. C., Krantz, S., Mendeloff, J., et al.: Exfoliative cytology and the early diagnosis of oral cancer. Cancer, *16*:160, 1963.
4. King, O. H., Jr., and Coleman, S. A.: Analysis of oral exfoliative cytologic accuracy by control biopsy technique. Acta Cytol., *9*:351, 1965.
5. McCarthy, P. L., and Shklar, G.: Diseases of the Oral Mucosa, 2nd ed. Philadelphia, Lea and Febiger, 1980.
6. Medak, H., McGrew, E. A., Burlakow, P., et al.: Atlas of oral cytology. U.S. Govt. Printing Office, Washington, D.C., 1970.
7. Montgomery, P. W., and von Haam, E.: A study of the exfoliative cytology in patients with carcinoma of the oral mucosa. J. Dent. Res., *30*:308, 1951.
8. Papanicolaou, G. M.: Diagnostic value of exfoliated cells from cancerous tissues. J.A.M.A., *131*:372, 1946.
9. Rovin, S.: An assessment of the negative oral cytologic diagnosis. J. Am. Dent. Assoc., *74*:759, 1967.
10. Sandler, H. C.: Cytological screening for early mouth cancer. Cancer, *15*:1119, 1962.
11. Sandler, H. C.: Reliability of oral exfoliative cytology for detection of oral cancer. J. Am. Dent. Assoc., *68*:469, 1964.
12. Sandler, H. C.: Errors of oral cytodiagnosis; report of follow-up of 1801 patients. J. Am. Dent. Assoc., *72*:882, 1966.
13. Sandler, H. C., Stahl, S. S., Cahn, L. R., et al.: Exfoliative cytology for detection of early mouth cancer. Oral Surg., *13*:994, 1960.
14. Selbach, G. J., and von Haam, E.: The clinical value of oral cytology. Acta Cytol., *7*:337, 1963.
15. Shklar, G., and Cataldo, E.: Histopathology and cytology of oral lesions of pemphigus. Arch. Dermatol., *101*:635, 1970.
16. Shklar, G., Cataldo, E., and Meyer, I.: Reliability of cytologic smear in diagnosis of oral cancer. A controlled study. Arch. Otolaryngol., *91*:158, 1970.
17. Shklar, G., Meyer, I., Cataldo, E., et al.: Correlated study of oral cytology and histopathology. Report on 2052 oral lesions. Oral Surg., *25*:61, 1968.
18. Silverman, S., Becks, H., and Farber, S. M.: The diagnostic value of intraoral cytology. J. Dent. Res., *37*:195, 1958.
19. Tiecke, R. W., and Blozis G. G.: Oral cytology. J. Am. Dent. Assoc., *72*:835, 1966.
20. Tzanck, A.: Le cytodiagnostic immediat en dermatologie. Ann. Dermatol. Syph., *8*:205, 1948.

Vital Staining

21. Mashberg, A.: Reevaluation of toluidine blue application as a diagnostic adjunct in the detection of asymptomatic oral squamous carcinoma: a continuing prospective study of oral cancer III. Cancer, *46*:758, 1980.
22. Niebel, H. H., and Chomet, B.: In vivo staining test for delineation of oral intraepithelial neoplastic change. J. Am. Dent. Assoc., *68*:801, 1964.
23. Richard, R. M.: Clinical staining test for in vivo delineation of dysplasia and carcinoma in situ. Am. J. Obstet. Gynecol., *86*:703, 1963.
24. Shedd, D. P., Hukill, P. B., and Bahn, S.: In vivo staining properties of oral carcinoma. Am. J. Surg., *110*:631, 1965.
25. Strong, M. S., Vaughan, C. W., and Incze, J. S.: Toluidine blue in the management of carcinoma of the oral cavity. Arch. Otolaryngol., *87*:101, 1968.

8

Epidemiology of oral cancer

CHESTER W. DOUGLASS, D.D.S., Ph.D.
MARILIE D. GAMMON, M.S.P.H.
WILLIAM J. HORGAN, D.D.S., M.P.H.

As shown throughout this text, oral cancer is the most serious threat to life of all oral diseases. However, a low level index of suspicion still exists among many clinicians. The challenge to the profession is to control what should be the preventable forms of oral cancer and, with early detection, improve the prognosis of those that are treatable. Success in this effort lies in the clinician's understanding of the variation in the frequency, distribution, and types of oral cancer, the personal characteristics of its victims, factors associated with the disease, and the reasons for these associations. These variables provide insight into possible etiologic hypotheses, that is, the *epidemiology* of the disease. Thus, knowledge of the epidemiology of oral cancer is of the utmost importance for clinicians, scientists, and public health dentists in their efforts to prevent, diagnose, and treat oral cancer.

Epidemiologic studies are undertaken to identify factors that are associated with a disease in order to help to explain its observed frequency and distribution and to provide clues to its possible etiology. The scientific basis for the prevention and improved diagnosis and treatment of oral cancer will be found therefore in a better understanding of these factors. With regard to oral cancer, the findings of these studies are not conclusive. The inconsistency in the definition and classification of oral neoplasms presents problems. Possible etiologic factors are confounded by closely related factors, such as personal characteristics, health behavior, environment, and a variety of oral habits. Thus, the classification of primary causal factors and contributing factors from possible confounding factors is a difficult task.

This chapter is organized into three sections. First, common epidemiologic terms are reviewed to enable readers to better understand the existing literature. Second, the incidence and prevalence of oral cancer in the United States and the world is described. In addition, the trends in the incidence and mortality rates of oral cancer are presented, with some hypotheses for interpreting the dynamics that underlie these trends. The final section provides the epidemiologic evidence that identifies the major known risk factors of oral cancer.

COMMON EPIDEMIOLOGIC MEASURES

Measures of the frequency and distribution of disease are useful in quantifying the occurrence and spread of disease among different populations or subgroups within the same population. In this manner, comparisons, which help to explain the pattern of disease and thus identify possible etiologic factors, can be made. The two most common measures of the frequency of a disease are incidence and prevalence.

Incidence and Prevalence

The incidence of a disease may be defined as the number of newly acquired cases during a specified period of time. The incidence rate (I) is the number of new cases reported for a specified population in a given period of time, and by convention this is usually expressed as new cases per 100,000 persons per year. The incidence rate is also used as an estimate of the probability that an individual will acquire a particular disease during a given period of time. For example, in Connecticut in 1968 there were 49 newly diagnosed cases of cancer of the tongue among the male population, which totalled 1,474,217.

$$I = 49 \text{ cases per } 1,474,217 \text{ men per year}$$

$$I = 3 \text{ cases per } 100,000 \text{ persons per year}$$

Prevalence (sometimes called *point prevalence*) is the frequency or number of all cases of a disease that can be identified within a population at a given point in time. The prevalence rate (point prevalence rate) (P) is the proportion of the population that has the disease at that point in time. Period prevalence refers to the number of all cases of a disease identified within a specified period of time and thus is the sum of point prevalence and incidence. As an example of point prevalence rate, in Connecticut in 1968 there were approximately 200 men still living who had been diagnosed as having tongue cancer.

$$P = 200 \text{ cases per } 1,474,217 \text{ men per year}$$

$$P = 0.01 \text{ percent per year}$$

Duration
Duration is the period of time from the onset of a disease to its termination. The termination of a disease is relatively easy to determine. The onset may be exceedingly more difficult to identify. One usually does not know the length of time between the instant of initiation and the point at which the disease is first detected either through examination, screening tests, or symptoms. It is clear that the specificity and sensitivity of the test that is being used as well as the level of awareness of the health care providers and the population they serve will significantly influence the observed duration of oral cancer. For this reason, data collected at varying times and places should be considered independently and critically before one attempts to make comparisons.

Incidence, prevalence, and duration are interrelated measures. The number of cases at any point in time is dependent upon not only the number of newly acquired cases but also the number of previous cases that are surviving. Thus, prevalence is a product of the incidence and duration of a disease.

Mortality Rate
The mortality rate (M) may be defined as the number of deaths resulting from a particular disease in a given population during a specified period of time. This rate should be distinguished from the *case fatality rate,* which is the number of deaths resulting from a disease in the population that has contracted the disease. If a disease has a short duration and a high fatality rate, the mortality rate is a fairly reliable measure of the incidence.

For example, in 1968 there were approximately 32 deaths related to tongue cancer among the male population in Connecticut.

$$M = 32 \text{ deaths per } 1,474,217 \text{ men per year}$$

$$M = 2.2 \text{ deaths per } 100,000 \text{ persons per year}$$

Relative Risk
Relative risk (RR) is a measure of the association between exposure to a particular factor and the risk of developing a disease. It is expressed as a ratio of the incidence or mortality of disease among those who are exposed to those who are not exposed. Populations under study may be divided into four groups based on the presence or absence of a particular disease among those who are exposed and those who are not exposed to a suspected etiologic factor as follows:

	DISEASE		
Exposure	Present	Absent	Total
Exposed	a	b	a + b
Unexposed	c	d	c + d
TOTAL	a + c	b + d	N

Therefore, the relative risk can be computed as:

$$RR = \frac{\text{rate in exposed population}}{\text{rate in unexposed population}}$$

$$= \frac{a}{a + b} \div \frac{c}{c + d} = \frac{a(c + d)}{c(a + b)}$$

Because the percentage of the population in which the disease develops is usually small in comparison with the population being studied, $(c + d)$ is approximately equal to d and $(a + b)$ is approximately equal to b. The formula then becomes:

$$\text{estimate of relative risk} = \frac{ad}{cb}$$

In case-control studies, the cases (i.e., those with the disease) and controls (i.e., individuals who have characteristics that are similar to the cases but who do not have the disease) represent unknown and usually different factions of those who have and those who do not have the disease in the population as a whole. Therefore, in a case-control study, the row totals (a + b or c + d) are not meaningful population estimates of exposed and unexposed individuals and cannot be used as such. Thus, when analyzing data from case-control studies, the estimate of relative risk, just given (more correctly known as the relative odds), is particularly useful.

The concept of relative risk can be seen in the risk of oral cancer associated with smoking. Data from a New York case-control study (Graham et al., 1977) concerning the association of tobacco and oral cancer is presented in Table 8–1.

Using the formula developed previously for the relative odds, the risk of developing oral cancer in heavy smokers compared with nonsmokers may be calculated as follows:

estimate of relative risk

$$= \frac{ad}{cb}$$

$$= \frac{189 \times 102}{20 \times 171} = 5.64$$

Risks are expressed relative to a risk of 1.0 for persons who are not exposed. Therefore, these data show that for this sample a heavy smoker has a 5.64 times higher risk of developing oral cancer than a nonsmoker.

Attributable Risk

Attributable risk (AR) is the incidence of a disease among exposed individuals due to exposure and is calculated by subtracting the incidence (or mortality) rate of the disease among unexposed individuals from the incidence (or mortality) rate among the exposed (AR = $I_e - I_0$). This measure assumes that factors other than the one being examined equally affect both the exposed and unexposed populations. For example, in a 10-year follow-up survey in rural India, Gupta and coworkers (1980) observed an age-adjusted oral cancer incidence rate of 37 cases per 100,000 population per year among reverse smokers compared with a zero rate among nonsmokers, yielding an attributable risk of 37 (37 minus 0) per 100,000 persons per year.

Table 8–1. RISK OF ORAL CANCER ASSOCIATED WITH SMOKING TOBACCO

Maximum Amount of Tobacco Smoked/Day	Cancer Patients No.	Percent	Control Patients No.	Percent	Risk
Heavy	189	45.1	171	33.1	5.64
Light	210	50.1	243	47.1	4.41
Never	20	4.8	102	19.8	1.00
TOTAL	419	100.0	516	100.0	

(From Graham, S., Dayal, H., Rohrer, T., et al.: Dentition, diet, tobacco, and alcohol in the epidemiology of oral cancer. J. Natl. Cancer Inst., *59*, 1611, 1977.)

The population attributable risk percent (PAR %) is a measure of the percentage of the disease incidence in the population as a whole due to exposure. The formula used is expressed as the total incidence (I) minus the incidence of the unexposed (I_0) divided by the total incidence

$$PAR\% = \frac{I - I_0}{I}$$

For a case-control study, the population attributable risk percent can be approximated without knowing the incidences in the entire population. The estimation of the incidence among the unexposed (I_0) is based on the relative risk for the exposure at issue and the proportions of the exposed and unexposed populations. For example, in a case-control study on the association between oral cancer and the joint exposure to smoking and alcohol, Rothman and Keller (1972) calculated the risk among the unexposed to be 0.24I. Therefore, the population attributable risk percent is I − 0.24I = 1 − 0.24 = 76 percent; that is, 76 percent of oral cancer observed in the male population in this study was caused by exposure to smoking and alcohol. The other 24 percent of oral cancer was caused by other, unknown factors.

EPIDEMIOLOGY OF ORAL CANCER IN THE UNITED STATES

Oral cancer is usually defined as neoplasms of the lip, tongue, and intraoral tissue, including the oropharynx. In the eighth revision of the International Classification of Disease (ICD), the various neoplastic sites are separated into 10 different categories (140 to 149), but the sites are often summarized together and referred to as cancer of the buccal cavity and pharynx.

In the United States, reliable incidence and mortality data are collected by the National Cancer Institute, currently under the Surveillance, Epidemiology, and End Results (SEER) Program. The project includes 11 geographically diverse population-based cancer registries within the United States, including Puerto Rico, Connecticut, Detroit, Iowa, Atlanta, New Orleans, New Mexico, Utah, Seattle-Puget Sound, San Francisco-Oakland, and Hawaii. The participants represent slightly more than 10 percent of the United States population and are fairly representative with respect to age. The population covered by SEER programs is somewhat younger and better educated with a higher mean family income than the United States population as a whole. In addition, rural populations, especially rural blacks, are underrepresented, whereas other minority populations (Chinese, Japanese, Hawaiians, and American Indians) and urban blacks are overrepresented (Greenberg et al., 1982). Nevertheless, the cancer mortality rate as reported by the SEER program is similar to the rates reported from other sources (Doll and Peto, 1981).

Incidence Data

The most recently available incidence rates from SEER include data from the years 1973 to 1977 and are presented in Table 8–2 (Young et al., 1981). The annual incidence rates for cancer of the buccal cavity and pharynx for both men and women and both races is 11.2 cases per 100,000 persons, which is 3.4 percent of all cancer cases (excluding Puerto Rico). The incidence of oral cancer varies substantially by site within the oral cavity, gender, and race. New cases of the disease at all oral sites are more common in men (17.4 per 100,000) than in women (6.2 per 100,000) for both whites and blacks. Overall, the incidence rate for buccal and pharyngeal cancer is slightly higher for blacks than for whites for both sexes; this is not true, however, at every site. For example, the incidence rate for cancer of the lip is much higher in whites than in blacks. In white males, the lip is the most common site of oral cancer, with an annual incidence rate of 3.9 per 100,000 persons, whereas the tongue is the most afflicted site in black males, with an incidence rate of 3.7 per 100,000 persons. In females, regardless of race, the most common site of oral cancer is the gum and other areas in the mouth (1.2 per 100,000 and 1.4 per 100,000 for white and black females, respectively).

The incidence rate for cancer of the buccal and pharyngeal cavity increases with age and

Table 8–2. U.S. AVERAGE ANNUAL AGE-ADJUSTED (1970 STANDARD) INCIDENCE RATES PER 100,000 POPULATION, 1973–1977

Cancer Site	Men			Women		
	All	*White*	*Black*	*All*	*White*	*Black*
Buccal cavity and pharynx	17.4	16.8	19.3	6.2	6.0	7.0
Lip	3.9	3.9	0.3	0.3	0.3	0.1
Tongue	3.0	2.9	3.9	1.2	1.2	1.3
Major salivary gland	1.1	1.1	1.0	0.8	0.8	0.8
Floor of mouth	2.0	1.9	2.8	0.7	0.7	0.6
Gum and other mouth	2.4	2.3	3.3	1.4	1.3	1.8
Nasopharynx	0.9	0.7	0.8	0.3	0.3	0.4
Tonsil	1.6	1.5	2.7	0.7	0.7	1.0
Oropharynx	0.5	0.5	0.8	0.1	0.1	0.0
Hypopharynx	1.7	1.6	2.8	0.4	0.4	0.6
Pharynx and buccal cavity	0.5	0.5	0.9	0.2	0.2	0.2

(From Young, J. L., Percy, C. L., Asire, A. J., et al.: Cancer incidence and mortality in the United States, 1973–1977. SEER–NIH Publication No. 81 (2330). National Cancer Institutes Monograph No. 57. Bethesda, MD, Public Health Service, 1981.)

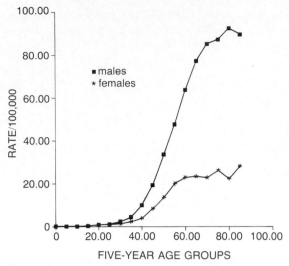

Figure 8–1. Average annual age-specific incidence rates per 100,000 U.S. population of cancer of the buccal cavity and pharynx, 1973–1977. (From Young, J. L., Percy, C. L., Asire, A. J., et al.: Cancer incidence and mortality in the United States, 1973–1977. SEER-NIH Publication No. 81 (2330). National Cancer Institute Monograph No. 57. Bethesda, MD., Public Health Service, 1981.)

peaks at various decades, depending upon the site. Figure 8–1 shows the age-specific rates for cancer of the buccal cavity and pharynx. As with most epithelial tumors (Doll, 1973), cancer of the oral cavity (all sites combined) increases progressively with age, with the oldest decades (more than 80 years) experiencing the highest incidence. For subsites such as the tongue, tonsil, oropharynx, hypopharynx, and pharynx, however, the incidence rates are usually more common at the slightly younger age of 70 to 74 in men and 60 to 70 in women (not shown).

The incidence of oral cancer varies geographically within the United States. If the 10 areas of the SEER program (excluding Puerto Rico) are viewed separately, between the years 1973 and 1977, New Orleans has the highest overall annual incidence rate (23.7 per 100,000) for males, and the San Francisco-Oakland area has the highest overall incidence rate (8.7 per 100,000) for females. If each subsite and geographic area are examined separately, Utah has the highest annual incidence rate in males for cancer of the lip (12.4 per 100,000); this is six times higher than the incidence rate in the rest of the western United States or in the United States as a whole (Smart et al., 1974). Atlanta has the highest annual incidence rate for cancer of the gum

and other mouth in females (2.2 per 100,000). Geographic variations cannot easily be explained by differences in ethnic mix, because the incidence of cancer of the oral cavity also varies geographically by ethnic group. For example, the age-adjusted incidence rates of cancer in the buccal cavity and pharynx as reported by SEER for 1973 to 1977 for Chinese women in the United States varied from 3.5 per 100,000 persons in Hawaii to 11.4 per 100,000 persons in the San Francisco-Oakland area; similar differences were reported for males. Thus, the incidence of cancer of the oral cavity varies substantially by geographic location and for each subsite.

Mortality Data

In a study by Percy and colleagues (1981), which evaluated the accuracy of cancer death certificates in the United States, it was reported that cancer of the buccal cavity and its components (cancer of the lip, tongue, salivary gland, and gum) are underreported on death certificates. Nevertheless, the SEER mortality rates for oral cancer within the United States (Young et al., 1981) are relatively high, with an overall rate of 3.8 per 100,000 persons for the years 1973 to 1977 (excluding Puerto Rico). Again, the rates vary by site, gender, race, age and geographic area. The annual mortality rate of 6.0 per 100,000 males from 1973 to 1977 is nearly triple the annual rate of 2.1 per 100,000 females. As with the incidence rate, the mortality rate for oral cancer of all sites is also higher in blacks than in whites, although this varies within each subsite. With regard to mortality rate in males, the same subsites are predominant as with the incidence rates: for white males, the highest mortality rate is for cancer of the lip (1.4 per 100,000), whereas death from cancer of the tongue is more frequent in black males (2.0 per 100,000). In females, however, the most predominant sites in mortality rates are not the same as the incidence rates; in white females, the major salivary gland is the most fatal site (0.5 per 100,000), whereas in black females, the pharynx and the buccal cavity is the most fatal site (0.6 per 100,000).

Mortality rates also vary geographically within the United States. Using SEER data (excluding Puerto Rico), New Orleans, again, has the highest overall rates of oral cancer for males, with an annual mortality rate of 11.7 per 100,000 persons, whereas the San Francisco-Oakland area has the highest rates for females, with an annual mortality rate of 3.2

per 100,000 persons. When each subsite and geographic area is considered separately, cancer of the tongue in New Orleans has the highest annual mortality rate for males (2.6 per 100,000), and cancer of the tongue in the San Francisco-Oakland area has the highest annual mortality rate for females (0.9 per 100,000). These are not the same cancer sites or geographical areas that predominate in the cancer incidence data.

Using cancer mortality data for the 20-year period from 1950 to 1969, Blot and Fraumeni (1977) reported on the geographic variation within 3056 counties of the contiguous United States for oral cancer (ICD sites 140–148, seventh revision). Of the variables considered, urbanization was the major indicator of death due to oral cancer in white males, with the highest rates occurring in the most heavily populated counties. In contrast, only slight increases were noted in the mortality rates in white females living in an urban area. With the confounding effect of urbanization removed, an increase in the mortality rate from oral cancer among white males in the North was no longer observed, whereas a predominance of deaths due to oral cancer persisted among white females in the South. Deaths due to oral cancer increased sharply with urbanization among nonwhite males, similar to the pattern for white males, with no North-South differences evident within population strata. In females, the increase with urbanization was greater among nonwhites than among whites, and the increase in deaths in the South for whites was not apparent for nonwhites. In the Tidewater Region of North Carolina, almost every county had elevated mortality rates, including some of the highest rates for white males and females. The counties involved were predominantly rural-farm areas, and few of the residents were of foreign origin.

In an analysis by Burmeister (1981), the mortality rates of Iowan farmers and nonfarmers were compared and perhaps could be interpreted as a comparison between selected rural and urban residents of Iowa. The author found the proportionate mortality rates to be significantly lower in farmers for cancers of the mouth other than the lip, whereas significantly higher mortality rates were noted in farmers for lip cancer. Thus, the significance of the urban/rural gradient on mortality rates due to oral cancer in the United States may be dependent upon the geographical area and the site of oral cancer.

EPIDEMIOLOGY OF ORAL CANCER IN THE WORLD

As within the United States, variations occur in the morbidity and mortality rates of oral cancer among various countries, cultures within countries, geographic areas, occupations, races, and genders. Some of the variations, however, may be caused by the changing status of the ICD disease classifications and the failure of various countries to employ the most recent system or to supply data that are comparable with the ICD. Thus, when examining data from different geographical areas, one should keep in mind the differences in the various classification systems and that only rates from similar time frames that use the same ICD codes are comparable.

Discrepancies observed among various countries may be the result of differences in the age distribution within each population. Although oral cancer is generally regarded as a disease of the aged (Pindborg, 1978), the age-specific risk of the disease varies. For instance, the age-specific incidence rate for lip cancer in Israel steeply increases, culminating at age 75 years, whereas in Newfoundland, there is a marked shift toward lip cancer in people in younger age groups. To improve the comparability of world cancer statistics, each nation's rates are usually standardized to a "world population" (Waterhouse et al., 1976; Segi et al., 1981); however, this procedure tends to mask important variations in the age-specific rates (Doll and Cooke, 1967).

Worldwide variations in the incidence or mortality rates of oral cancer may be caused by differences in the methods of collecting data from country to country. Not all countries have cancer registries that require the reporting of cancer cases to a central agency (either regional or national). Instead, information may come from cancer hospitals, departments of pathology, or death certificates. In addition, the care-seeking behavior of cancer patients varies among cultures, according to socioeconomic status, age, gender, and race. Such variations in behavior influence the probability of the disease being detected and diagnosed accurately, the stage of the disease at diagnosis, the subsequent treatment and prognosis, and, ultimately, whether the case is recorded. Nevertheless, gross worldwide variations in oral cancer may suggest plausible etiologic hypotheses.

Incidence Data

Age-adjusted incidence rates for oral cancer sites 140 to 145 (ICD eighth revision) in males from many diverse countries as reported by Waterhouse and colleagues in 1976 are shown in Table 8–3. Incidence rates for oral cancer vary geographically with each site of cancer, with no single geographical location being predominant for each site, suggesting that there may be different etiologic agents for various sites. For instance, cancer of the lip has a wide geographical variation, from a low incidence rate of 0.1 per 100,000 persons in Bulawayo and Japan to a high incidence rate of 27.1 per 100,000 persons in Newfoundland, and new cases of cancer of the tongue are found infrequently in both Rumania and Bulawayo (0.3 per 100,000) but are very common in Bombay (12.6 per 100,000). Cancer of the salivary gland has a low incidence rate throughout the world, with only a slight variation of 0.2 per 100,000 persons in Hungary and Rumania to a slightly elevated rate of 1.9 per 100,000 persons in Nigeria. All cancers of the mouth (ICD 143–145) range from a low incidence rate of 0.7 per 100,000 persons in Finland to a high incidence rate of 7.8 per 100,000 persons in Puerto Rico.

The relative significance of the incidence rate of oral cancer compared with total incidence of cancer also varies among nations and cultures. For example, in India and Sri Lanka, oral cancer cases constitute almost 30 to 50 percent of all cases of cancer in males (Jussawalla, 1976; Nissanga, 1976), whereas in most western countries, oral cancer accounts for only 2 to 6 percent of all cancer (Pindborg, 1977). Similarly, the predominant site of the tumor within the oral cavity varies geographically. In Canada and Israel and in all but three of the European countries listed in Table 8–3, the predominant site of oral cancer among males was the lip. In contrast, in England, Switzerland, Zimbabwe, Brazil, Connecticut, Puerto Rico, and Sri Lanka (not shown), the predominant site of oral cancer was the mouth (Waterhouse et al., 1976; Nissanga, 1976).

Comparatively speaking, the incidence rates for oral cancer at most subsites in women are low, with the mouth (ICD sites 143–145) being the more predominant site. Thus, throughout the world, as in the United States, oral cancer

Table 8–3. WORLDWIDE INCIDENCE BY SITE, MALES (AGE-ADJUSTED TO THE WORLD POPULATION)

ICD (8th Revision)	Lip (Site 140)	Tongue (Site 141)	Salivary Gland (Site 142)	Mouth (Sites 143–145)
Africa and Asia				
Nigeria (Ibadan)	0.4	0.6	1.9	1.2
Zimbabwe (Bulawayo)	0.1	0.3	0.4	4.1
India (Bombay)	0.3	12.6	0.3	6.7
Israel (All Jews)	4.2	0.5	1.0	0.6
Japan (Osaka)	0.1	1.3	0.3	0.7
Americas				
Brazil (Sao Paulo)	6.2	5.7	0.7	7.0
Canada—Br. Columbia	4.7	1.6	0.9	1.9
—Newfoundland	27.1	1.2	0.5	1.6
Colombia (Cali)	0.6	1.9	1.1	1.7
Cuba	2.6	4.2	0.7	3.7
United States—Connecticut	2.1	2.8	1.1	4.3
—Puerto Rico	1.5	7.5	0.4	7.8
Europe				
Finland	5.8	0.8	0.9	0.7
West Germany (Saarland)	1.3	2.0	1.5	1.8
Hungary (Szaboks)	12.1	0.6	0.2	0.9
Malta	13.0	1.9	1.2	2.0
Norway	4.2	0.8	0.6	1.3
Poland (Cracow)	7.6	0.7	0.9	1.0
Rumania (Timis)	6.0	0.3	0.2	1.4
Spain (Zaragoza)	8.0	2.2	0.4	1.1
Sweden	2.7	0.6	0.7	1.1
Switzerland (Geneva)	0.2	2.9	0.5	3.0
United Kingdom (Birmingham)	1.2	1.0	1.0	1.5
Yugoslavia (Slovenia)	4.7	2.0	0.5	2.2

(From Waterhouse, J., Muir, C., Correa, P., et al.: Cancer Incidence in Five Continents. Vol. III. Lyon, International Agency for Research on Cancer, 1976.)

usually affects males more frequently than females. The magnitude of the male to female ratio, however, varies depending upon the tumor site and the population. For instance, in Newfoundland, the age-adjusted incidence rate of cancer of the lip in females is 0.8 per 100,000 persons compared with the male incidence rate of 27.1 per 100,000 persons, whereas in Cali, Colombia, the incidence rates for lip cancer are equal for men and women (0.6 per 100,000) (Waterhouse et al., 1976). The exception to this general rule is in Singapore, where Indian women have elevated annual rates for cancer of the mouth of 16.9 per 100,000 persons compared with rates of 8.6 per 100,000 persons for Indian men. (In India, however, males have a higher incidence rate than do females.) Similarly, in El Paso, Texas, women of Spanish descent have slightly higher incidence rates for cancer of the mouth (2.2 per 100,000) than do men of Spanish descent (1.3 per 100,000) (Waterhouse et al., 1976). These last two examples are definitely exceptions to the rule, because men are more likely to have oral cancer than are women.

The effects of racial and ethnic variations in the incidence rates of cancer of the buccal cavity and the pharynx occur worldwide. In New Zealand, both males and females in the non-Maori population experienced higher incidence rates for cancers of the lip, tongue, and mouth than the Maori population (not shown). Ethnic differences were highly evident in Singapore, where Indian males and females experienced substantially higher incidence rates of mouth cancer (ICD sites 143 to 145) than either the Malaysians or the Chinese. On the other hand, Malaysian males and Chinese females had higher incidence rates of cancer of the lip than the others.

In many countries, a notable variation occurs between urban and rural areas and among the sites of oral cancer. Lindquist and Teppo (1978), using a national population-based tumor registry, reported that the mean annual age-adjusted incidence rate of lip cancer from 1966 to 1970 in Finland was significantly higher in rural areas (7.2 per 100,000) than in urban areas (3.8 per 100,000). Similarly, urban/rural differences in the incidence of lip cancer have been reported for Poland (Warsaw and environs) and Norway (Waterhouse et al., 1976). In contrast, for cancers of the tongue, salivary gland, and mouth in Poland and Norway, higher incidence rates occurred in urban areas than in rural areas.

Mortality Data

Variations in the 1975 worldwide mortality rates for cancer of the buccal cavity and pharynx as reported by Segi and coworkers (1981) are shown in Table 8–4. Countries with a high incidence of age-adjusted death rates are not restricted to one geographic location or ethnic group but are spread throughout the world. They include Hong Kong (20.25 per 100,000), France (14.75 per 100,000), Martinique (14.59 per 100,000), and Singapore (14.12 per 100,000). Countries with fairly high incidence rates include Puerto Rico (8.73 per 100,000), Cuba (7.02 per 100,000), and Switzerland (6.05 per 100,000). Countries with low mortality rates include Honduras (0.51 per 100,000), Israel (1.03 per 100,000), and Greece (1.23 per 100,000).

The wide disparities observed in the mortality rates of oral cancer may reflect variations in the etiology of the disease. On the other hand, variations in care-seeking behavior of the poor population, that is, the tendency for some people, especially the elderly, to disregard symptoms and to seek care only when the disease is almost beyond treatment, may be one reason for the wide variations in mortality. Nevertheless, the mortality rates coupled with the incidence rates indicate that oral cancer has a comparatively high case fatality rate.

TRENDS IN ORAL CANCER

Assessment of disease trends is a useful mechanism that is used to help develop etiologic hypotheses. A trend, however, represents a spectrum of many changes, and thus, changes in the disease incidence and mortality rates within the same geographic population should be interpreted cautiously. Any changes that are observed may be caused by variations in the definition of the disease, diagnostic capabilities, patient survival and mortality rates, and cohort effects. For example, minor salivary glands are no longer included under the category "salivary" gland tumor but rather are recorded according to the site of cancer within the mucosa (Waterhouse et al., 1976). Problems associated with the analysis of cancer trends have been reviewed in detail elsewhere (Magnus, 1982). When analyzing time trends, the many limitations must be kept in mind; nevertheless, trend analysis can often elicit important factors for further study.

Incidence Data

Until recently, data on the morbidity rate of

Table 8–4. ANNUAL AGE-ADJUSTED MORTALITY RATES FOR CANCER OF BUCCAL CAVITY AND PHARNYX IN MALES IN THE WORLD, 1975

	Rate per 100,000		Rate per 100,000
Americas		Europe	
Martinique	14.59	France	14.75
Puerto Rico	8.73	Switzerland	6.05
Cuba	7.02	Hungary	5.57
Uruguay	5.78	Poland	14.95
United States	4.73	Portugal	4.87
Canada	4.7	Spain	3.94
Costa Rica	4.03	Ireland	3.89
Paraguay	3.7	Austria	3.8
Trinidad and Tobago	2.9	Czechoslovakia	3.75
Chile	2.89	Belgium	3.51
Dominican Republic	1.98	Yugoslavia	3.42
Nicaragua	1.2	Scotland	3.21
Honduras	0.51	England and Wales	2.75
Asia		West Germany	2.71
Hong Kong	20.25	Norway	2.55
Singapore	14.12	Iceland	2.47
Phillipines	4.11	Sweden	2.36
Thailand	2.53	Finland	2.32
Japan	1.71	Bulgaria	1.98
Israel	1.03	Denmark	1.8
Oceania		Northern Ireland	1.64
Australia	4.32	Greece	1.23
New Zealand	3.63		

(From Segi, M., Tomihaga, S., Aoki, K., et al.: Cancer mortality and morbidity statistics. GANN Monograph on Cancer Research, No. 26. Tokyo, Japan Scientific Societies Press, 1981.)

cancer in this country had been collected only sporadically through periodic surveys in selected areas. Before the initiation of the SEER program, the National Cancer Institute (NCI) completed three National Cancer Surveys (NCS): the first in 1937–1939 (FNCS) (Dorn, 1944), the second in 1947–1948 (SNCS) (Dorn and Cutler, 1959), and the third in 1969–1971 (TNCS) (Cutler and Young, 1975). In the first survey, prevalence data was collected, whereas in the other two surveys, primarily incidence data was collected. In the first two surveys, data was compiled concerning 10 cities, 9 of which were common to each survey. The sampling areas were not meant to be representative of the United States population but were, instead, restricted to large metropolitan regions where better diagnostic information was available. Because of the lack of data in rural areas, where cancer is less prevalent, the occurrence of cancer as reported in the SNCS was estimated to be about 10 percent higher than that for the United States as a whole (Greenberg et al., 1982). Those who undertook the TNCS tried to improve its coverage of the United States by broadening the areas included in 7 of the original 10 cities and added a rural population, for a total of 10 geographic areas.

In 1978, Devesa and Silverman used the data from the three national cancer surveys for a trend analysis. The original data tapes were used to compile information for the seven common areas included in each of the three surveys. The changes in the nomenclature of cancer sites were accounted for to improve the comparability of the surveys. In addition, the incidence of cancer morbidity was proportionately estimated from the prevalence data originally collected during the FNCS (1937 to 1939). The rates for all three surveys were standardized by age according to the population of the United States in 1950.

In the first three columns of Tables 8–5, 8–6, and 8–7, the oral cancer findings from the Devesa and Silverman (1978) analysis are listed. In the last two columns, the geographic areas in TNCS are compared with the geographic areas in SEER. Although the FNCS, SNCS, and TNCS have seven common geographic areas, the TNCS and SEER have only four geographic areas in common and thus must be interpreted with care. Note that the TNCS incidence rates for oral cancer in the

Table 8–5. TRENDS IN THE ANNUAL AGE-ADJUSTED INCIDENCE RATES (1950 STANDARD) FOR BOTH SEXES AND RACES, UNITED STATES

Site	7 Common Areas*			All 10 Areas†	
	FNCS‡ 1937–1939	SNCS 1947–1948	TNCS 1969–1971	TNCS 1969–1971	SEER 1973–1977
Buccal cavity and pharynx	15.1	14.0	10.1	10.0	10.8
Lip		4.0	1.2	1.7	1.7
Tongue		2.3	2.1	1.9	1.8
Salivary gland		2.4	1.0	1.0	0.9§
Floor of mouth					1.3
Gum and mouth		2.8	2.8	2.6	1.8‖
Pharynx	1.1	2.6	3.0		
Other buccal cavity	14.0				
Nasopharynx				0.6	0.6
Tonsil				1.1	1.0
Other pharynx				1.4	
Oropharynx					0.3
Hypopharynx					1.0
Pharynx and other buccal cavity					0.4

*These national survey rates are restricted to 7 common geographic areas of the 10 areas surveyed: Atlanta, Birmingham, Dallas, Denver, Detroit, Pittsburgh, and San Francisco-Oakland (Devesa and Silverman, 1978).
†These rates apply to all 10 areas included in each program; only 4 areas were common to each: Atlanta, Iowa, Detroit, and San Francisco-Oakland (Culter and Young, 1975; Young and coworkers, 1981).
‡Estimated incidence.
§Rates are for "major salivary gland."
‖Rates are for "gum and other mouth."

Table 8–6. TRENDS IN THE ANNUAL AGE-ADJUSTED INCIDENCE RATES FOR U.S. MALES

Site	7 Common Areas*						All 10 Areas†			
	1937–1939		1947–1948		1969–1971		1969–1971		1973–1977	
	W‡	NW§	W	NW	W	NW	W	B‖	W	B
Buccal cavity and pharynx	25.4	6.4	22.4	9.4	16.0	13.0	17.2	13.4	15.9	20.7
Lip			7.8	0.7	2.6	0.3	4.1	0.3	3.4	0.5
Tongue			3.8	1.5	3.3	3.1	3.1	3.5	2.6	3.1
Salivary gland			2.1	2.8	1.1	1.2	1.3	1.2	1.1¶	0.5¶
Floor of mouth									1.8	3.8
Gum and mouth			4.4	1.4	4.0	3.4	3.9	3.9	2.2**	3.5**
Pharynx	1.9	1.2	4.3	3.0	4.8	4.0				
Other buccal cavity	23.5	5.2								
Nasopharynx							0.7	0.5	0.7	0.8
Tonsil							1.7	1.7	1.4	2.9
Other pharynx							2.4	2.3		
Oropharynx									0.5	0.9
Hypopharynx									1.6	0.6
Pharynx and other buccal cavity									0.6	1.2

*1950 Standard Population (Devesa and Silverman, 1978).
†1970 Standard Population (Cutler and Young, 1975; Young and coworkers, 1981).
‡W—whites.
§NW—nonwhites.
‖B—Blacks.
¶Rates for "major salivary gland."
**Rates for "gum and other mouth."

Table 8–7. TRENDS IN THE ANNUAL AGE-ADJUSTED INCIDENCE RATES FOR U.S. FEMALES

| | 7 Common Areas* | | | | | | All 10 Areas† | | | |
| | 1937–1939 | | 1947–1948 | | 1969–1971 | | 1969–1971 | | 1973–1977 | |
Site	W‡	NW§	W	NW	W	NW	W	B‖	W	B
Buccal cavity and pharynx	6.9	5.3	7.6	5.9	5.3	4.9	5.6	5.2	5.8	5.9
Lip			1.2		0.2	0.1	0.3	0.1	0.3	
Tongue			1.1	0.3	1.1	1.1	1.1	1.3	1.2	0.9
Salivary gland			2.4	3.8	0.9	1.0	1.0	0.9	0.7¶	0.9¶
Floor of mouth									0.7	0.4
Gum and mouth			1.7	0.5	1.8	1.4	1.9	1.6	1.3**	1.6**
Pharynx	0.6	0.1	1.2	1.3	1.4	1.3				
Other buccal cavity	6.3	5.2								
Nasopharynx							0.3	0.3	0.2	0.5
Tonsil							0.6	1.1	0.5	0.9
Other pharynx							0.5	1.3		
Oropharynx									0.2	
Hypopharynx									0.5	0.6
Pharynx and other buccal cavity									0.2	0.1

*1950 Standard Population (Devesa and Silverman, 1978).
†1970 Standard Population (Cutler and Young, 1975; Young and coworkers, 1981).
‡W—whites.
§NW—nonwhites.
‖B—Blacks.
¶Rates for "major salivary gland."
**Rates for "gum and other mouth."

seven areas in common is essentially the same as for all 10 areas surveyed. Blank spaces indicate that at a specific time, those particular site classifications were not separately categorized.

Between the 1937–1939 and 1969–1971 surveys, the overall incidence of cancer of the buccal cavity and pharynx decreased from 15.1 per 100,000 persons to 10.1 per 100,000 persons. This decrease was mainly the result of the decline in the incidence rate of lip cancer between the second and third surveys (see Table 8–5). The decrease in the incidence rate for males was more substantial than for females and was restricted mainly to whites (see Tables 8–6 and 8–7). Between the 1969–1971 TNCS survey and the 1973–1977 SEER program, the rates changed little, and if anything, increased slightly. Closer examination of the changes by gender and race indicates that the overall decrease in the incidence of oral cancer in white males seen since the 1937–1939 survey continued; progressively more favorable rates were observed for cancers of the lip, tongue, and salivary gland. For black males, however, the incidence rates have continued to increase, with the largest increase seen for cancers of the gum, mouth (including floor of mouth), and pharynx (all sites). In females of all races, the incidence rates continue to fluctuate between surveys, sometimes increasing and sometimes decreasing, with no clear pattern emerging.

Mortality Data

The national mortality rate for cancer is published annually by the National Center for Health Statistics and is derived from death certificates for all persons in the United States. Primary neoplastic sites are designated on the death certificates according to the ICD rules of disease classification. Thus, one would conclude that information on the occurrence of cancer as measured by mortality statistics is more complete and is a better representation of the United States population than incidence data. Nevertheless, there may be some inconsistencies with death certificates, such as changes in diagnostic procedures, changes in the procedures for listing cause of death, and disease misclassification, when trying to determine disease trends over a period of time. To ensure a greater accuracy for trend analysis, one hopes that the amount and type of disease misclassification have been random over time.

Several investigators (Gordon et al., 1961; Cutler and Devesa, 1973; Devesa and Silverman, 1978; Pollack and Horm, 1980) have reported on the trends in the mortality rate of cancer; the analysis by McKay and colleagues in 1982 is the most recent. Their analysis of the mortality rate of cancer in the United States from 1950 to 1977 used NCHS annual data from death certificates. As shown in Figure 8–2, the age-adjusted mortality rates for cancer of the buccal cavity plus oral pharynx in women of all races have remained fairly

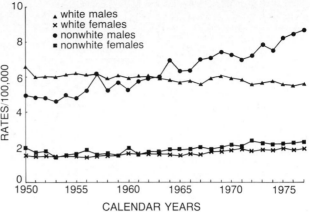

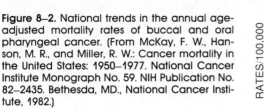

Figure 8–2. National trends in the annual age-adjusted mortality rates of buccal and oral pharyngeal cancer. (From McKay, F. W., Hanson, M. R., and Miller, R. W.: Cancer mortality in the United States: 1950–1977. National Cancer Institute Monograph No. 59. NIH Publication No. 82–2435. Bethesda, MD., National Cancer Institute, 1982.)

stable, with only a suggestion of a slight increase. In white males, the mortality rates also remained stable, with a slight decline noted over the 27-year period, whereas for nonwhite males, a dramatic increase occurred.

The mortality rate for cancer of the lip (Fig. 8–3) showed a definite and substantial decline, ranging from 0.78 per 100,000 persons to 0.20 per 100,000 persons between 1950 and 1965 for white males, followed by a relatively stable period clustered around the latter rate. In others, the rate dropped slightly between 1950 and 1965 and has remained very low since that time. The mortality rate for cancer of the tongue (not shown) showed a slight decline in white males, whereas in nonwhite males, the rate have generally increased. Mortality rates for females, however, have remained stable.

In contrast, the national trends in the age-adjusted mortality rates for cancers of the floor of the mouth and oral mesopharynx in males increased. The rates for nonwhite males have risen dramatically over the 27-year period for both sites. In white males, the increase was

slight but steady over the entire period studied for cancer of the oral mesopharynx, whereas only a slight increase occurred between 1950 and 1965 for cancer of the floor of the mouth. The rates in females, though variable, have remained fairly stable throughout the entire period.

Thus, the overall increase noted in the age-adjusted mortality rates for cancers of the buccal cavity and oral pharynx in nonwhite males was seen for every oral subsite. In contrast, the overall slight decrease in the age-adjusted mortality rates in white males was due to the substantial decline in lip cancer and the slight decrease in cancer of the tongue, whereas cancers located in the floor of the mouth and oral mesopharynx actually increased. In females of all races, the age-adjusted mortality rates have remained fairly constant.

Survival Rates

The trends in the survival rates of white patients who have cancer are presented in Table 8–8. The 1960–1963 data were collected

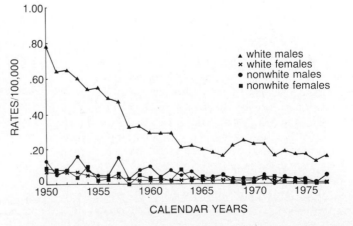

Figure 8–3. National trends in the annual age-adjusted mortality rates of lip cancer. (From McKay, F. W., Hanson, M. R., and Miller, R. W.: Cancer mortality in the United States: 1950–1977. National Cancer Institute Monograph No. 59. NIH Publication No. 82–2435. Bethesda, MD., National Cancer Institute, 1982.)

Table 8–8. TRENDS IN SURVIVAL RATES FOR ORAL CANCER PATIENTS

| | 5-Year Relative Survival Rates (%) | | | |
| | White Men | | White Women | |
Site	1960–1963	1970–1973	1960–1963	1970–1973
Lip	84	87	88	Too few cases
Tongue	23	32*	44	46
Salivary gland	55	53	82	85
Mouth	42	40	50	51
Pharynx	21	27*	35	31

*Increase in survival statistically significant at the 0.05 level. (From National Institute of Health: Cancer Patient Survival Experience. Trends in Survival 1960–1963 to 1970–1973. Comparison of Survival for Black and White Patients. Long Term Effects of Cancer. Public Health Service. DHHS (NIH) Publication No. 80–2148, U.S. Department of Health and Human Services, 1980.)

by the now defunct End Results Program. The 1970–1973 data are part of the ongoing SEER program (National Institute of Health, 1980). Cancer of the lip has the best 5-year relative survival rate, with over 80 percent of both men and women surviving. Patients who have cancer of the pharynx have the worst prognosis, with less than 35 percent surviving the 5-year period. In general, women have better survival rates than do men. Perhaps this is because they are diagnosed at an earlier stage, which improves a patient's prognosis (Keller, 1969; Mashberg and Meyers, 1976; National Institute of Health, 1980). Other factors such as the patient's race, religion, marital status, occupation, and residence have not been found to significantly alter survival (Keller, 1969). Between 1960–1963 and 1970–1973, the relative survival rates have not significantly changed. For most of the subsites, the survival rates have improved slightly, and those for the tongue and pharynx have improved significantly (National Institute of Health, 1980).

RISK FACTORS

Tobacco and Alcohol

For almost a century, investigators have suspected that heavy tobacco smoking is a major etiologic factor in cancer of the mouth (Clemmesen, 1965; Vogler et al., 1962). More recently, the carcinogenic risk of alcohol consumption has been investigated, despite earlier studies that failed to find an association between oral cancer and alcohol (Vogler et al., 1962; Anderson and Lewis, 1970) or alcoholism (Keller, 1963). Within the last few decades, epidemiologic studies have overwhelmingly verified heavy tobacco smoking and heavy alcohol consumption as significant risk factors for oral cancer (Wynder et al., 1957; Vincent and Marchetta, 1963; Keller and Terris, 1965; Martinez, 1969; Feldman et al., 1975; Bross and Coombs, 1976; Keller, 1977; Williams and Horm, 1977; Wynder and Stellman, 1977; Graham, et al., 1977; Hinds et al., 1980; Herity et al., 1981; Mashberg et al., 1981). Thus, current epidemiologic research is no longer directed toward determining whether exposure to these factors increases a person's risk of oral cancer. It is now concerned with whether the combined effect is the result of factors acting independently, antagonistically, or synergistically; with which factor poses the greater risk of oral cancer; and with the importance of the type, amount, and duration of each exposure variable.

Assessing the risk of the combined exposure to alcohol and tobacco for oral cancer is confounded by the strong association between the two exposure variables. For example, drinkers often are heavy smokers (Wynder et al., 1957; Rothman and Keller, 1972; Hinds et al., 1980), and few oral cancer patients either only smoke or only drink (Mashberg et al., 1981). Nevertheless, several investigators have attempted to determine whether the effect of the combined exposure to the two variables is independent or interactive. Rothman and Keller (1972) estimated the relative risk of oral cancer in heavy smokers (without consumption of alcohol) as 2.43, whereas the risk of oral cancer associated with heavy alcohol consumption (without tobacco exposure) as 2.33. The estimated relative risk of oral cancer for people who both smoked and consumed alcohol was 15.5 (see Table 8–9). The authors concluded that this was suggestive of a combined effect

Table 8–9. RELATIVE RISK* OF ORAL CANCER ACCORDING TO LEVEL OF EXPOSURE TO SMOKING AND ALCOHOL

| Alcohol (ounces per day) | Smoking (cigarette equivalents/day) | | | |
	0	<20	20–39	40+
0	1.00	1.52	1.43	2.43
<0.4	1.40	1.67	3.18	3.25
0.4–1.5	1.60	4.36	4.46	8.21
1.6+	2.33	4.13	9.59	15.5

*Risks are expressed relative to a risk of 1.00 for persons who neither smoked nor drank. (From Rothman, D., and Keller, A.: The effect of joint exposure to alcohol and tobacco on risk of cancer of the mouth and pharynx. J. Chron. Dis., 25:711, 1972.)

equal to the sum of two strong individual effects plus a synergistic component. Similarly, Mashberg and colleagues (1981) reported that their data also supported the hypothesis of the synergistic effects of alcohol and tobacco. Feldman and coworkers (1975) stated that their data suggested a possible synergy between smoking and drinking but that the interaction was not statistically significant. However, Graham and colleagues (1977), Hinds and coworkers (1980), and Herity and colleagues, (1981) found that the increased risk of oral cancer from the combined effect of heavy smoking and heavy alcohol consumption showed no synergy. In contrast, Wynder and coworkers (1957), found that the risks of oral cancer from tobacco and alcohol operated independently, that is, neither synergism nor antagonism was present.

Whether exposure to one is a greater threat to the risk of oral cancer than exposure to the other is also not clear. Self-reported cigarette smoking is usually regarded as more accurate than self-reported alcohol consumption, which is probably underestimated because of the social stigma attached to excessive drinking (Keller and Terris, 1965). Undoubtedly, inaccurate responses obscure the comparisons between the two variables and their association with oral cancer. Several investigators (Vogler et al., 1962; Feldman et al., 1975; Graham et al., 1977; Wynder et al., 1977; Herity et al., 1981; and Williams and Horm, 1977 [for women only]) found that tobacco smoking is a more important risk factor than is alcohol consumption, whereas other researchers (Martinez, 1969; Williams and Horm, 1977 [for men], Mashberg et al., 1981) reported the opposite.

Information reported on the critical type and amount of either risk factor is variable as well. In earlier reports (Wynder et al., 1957; Vogler et al., 1962), it was stated that those who smoked cigars and pipes had an increased risk of oral cancer, whereas in more recent reports, researchers (Martinez, 1969; Williams and Horm, 1977; Hinds et al., 1980) have found that cigarettes are a more important risk factor. For lip cancer in Newfoundland, however, a slightly elevated risk was observed among pipe-smokers but not among tobacco users in general (Spitzer et al., 1975). In addition, the relatively infrequent smoking of pipes and cigars by either patients or control subjects (Wynder and Stellman, 1977; Herity et al., 1981) impedes risk assessment. Similar problems develop when one tries to determine which type of alcohol is a greater risk factor of oral cancer. Whiskey or mixed drinks were often cited as the stronger risk factors compared with wine and beer (Wynder et al., 1957; Martinez, 1969; Feldman et al., 1975). However, in more recent studies, it has been reported that the greater risk may be associated with beer (Williams and Horm, 1977; Hinds et al., 1980; Herity et al., 1981) or beer and wine (Mashberg et al., 1981) consumption (see Table 8–10). Additionally, constituents of alcoholic beverages other than alcohol per se may be important. In many studies, the issue has been simplified by combining types (i.e., all tobacco or all alcohol) and by classifying only according to amount per day. Most investigators have found a linear dose-response relationship between increased risk of oral cancer and either increased consumption of alcohol or increased tobacco smoking, with the highest elevated risk associated with "heavy" use, regardless of the definition used for "heavy." Similarly, ex-smokers have been found to have a decreased risk of oral cancer compared with current smokers (Wynder and Stellman, 1977).

Thus, both tobacco smoking and alcohol consumption have repeatedly been shown to be significantly associated with the risk of oral cancer, especially in males. To improve tertiary prevention measures, the emphasis of further research should be on defining the interactive relationships between the two exposure variables and oral cancer. In addition, the type and critical doses of tobacco and alcohol that increase the risk of oral cancer should be determined.

Chewing Habits

As mentioned previously, there is a relatively high frequency of oral cancer in India, Sri Lanka, and most countries of Southeast

Table 8–10. RELATIVE RISKS FOR WHISKEY DRINKERS AND BEER OR WINE DRINKERS

	WE*/day	Relative Risk
Whiskey drinkers	less than 6	1.5
	6 to 9	7.3
	10 or more	7.3
Beer/wine drinkers	less than 6	4.2
	6 to 9	24.7
	10 or more	20.4

*One Whiskey Equivalent (WE) was defined as that amount of alcohol contained in 1 oz of 86-proof whiskey. Using this standard, approximately 12 oz of beer or 4 oz of dry wine equals 1 WE. (From Mashberg, A., Garfinkel, L., and Harris, S.: Alcohol as a primary risk factor in oral squamous carcinoma. CA, *31*:146, 1981.)

Asia. With one exception (Burton-Bradley, 1979), many investigators have associated the elevated risk of oral cancer in Asia to the widespread use of chewing betel quid, a popular mixture of areca nut, tobacco, and lime wrapped in a betel leaf (Hirayama, 1966; Mehta et al., 1972; Wahi, 1976; Mahboubi, 1977; Henderson and Aiken, 1979; Gupta et al., 1980; Mehta et al., 1981). For example, in a case-control study in Sri Lanka by Hirayama (1966), tobacco chewing was more common among the group that had oral cancer than among the control group, whereas no significant difference was found in the smoking habits of the two groups. Similar studies in India, Central Asia, and Malaya conducted by the same investigator produced results resembling those of the studies in Sri Lanka (Hirayama, 1966). In a 10-year follow-up study in India conducted by Gupta and coworkers (1980), the annual incidence of oral cancer in the Ernakulam district was 23 per 100,000 among those who had a chewing habit, zero for smokers (mostly "bidi" smokers), 32 per 100,000 among those who both smoked and chewed, and zero for those who had no smoking or chewing habits. At the present time, the exact carcinogenic agent of the betel quid has not been defined. Nevertheless, the high risk of oral cancer among betel quid chewers has firmly been established, and the additional risk of "bidi" smoking should not be overlooked.

In the United States where oral cancer mortality rates are elevated among southern women, Blot and Fraumeni (1977) reported that this was consistent with the relatively frequent use of snuff among females who have oral cancer. Because of the relatively infrequent use of chewing tobacco or snuff in the United States, it is difficult to test the hypothesis (Wynder et al., 1957; Wynder and Stellman, 1977). For instance, the association between the use of snuff and oral cancer has not been validated in a prospective study by one group of investigators (Smith et al., 1970; Smith, 1975). However, the findings of most retrospective studies in the southern United States have consistently supported the hypothesis (Christen, 1980; Peacock et al., 1960; Rosenfeld and Calloway, 1963; Vincent and Marchetta, 1963). For example, in a case-control study in North Carolina, a four-fold increase of cancers of the gum and buccal mucosa was found among rural women who used snuff compared with nonusers (Winn et al., 1981).

Oral Health Status

Inadequate dental health has been suspected of increasing the risk of oral cancer (Binnie, 1976), yet few investigators have been able to validate such an association (Smith, 1972). Using the prevalence of edentulousness or denture wearing as a measure of oral health status, most studies have found no statistically significant differences between case and control subjects (Wynder et al., 1957; Vogler et al., 1962; Vincent and Marchetta, 1963; Martinez, 1969; and Whitaker et al., 1979). In addition, in a prospective study Mashberg and Meyers (1976) found that gingival trauma was generally not located at the disease site. In contrast, in two recent studies a difference was found in dental conditions between patients with oral cancer and control groups (Graham et al., 1977; Herity et al., 1981). In a case-control study of oral cancer and several exposure variables, Graham and colleagues (1977) used a more detailed index of oral health, a composite score that measured the number of septic and missing teeth and the condition of dentures and the periodontium. The investigators found that heavy smokers and heavy drinkers who had poor dentition had a substantially higher risk of oral cancer than those who had adequate dentition (see Table 8–11). Although Graham's work has resulted in some convincing data, most other investigators have not reported similar results. Thus, further research with better dental health indices is needed.

Table 8–11. RELATIVE RISKS OF ORAL CANCER FOR WHITE MALES POSSESSING VARIOUS COMBINATIONS OF HIGH-RISK TRAITS

High-Risk Trait	Relative Risk
Dentition adequate	
Smoking, light	
Drinking, light	1.00
Drinking, heavy	1.91
Smoking, heavy	
Drinking, light	2.06
Drinking, heavy	2.29
Dentition inadequate	
Smoking, light	
Drinking, light	2.97
Drinking, heavy	6.72
Smoking, heavy	
Drinking, light	6.00
Drinking, heavy	7.68

From Graham, S., Dayal, H., Rohrer, T., et al.: Dentition, diet, tobacco, and alcohol in the epidemiology of oral cancer. J. Natl. Cancer Inst., 59:1611, 1977.)

Diet

The association between an inadequate diet and oral cancer has been examined by several investigators during the last few decades. In a retrospective study in India, Hirayama (1966) found that the relative risk of developing oral cancer was more than three times higher among non–tobacco chewing vegetarians than among nonvegetarians. The investigator attributed this effect to malnutrition. In addition, in a large community-based case-control study Martinez (1969) found that meals for case subjects were fewer, scantier, and more irregular than for control subjects, yet both case and control subjects had diets deficient in fresh vegetables, fruit, milk, eggs, and meat. However, the results of most studies have not indicated any relationship between diet and oral cancer (Wynder et al., 1957; Vogler et al., 1962; Feldman et al., 1975; Graham et al., 1977), which may be due to the inadequate assessment of dietary intake. For example, in a more detailed re-examination of their earlier data, Marshall and colleagues (1982) found that the risk of oral cancer increased in a dose-response fashion as intake of vitamin A or vitamin C decreased, even when smoking and alcohol ingestion was controlled.

Dietary research is becoming more sophisticated, with its ability to accurately classify patients and control groups with regard to nutritional intake, resulting in easier assessment of the role of diet in cancer etiology. However, the nutritional influence on the risk of oral cancer needs to be further studied, using more accurate assessment and classification methods.

Sunlight

The relationship between actinic radiation and cancer of the lower lip has been considered to be causal for a long period of time (Wynder et al., 1957; Stoddart, 1964; Ratzkowski, et al., 1966; Anderson, 1971; Smith, 1972; Ju, 1973; Binnie, 1976). Most of the evidence that implicates sunlight as an etiologic factor, however, is based on analyses that used indirect measures of solar exposure such as geographic residence and employment in an outdoor occupation. Furthermore, many investigators who have concluded that lip cancer is caused by sunlight based their reports on pathologic case series (Clemmensen, 1965). This type of analysis lacks a control group, and, therefore, observations from a case series study cannot be construed as providing proof of a causal relationship.

Many better controlled studies have found lip cancer to be associated with either rural residence or an outdoor occupation. For instance, a greater incidence of lip cancer in rural areas has been well documented throughout the world (Anderson and Lewis, 1970; Waterhouse et al., 1976; Lindqvist and Teppo, 1978). Similarly, increased risk of lip cancer has been recorded among white, male residents of the southern United States (Dorn and Cutler, 1959; Keller, 1970), yet results of studies have not shown a high risk consistently in all western states (Keller, 1970; Smart et al., 1974). In addition, in a case-control study of 74 men who had lip cancer Wynder and colleagues (1957) found a significantly higher proportion of the cancer patients to be laborers than were patients in the control group. More recent investigations have resulted in reports of increased lip cancer in farmers (Keller, 1970; Burmeister, 1981; Lindqvist et al., 1981) and in fishermen in Newfoundland (Spitzer et al., 1975) and Finland (Lindqvist et al., 1981). Additional support for the actinic radiation–lip cancer hypothesis was provided by the association of skin cancer of the head, face, and neck with lip cancer (Keller, 1970).

In contrast, the results of more recent studies have been unable to link sunlight with lip cancer using the traditional surrogate measures of geography and occupation. Most noteworthy is the recent analysis of the TNCS data by Szpak and colleagues (1977), which found that the incidence of lip cancer did not correlate with geographic latitude nor with the incidence of skin cancer. Similarly, the rate observed for the western region of the United States is a fraction of Utah's very high incidence of lip cancer (Smart et al., 1974). These data do not support the actinic radiation hypothesis.

In addition, in a case-control study in Newfoundland, fishermen had a higher risk of lip cancer, but this was not true for skin cancer of the head and neck (Spitzer et al., 1975). The authors concluded that it was not possible to attribute the higher risk of lip cancer to the particular work activity of fishermen, and no specific carcinogen was identified.

Lindqvist and Teppo (1978) compared the incidence rates of lip cancer in Finland with the variation of mean annual solar radiation throughout the nation and found an inverse correlation rather than the expected positive correlation. In an analysis comparing the incidence of lip cancer with that of skin cancer,

Lindqvist (1979a) found no correlation between geographic distribution or secular trend pattern. In a Finnish case-control study by Lindqvist (1979b), patients who had lip cancer were found to be at an increased risk if they both smoked and were employed in an outdoor occupation; however, neither factor alone was associated with an increased risk of lip cancer.

Both employment in an outdoor occupation and rural residence are risk factors for lip cancer in white males. It has always been assumed that these variables indicate prolonged exposure to actinic radiation. However, in reviewing the literature on the association of actinic radiation and lip cancer, the case for a causal association appears to be equivocal. The earlier literature is not entirely convincing, considering the inadequate study designs that were used and the inability of the more recent analyses, which have better study designs, to validate the conclusions from the more dated research. Thus, the role of sunlight as a risk factor for lip cancer must be re-evaluated, and its relative importance as an etiologic agent or cocarcinogen should be better defined (Smith, 1979; Szpak et al., 1977; Lindqvist and Teppo, 1978; Lindqvist, 1979a,b).

Occupation

Although outdoor occupations such as fishing (Spitzer et al., 1975) and farming (Burmeister, 1981) have been implicated as risk factors for lip cancer, other, more industrially related occupations have been linked to the elevated risk of cancers of the oral cavity.

In a survey of the mortality rates of cancer of the buccal cavity and pharynx in the United States, Blot and Fraumeni (1977) found elevated rates of oral cancer in counties in which leather, paper, and chemical manufacturing industries (in males who lived in the North) and apparel and textile industries (in females who lived in the South) were located. In addition, in a case-control study in Atlanta, Georgia, an association between female textile workers and oral cancer was observed, but no association between occupation and oral cancer was observed in males (Vogler et al., 1962).

Similarly, a high incidence in both the mortality and morbidity rates from oral and pharyngeal cancer was noted among textile workers in England and Wales (Binnie et al., 1972; Moss and Lee, 1974). However, in a case-control study of textile workers in England, only the women in one of the two regions had significantly more textile workers in the case group than in the control group. The authors concluded that their results did not confirm a positive association between the mortality rate of oral cancer and textile workers. Investigation into this possible relationship should be explored further.

Socioeconomic Status

Income and education have often been cited, with little data verification, as risk factors for oral cancer (Smith, 1979). However, some interesting relationships have been reported. For example, from United States' mortality data from 1950 to 1969, Hoover and colleagues (1975) found that lip cancer in males and females and mouth-throat cancers in females were inversely related to social class. Using TNCS incidence data, Williams and Horm (1977) confirmed the inverse relationship between invasive neoplasms of the lip and tongue and college education and high income. The relative significance of these associations is clouded by the fact that each of these socioeconomic variables is correlated with other possible risk factors such as heavy alcohol consumption and heavy tobacco smoking, dental health, urban or rural residence, and occupation (Wynder and Stellman, 1977).

SUMMARY

The risk of buccal cavity and pharyngeal cancer differs substantially from country to country throughout the world and varies by site, gender, age, and ethnic background. In some countries such as India or Sri Lanka, oral cancer and its various components constitute about 30 to 50 percent of all cancers in males, whereas in most western countries it accounts for only 2 to 6 percent. Generally, incidence rates of oral cancer increase with age and are more common in males than females. The morbidity and mortality rates of oral cancer vary with ethnic background but are dependent upon the country in which one lives.

In the United States, the majority of cases of oral cancer occur among whites, but with the exception of lip cancer, incidence rates are generally higher in blacks. Low socioeconomic status has been linked to an increased risk of oral cancer, especially in males. In addition, geographic location has an influence on the variable risk of oral cancer; lip cancer is more common in rural areas than in urban areas, whereas cancers of the mouth other than the lip are more common in urban areas.

National trends in morbidity and mortality rates of oral cancer indicate an overall decrease in 1937–1939 to 1969–1971, which is mainly attributable to a decrease in lip cancer among white males. Between 1969–1971 and 1973–1977, the combined rates of all sites remained constant. On the other hand, if the rates are broken down by gender and race, different patterns emerge. Although rates for white males declined, rates for black males increased, yet rates for females were fairly stable regardless of race.

Tobacco and alcohol are two well-established high risk factors for oral cancer. Usually, when rates were adjusted for one exposure variable, the other remained positively associated with oral cancer. The relative effect of smoking and alcohol consumption on the risk of oral cancer (i.e., is it synergistic, antagonistic, or independent) is obscured by the confounding relationship between the two exposure variables. Additional research is needed to assess the risk of oral cancer and the various types of smoking habits and alcoholic beverages ingested and the critical dose and duration of each.

In India and Sri Lanka, betel quid chewing is associated with an increased risk of oral cancer. Whether cigarette smoking is a cocarcinogen or an additional risk of oral cancer in this area of the world is not clear. Similarly, in the United States, the use of snuff and chewing tobacco has been associated with oral cancer in several retrospective studies.

Risk factors for lip cancer include outdoor occupations and rural residence. Investigators have traditionally interpreted this as a causal association between lip cancer and exposure to actinic radiation. The results of more recent investigations have not entirely supported this hypothesis; thus, further research is needed to more clearly define the etiologic relationship between lip cancer and outdoor occupation and rural residence.

Other less well-established associations with oral cancer include inadequate dentition, poor diet, and employment in the textile industries. With an improvement in the methodology of assessing these exposure variables, investigators should be able to clarify their relationship with oral cancer.

REFERENCES

1. Anderson, D. L.: Cause and prevention of lip cancer. J. Can. Dent. Assoc., *37*:138, 1971.
2. Anderson, D. L., and Lewis, D. W.: Male oral cancer: correlation of incidence with mortality and population characteristics. J. Can. Dent. Assoc., *36*:26, 1970.
3. Binnie, W. H.: Epidemiology and aetiology of oral cancer in Britain. Proc. R. Soc. Lond., *69*:737, 1976.
4. Binnie, W. H., Cawson, R. A., Hill, G. B., et al.: Oral Cancer in England and Wales. Studies on Medical and Population Subjects, No. 23, London, Her Majesty's Stationary Office, 1972.
5. Blot, W. J., and Fraumeni, J. F.: Geographic patterns of oral cancer in the United States: etiologic implications. J. Chron. Dis., *30*:745, 1977.
6. Bross, I. D., and Coombs, J.: Early onset of oral cancer among women who drink and smoke. Oncology, *33*:136, 1976.
7. Burmeister, L. F.: Cancer mortality in Iowa farmers, 1971–1978. J. Natl. Cancer Inst., *66*:461, 1981.
8. Burton-Bradley, B. G.: Is "betel chewing" carcinogenic? (letter). Lancet, *2*:903, 1979.
9. Christen, A. G.: The case against smokeless tobacco: five facts for the health professional to consider. J. Am. Dent. Assoc., *101*:464, 1980.
10. Clemmesen, J.: Statistical studies in the aetiology of malignant neoplasms. I. Review and results. Supplement 174. Acta Path. Microbiol. Scand., *1*:543, 1965.
11. Cutler, S. J., and Devesa, S. S.: Trends in cancer incidence and mortality in the USA. *In*: Doll, R., and Vodopija, I. (eds.): Host Environment Interactions in the Etiology of Cancer in Man. IARC Scientific Publication No. 7. Lyon, International Agency for Research in Cancer, 1973.
12. Cutler, S. J., and Young, J. I. (eds.): Third National Cancer Survey: Incidence Data. DHEW Publication No. (NIH) 75–787, National Cancer Institute Monograph No. 41. Bethesda, MD, Public Health Service, 1975.
13. Devesa, S. S., and Silverman, D. T.: Cancer incidence and mortality trends in the United States: 1935–1974. J. Natl. Cancer Inst., *60*:545, 1978.
14. Doll, R.: Age. *In*: Doll, R. and Vodopija, I.: Host Environment Interactions in the Etiology of Cancer in Man. IARC Scientific Publication No. 7. Lyon, International Agency for Research on Cancer, 1973.
15. Doll, R., and Cooke, P.: Summarizing indices for comparison of cancer incidence data. Int. J. Cancer, *2*:269, 1967.
16. Doll, R., and Peto, R.: The causes of cancer: quantitative estimate of avoidable risks of cancer in the United States today. J. Natl. Cancer Inst., 66:1191, 1981.
17. Dorn, H. F.: Illness from cancer in the United States. Public Health Rep., *59*:33, 65, 97, 1944.
18. Dorn, H. F., and Cutler, S. J.: Morbidity from cancer in the United States. I-II. Public Health Monograph No. 56. Washington, DC, 1959.
19. Feldman, J. G., Hazan, M., Nagarajan, M., et al.: A case control investigation of alcohol, tobacco, and diet in head and neck cancer. Prev. Med., *4*:444, 1975.
20. Gordon, T., Crittenden, M., and Haenzel, W.: Cancer mortality trends in the United States, 1930–1955. End Results and Mortality Trends in Cancer, Part II. National Cancer Institute Monograph No. 6. Washington, DC, Public Health Service, 1961.
21. Graham, S., Dayal, H., Rohrer, T., et al.: Dentition, diet, tobacco, and alcohol in the epidemiology of oral cancer. J. Natl. Cancer Inst., *59*:1611, 1977.
22. Greenberg, E. R., Colton, T., and Bagne, C.: Measurement of cancer incidence in the United States: sources and uses of data. J. Natl. Cancer Inst., *68*:743, 1982.
23. Gupta, P. C., Mehta, T. S., Daftary, D. K., el al.: Incidence rates of oral precancerous lesions in a 10-

year follow-up study of Indian villages. Community Dent. Oral Epidemiol., *8*:287, 1980.

24. Henderson, B. E., and Aiken, G. H.: Cancer in Papua New Guinea. *In*: Second Symposium on Epidemiology and Cancer Registries in the Pacific Basin. National Cancer Institute Monograph No. 53. NIH Publication No. 79–1864. Bethesda, MD, Public Health Service, 1979.

25. Herity, B., Moriarty, M., Bourke, G. J., et al.: A case-control study of head and neck cancer in the Republic of Ireland. Br. J. Cancer, *43*:177, 1981.

26. Hinds, M. W., Kolonel, N., Lee, J., et al.: Associations between cancer incidence and alcohol/cigarette consumption among five ethnic groups in Hawaii. Br. J. Cancer, *41*:929, 1980.

27. Hirayama, T.: An epidemiological study of oral and pharyngeal cancer in Central and Southeast Asia. Bull. WHO, *34*:41, 1966.

28. Hoover, R., Mason, T. J., McKay, F. W., et al.: Geographic patterns of cancer mortality in the United States. *In* Fraumeni, J. F. (ed.): Persons at High Risk of Cancer. New York, Academic Press, Inc., 1975, Chapter 20.

29. Ju, D. M. C.: On the etiology of cancer of the lower lip. Plast. Reconstr. Surg., *52*:151, 1973.

30. Jussawalla, D. J.: The problem of cancer in India: an epidemiological assessment. *In* Hirayama, T. (ed.): Cancer in Asia. GANN Monograph on Cancer Research, No. 18. Tokyo, Japan Scientific Societies Press, 1976.

31. Keller, A. Z.: The epidemiology of lip, oral and pharyngeal cancers, and the association with selected systemic diseases. Am. J. Public Health, *53*:1214, 1963.

32. Keller, A. Z.: Survivorship with mouth and pharynx cancers and their association with cirrhosis of the liver, marital status, and residence. Am. J. Public Health, *59*:1139, 1969.

33. Keller, A. Z.: Cellular types, survival, race, nativity, occupations, habits, and associated diseases in the pathogenesis of lip cancer. Am. J. Epidemiol., *91*:486, 1970.

34. Keller, A. Z.: Alcohol, tobacco, and age factors in the relative frequency of cancer among males with and without liver cirrhosis. Am. J. Epidemiol., *106*:194, 1977.

35. Keller, A. Z., and Terris, M.: The association of alcohol and tobacco with cancer of the mouth and pharynx. Am. J. Public Health, *10*:1578, 1965.

36. Lindqvist, C.: Risk factors of lip cancer: a critical evaluation based on epidemiological comparisons. Am. J. Public Health, *69*:256, 1979a.

37. Lindqvist, C.: Risk factors in lip cancer: a questionnaire survey. Am. J. Epidemiol., *109*:521, 1979b.

38. Lindqvist, C., and Teppo, L.: Epidemiological evaluation of sunlight as a risk factor of lip cancer. Br. J. Cancer, *37*:983, 1978.

39. Lindqvist, C., Teppo, L., and Pukkala, E.: Occupations with low risk of lip cancer show high risk of skin cancer of the head. Community Dent. Oral Epidemiol., *9*:247, 1981.

40. McKay, F. W., Hanson, M. R. and Miller, R. W.: Cancer mortality in the United States: 1950–1977. National Cancer Institute Monograph No. 59, NIH Publication No. 82-2435. Bethesda, MD, National Cancer Institute, 1982.

41. Magnus, K. (ed.): Trends in Cancer Incidence. New York, Hemisphere Publishing Corp., 1982.

42. Mahboubi, E.: The epidemiology of oral cavity, pha-

ryngeal, and esophageal cancer outside of North America and Western Europe. Cancer, *40*:1879, 1977.

43. Marshall, J., Graham, S., Mettlin, C., et al.: Diet in the epidemiology of oral cancer. Nutr. Cancer, *3*:145, 1982.

44. Martinez, I.: Factors associated with cancer of the esophagus, mouth, and pharynx in Puerto Rico. J. Natl. Cancer Inst., *42*:1069, 1969.

45. Mashberg, A., Garfinkel, L., and Harris, S.: Alcohol as a primary risk factor in oral squamous carcinoma. CA, *31*:146, 1981.

46. Mashberg, A., and Meyers, H.: Anatomical site and size of 222 early asymptomatic oral squamous cell carcinomas. A continuing prospective study of oral cancer. II. Cancer, *37*:2149, 1976.

47. Mehta, F. S., Gupta, P. C., Daftary, K. K., et al.: An epidemiology study of oral cancer and precancerous conditions among 101,761 villagers in Maharashtra, India. Int. J. Cancer, *10*:134, 1972.

48. Mehta, F. S., Gupta, P. C., and Pindborg, J. J.: Chewing and smoking habits in relation to precancer and oral cancer. J. Cancer Res. Clin. Oncol., *99*:35, 1981.

49. Moss, E., and Lee, W. R.: Occurrence of oral and pharyngeal cancers in the textile workers. Br. J. Ind. Med., *31*:224, 1974.

50. National Institute of Health: Cancer Patient Survival Experience, Trends in Survival 1960–1963 to 1970–1973. Comparison of Survival for Black and White Patients. Long Term Effects of Cancer. Public Health Service. DHHS (NIH) Publication No. 80–2148, US Department of Health and Human Services, 1980.

51. Nissanga, S.: Incidence and pattern of cancer in Sri Lanka. *In*: Hirayama T. (ed.): Cancer in Asia. GANN Monograph on Cancer Research, No. 18. Tokyo, Japan Scientific Societies Press, 1976.

52. Peacock, E. E., Greenburg, B. G., and Brawley, B. W.: The effect of snuff and tobacco on the production of oral carcinoma. Ann. Surg., *151*:242, 1960.

53. Percy, C., Staneh, E., and Gloeckler, L.: Accuracy of cancer death certificates and its effect on cancer mortality statistics. Am. J. Public Health, *71*:242, 1981.

54. Pindborg, J. J.: Epidemiological studies of oral cancer. Int. Dent. J., *27*:172, 1977.

55. Pindborg, J. J.: Oral cancer and precancer as diseases of the aged. Community Dent. Oral Epidemiol., *6*:300, 1978.

56. Pollack, E. S., and Horm, J. H.: Trends in cancer incidence and mortality in the United States, 1969–1976. J. Natl. Cancer Inst., *64*:1091, 1980.

57. Ratzkowski, E., Hochman, A., Buchner, A., et al.: Causes of cancer of the lip. Review of 167 cases. Oncologia, *20*:129, 1966.

58. Rosenfeld, L., and Callaway, J.: Snuff-dipper's cancer. Am. J. Surg., *106*:801, 1963.

59. Rothman, D. and Keller, A.: The effect of joint exposure to alcohol and tobacco on risk of cancer of the mouth and pharynx. J. Chron. Dis., *25*:711, 1972.

60. Segi, M., Tomihaga, S., Aoki, K., et al.: Cancer mortality and morbidity statistics. GANN Monograph on Cancer Research No. 26. Tokyo, Japan Scientific Societies Press, 1981.

61. Smart, C. R., Lyon, J. L., Skolnick, M., et al.: Cancer of the head and neck in Utah. Am. J. Surg., *128*:463, 1974.

62. Smith, C. J.: Global epidemiology and aetiology of oral cancer. Int. Dent. J., *23*:82, 1972.

63. Smith, E. M.: Epidemiology of oral and pharyngeal

cancers in the United States: review of recent literature. J. Natl. Cancer Inst., *63*:1189, 1979.
64. Smith, J. F.: Snuff-dippers lesion. A ten-year follow-up. Arch. Otolaryngol., *101*:276, 1975.
65. Smith, J. F., Mincer, H. A., Hopkins, K. P., et al.: Snuff-dippers lesion: a cytological and pathological study in a large population. Arch. Otolaryngol., *92*:450, 1970.
66. Spitzer, W. O., Hill, G. B., Chambers, L. W., et al.: The occupation of fishing as a risk factor in cancer of the lip. New Engl. J. Med., *293*:419, 1975.
67. Stoddart, T. G.: Conference on cancer of the lip. Can. Med. Assoc. J., *90*:666, 1964.
68. Szpak, C., Stone, M., and Frenkel, E.: Some observations concerning the demographic and geographic incidence of carcinoma of the lip and buccal cavity. Cancer, *40*:343, 1977.
69. Vincent, R. J., and Marchetta, F.: The relationship of the use of tobacco and alcohol to cancer of the oral cavity, pharynx, or larynx. Am. J. Surg., *106*:501, 1963.
70. Vogler, W. R., Lloyd, J. W., and Milmore, B. K.: A retrospective study of etiological factors in cancer of the mouth, pharynx, and larynx. Cancer, *15*:246, 1962.
71. Wahi, P. N.: Oral and oropharyngeal tumors. *In*: Hirayama, T. (ed.): Cancer in Asia. GANN Monograph on Cancer Research, No. 18. Tokyo, Japan Scientific Societies Press, 1976.
72. Waterhouse, J., Muir, C., Correa, P., et al. (ed.): Cancer Incidence in Five Continents. Vol. III. Lyon, International Agency for Research on Cancer, 1976.
73. Whitaker, C. J., Moss, E., Lee, W. R., et al.: Oral and pharyngeal cancer in the Northeast and West Yorkshire regions of England, and occupation. Br. J. Ind. Med., *36*:292, 1979.
74. Wiliams, R., and Horm, J.: Association of cancer sites with tobacco and alcohol consumption and socioeconomic status of patients. Interview study of the Third National Cancer Survey. J. Natl. Cancer Inst., *58*:525, 1977.
75. Winn, D. M., Blot, W. J., Shy, C. M., et al.: Snuff-dipping and oral cancer among women in the southern United States. N. Engl. J. Med., *304*:745, 1981.
76. Wynder, E. L., Bross, I. J., and Feldman, R. M.: A study of the etiology factors in cancer of the mouth. Cancer, *10*:1300, 1957.
77. Wynder, E. L., Mushinski, M. H., and Spivak, J. C.: Tobacco and alcohol consumption in relation to the development of multiple primary cancers. Cancer, *40*:1972, 1977.
78. Wynder, E. L., and Stellman, S. D.: Comparative epidemiology of tobacco related cancers. Cancer Res., *37*:4608, 1977.
79. Young, J. L., Perry, C. L., Asire, A. J., et al.: Cancer incidence and mortality in the United States, 1973–1977. SEER-NIH Publication No. 81(2330). National Cancer Institute Monograph No. 57. Bethesda, MD, Public Health Service, 1981.

9

Screening for oral cancer

EDWARD C. MALOOF, D.D.S., M.P.H.

Both the medical and dental professions have a major responsibility for the early detection and diagnosis of malignancies of the oral cavity and for the prevention of these diseases. Malignant tumors of the mouth often occur in people who are otherwise apparently healthy. Many patients who have oral cancer in its early stage may not consult a physician for a complaint that would require a thorough examination of the oral cavity. Therefore, the medical profession is often not able to provide early diagnosis and prophylaxis against oral cancer in this group of people. Many people do not see a dentist routinely and hesitate to make an appointment about a "minor" sore in their mouth.

In fact, the "challenge" of oral cancer should be both intriguing and frustrating to those in the dental and medical professions. The paradox is that one looks for a lesion that is easily accessible to the visual and tactile senses, as well as being relatively simple to recognize and diagnose. With these facts, how can the professions countenance a disease that accounts for 9000 deaths annually, or 8 percent of all deaths due to cancer?

Of more importance, however, is the great and devastating impact of oral cancer on the patient. Such an impact is exceeded by few other diseases. Treatment for an advanced oral cancer is mutilating, and this mutilation is most difficult to hide or correct. One can cover the scars from cancer of most other areas so that only the patient, the immediate family, and close friends know what type of operation the patient has undergone. Generally, defects caused by the treatment of extensive cancer of the oral regions cannot be hidden, and although the disability can be reduced by plastic surgery or by a prosthesis, function and esthetics are not completely satisfactory. Gen-

erally, a patient who has an extensive oral cancer that has been "successfully" treated can look forward only to extreme difficulty in eating and in communicating with those people who do not turn their heads away. In comparison, one man who had poliomyelitis, which was rightfully considered to be one of the most dreaded diseases, was able to communicate so well with his countrymen that he was elected President of the United States for an unprecedented four terms.

SCREENING

Screening for cancer has received renewed interest in recent years as a simple and effective means of controlling the high mortality and notable morbidity of many forms of cancer.[3] On the assumption that therapeutic techniques for advanced cancer may not improve significantly in the future, it is logical to support programs that will help to find cancers in their early stage of development, when they are small localized lesions and metastatic spread has not occurred. The finding of known precancerous lesions would be an added bonus. The results of screening programs for breast cancer and cervical cancer have generally been positive in providing evidence that early detection can lead to a reduction in mortality.[1, 2, 7, 8] However, results from screening for colorectal cancer and lung cancer have not been as encouraging.

Results on screening for oral cancer are not readily available, since oral cancer has a relatively low incidence and few screening programs have reported results. However, it can be assumed that screening for oral cancer would afford an opportunity of finding small, early asymptomatic lesions that could be effectively treated.[5, 6] Oral lesions are easily seen on examination and simple, reliable tests exist for their diagnosis. Furthermore, a high risk population for oral cancer has been defined,[4] and precancerous oral lesions are well understood and easily discernible upon oral examination.[7]

The goals of a screening program include documentation of both precancerous and cancerous lesions, health education, and public relations. Also to be considered is the recruitment of patients or improving the access of a particular population to medical and dental care. Elderly patients, especially those who live in nursing homes, fall into this group. If public relations is a goal, the program will want to attract as many patients as possible.

Anyone who undertakes a screening program should be perfectly clear about the program objective and should be aware of any potential "trade-offs" between achieving the maximum possible number of cases and other nonscreening goals.

Oral cancer is a lesion that is ideal for screening for the following reasons:

1. The mouth is easily accessible to careful visual examination.

2. Oral cancer is easily discernible as a lesion, even in its early stages of development.

3. There are simple, reliable tests for the diagnosis of oral cancer.

4. The high risk population can be identified.

5. Cost of screening for oral cancer is minimal.

6. Benefit of early diagnosis has clearly been shown in terms of decreased mortality and morbidity.

7. Early diagnosis usually results in more simplified therapy and less cost of rehabilitation.

8. Early diagnosis indicates better cosmetic results.

9. Current 5-year survival figures for oral cancer are poor.

PROGRAM PLANNING

There are three main considerations to be contemplated before a program is planned. The first consideration is to try to direct the screening toward the population at risk. In oral cancer, the program should be directed at the elderly and low income groups, those most likely to have poor nutrition and inadequate dental care. A more highly specific focus would be, if possible, to select the heavy smokers and drinkers from that population. This is very difficult because often the members of this population, who are at highest risk for oral cancer, do not believe in doctors and tend not to participate in any type of screening program.

The responsibility for a specific referral and follow-up arrangement for those individuals who are found to have a lesion is too often overlooked. It is harmful and useless to identify potential asymptomatic cases of cancer if they are not also diagnosed and treated early. Yet often, screening programs rely on the person who is screened to make arrangements for the follow-up. Some patients who have a lesion may not do anything at all, believing that if the follow-up were important the screening program would "take care of it." Other patients may believe that their own doctor might have limited interest in pursuing the result of a screening examination in which he or she did not participate. At least, the patient's dentist and physician should receive a full report of the results of the screening test. However, there should be a designated individual from the screening program who has the responsibility of referral or follow-up or both.

Finally, it is very important to review the data and to evaluate the number of people screened and lesions detected by the examiners. The technical skills of the examiner may also be described as a process measure.

PROGRAM IMPLEMENTATION

In setting up the operational program, there are several vital protocolar procedures to be followed. First, one must assess the available personnel and maximize, motivate, and coordinate their efforts.

In the case of oral cancer programs, voluntary agencies that should be contacted include the American Cancer Society, the local Dental Society or Medical Society, the local public health agency, and the neighboring educational or hospital institution (for the interpretation of the biopsies or slides). At the meeting of representatives from these groups, a program director should be appointed and areas of responsibility should be designated. At this time, it should be decided who the program director will be, who will obtain supplies, who the examining dentists or physicians, assistants, and volunteers will be, and who will be in charge of follow-ups or referrals and public relations.

It is of utmost importance to meet with the representatives of the targeted group (e.g., occupants of a nursing home, employees of a bank or insurance company) to discuss in depth the exact modus operandi of the program. The room in which the examinations are to be carried out should be visited, and a schematic layout for the chairs, and so on, should be agreed upon. If possible, a room with a sink should be selected. When gloves are used, it is especially important to let the new patient watch you discard the gloves from the previous patient and put on a fresh pair. Another important aspect is to provide some privacy for each patient, at least with portable screens. Many patients who have partial or full dentures do not want their fellow employees to know that they have dentures. This privacy must be respected. The pattern of the patient "flow" and the number of patients to be examined each hour should be decided on at this time. Examination time for each patient should be about 10 minutes, and assuming that the facility had four chairs, that would mean 24 patients per hour or 12 patients every 30 minutes. It has been agreed that for maximum effectiveness there should be 12 patients at the clinic area 10 minutes before the half-hour. Two or three portable tables or desks should be placed outside the examination room door so that the patients can fill out their record and history chart prior to their examination.

PATIENT RECORD AND HISTORY CHART

A major portion of the patient's record and history chart can be filled out by the patient or by volunteers from the group to be examined. The patient's history should be brief, and the record should include a chart or diagram to facilitate the listing of the examiner's findings. An excellent type of chart for oral cancer screening purposes is one developed in cooperation with the American Cancer Society, Massachusetts Division and widely used by us in screening programs in the New England Area. The chart has four copies (Fig. 9–1), one each of which is sent to the patient's dentist and physician if they are named. If there is no regular dentist or physician and the patient goes to a clinic or hospital for his or her health needs, a copy could be sent there to be included in the patient's record.

A leader-type member of the target group should be designated as the "doorkeeper" or traffic director, making sure that the patient flow is kept steady. If possible, the individual should call an hour ahead of time to alert the

various employees of their approaching examination appointments.

In a typical set-up, an adjoining room or a small section of the examining room is isolated for privacy and is used by the oral pathologist for oral cytological smears and for consultations with the examiners and patients who have some abnormality that the examiner deems worthy of a second opinion. With this special type of set-up, there will be no interruption in the flow of patients, because two or three patients may be seen by the consultant at the same time. In order that these patients not be alarmed, we explain to them that there is a slight abnormality about which we want the consultant to render a second opinion.

Of seemingly minor importance but of great concern (as expressed by many examiners) is the procuring of straight back chairs of good height for the patients to sit in. Whenever volunteers are called for this program, the first question often asked is: "What kind of chair will be used? The low chairs give me a back ache at the end of the session." It should be determined whether the clinic or facility has any gooseneck type of lamp for illumination during the examination. If not, flashlights or head lamps should be obtained. Disposable pen lights are effective and relatively inexpensive.

A meeting of the program director and other key workers should then be held to hear the report on the site and to decide the thrust of the public relations campaign.

If the program is to be held within an industry, campaign posters that indicate time and place and the fact that screening consists of a simple, quick, private, and painless examination should be displayed. If possible, the program director or his or her representative should attend a staff meeting of the supervisors of the industry and brief them about the examination. The program director's presentation should include slides, be short, and be spoken in terms understood by lay persons. If the business has a company newsletter, an article about the program should be published in two successive issues just prior to the examination date. If the company has a union, the stewards should be involved in the planning and execution of the program and attempts should be made to get a charismatic speaker to address the regular union meeting. At such a meeting, the presentation should be short and slides of the program are essential to ensure successful communication.

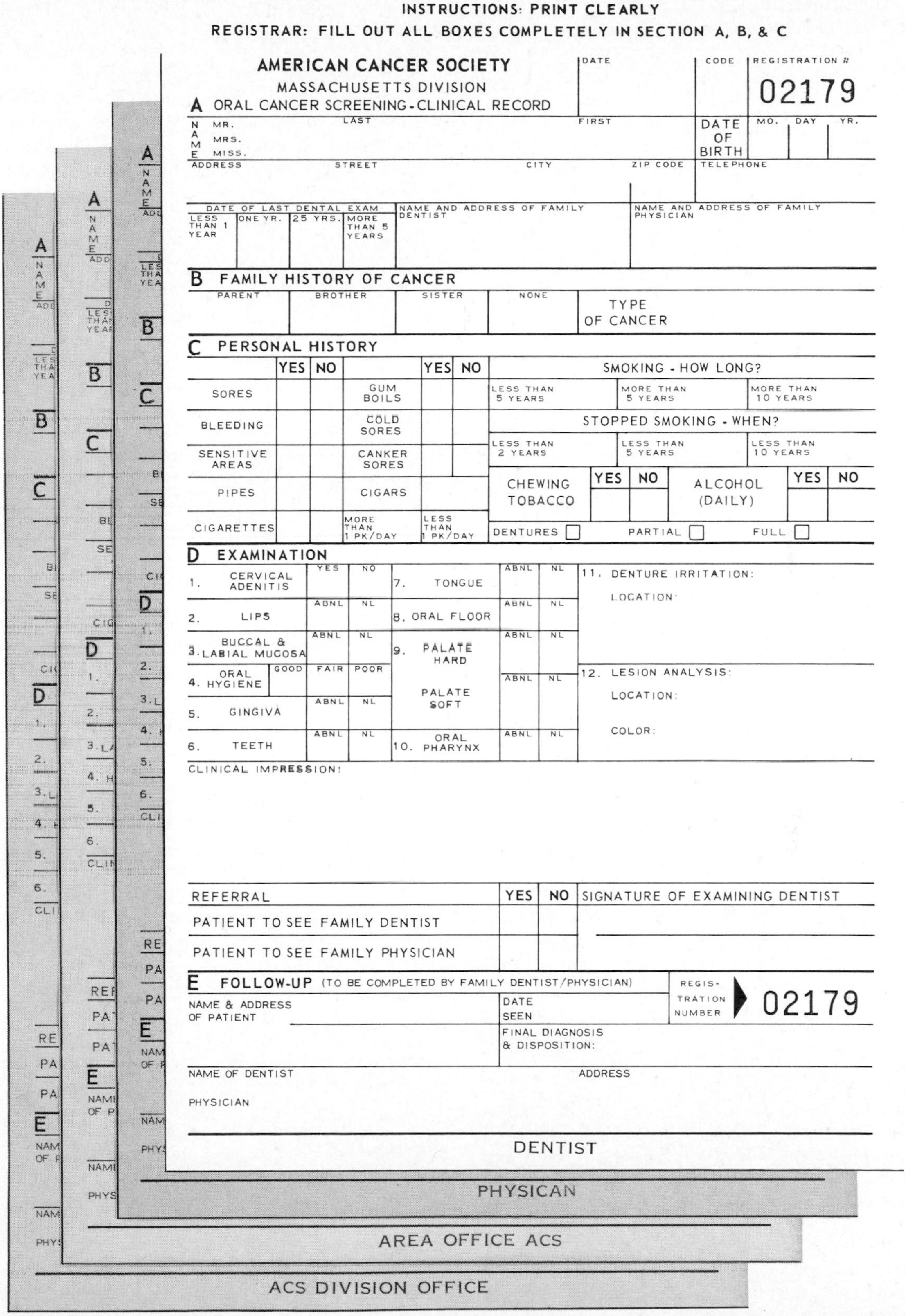

INSTRUCTIONS: PRINT CLEARLY
REGISTRAR: FILL OUT ALL BOXES COMPLETELY IN SECTION A, B, & C

AMERICAN CANCER SOCIETY
MASSACHUSETTS DIVISION
A ORAL CANCER SCREENING - CLINICAL RECORD

| DATE | CODE | REGISTRATION # |
| | | 02179 |

| NAME | MR. / MRS. / MISS. | LAST | FIRST | DATE OF BIRTH | MO. DAY YR. |

ADDRESS STREET CITY ZIP CODE TELEPHONE

| DATE OF LAST DENTAL EXAM | | | | NAME AND ADDRESS OF FAMILY DENTIST | NAME AND ADDRESS OF FAMILY PHYSICIAN |
| LESS THAN 1 YEAR | ONE YR. | 25 YRS. | MORE THAN 5 YEARS | | |

B FAMILY HISTORY OF CANCER

| PARENT | BROTHER | SISTER | NONE | TYPE OF CANCER |

C PERSONAL HISTORY

	YES	NO		YES	NO	SMOKING - HOW LONG?		
SORES			GUM BOILS			LESS THAN 5 YEARS	MORE THAN 5 YEARS	MORE THAN 10 YEARS
BLEEDING			COLD SORES			STOPPED SMOKING - WHEN?		
SENSITIVE AREAS			CANKER SORES			LESS THAN 2 YEARS	LESS THAN 5 YEARS	LESS THAN 10 YEARS
PIPES			CIGARS			CHEWING TOBACCO	YES NO	ALCOHOL (DAILY) YES NO
CIGARETTES			MORE THAN 1 PK/DAY	LESS THAN 1 PK/DAY		DENTURES ☐	PARTIAL ☐	FULL ☐

D EXAMINATION

	YES	NO			ABNL	NL	11. DENTURE IRRITATION:
1. CERVICAL ADENITIS			7. TONGUE				LOCATION:
2. LIPS	ABNL	NL	8. ORAL FLOOR		ABNL	NL	
3. BUCCAL & LABIAL MUCOSA	ABNL	NL	9. PALATE HARD		ABNL	NL	
4. ORAL HYGIENE	GOOD	FAIR	POOR				12. LESION ANALYSIS:
				PALATE SOFT	ABNL	NL	LOCATION:
5. GINGIVA	ABNL	NL					
6. TEETH	ABNL	NL	10. ORAL PHARYNX		ABNL	NL	COLOR:

CLINICAL IMPRESSION:

REFERRAL	YES	NO	SIGNATURE OF EXAMINING DENTIST
PATIENT TO SEE FAMILY DENTIST			
PATIENT TO SEE FAMILY PHYSICIAN			

E FOLLOW-UP (TO BE COMPLETED BY FAMILY DENTIST/PHYSICIAN)

| REGISTRATION NUMBER | ▶ 02179 |

NAME & ADDRESS OF PATIENT	DATE SEEN
	FINAL DIAGNOSIS & DISPOSITION:
NAME OF DENTIST	ADDRESS
PHYSICIAN	

DENTIST

PHYSICAN

AREA OFFICE ACS

ACS DIVISION OFFICE

Figure 9-1. A chart for oral cancer screening purposes. The chart consists of four copies. One copy is sent to the patient's dentist, and one is sent to the patient's physician.

The American Cancer Society is very cooperative and successful in the public relations aspect of cancer screening programs. They have many contacts in the newspaper industry and in other media. It is very important to involve their representative in all aspects of the program from its inception.

In reviewing the public relations aspect of the screening process, the objective must always be kept in sight. Mass screening programs for oral cancer have only had fair results because of their failure to reach those individuals—often isolated, unemployed, and alcoholic—who are at greatest risk.

In our experience, about 80 percent of the patients who participate in an oral cancer program, except for those from nursing homes, have seen a dentist less than one year prior to their being examined in our program.

The challenge is then to motivate or beguile those individuals who are truly at risk to attend the oral cancer program so that they can be examined.

In two programs, different approaches were used to reach the people who were at risk. In one program, during a union meeting that was attended by about 650 members, an oral cancer clinic was set up in the business offices, which were next to the meeting hall. During the meeting, the president of the union instructed each row to leave the meeting to attend the oral cancer clinic. There were a few mild objections, but due to peer pressure, there was almost 100 percent attendance, with outstanding results. Thirty-two lesions were discovered, three of which proved to be cancerous.

In another program, the administration of a large New England city was persuaded to distribute the paychecks of the police and firefighters at one central location. An oral cancer screening clinic was set up next to the paymaster. As the police or firefighters were paid, we had them go through the screening clinic. But somehow, by midmorning word had gotten out about the screening clinic, and there was a tremendous drop in attendance.

Another effort to reach the target population was used in conjunction with a glaucoma screening program. Glaucoma has a high incidence rate in older people, as has oral cancer. In one city, the Lions Club was conducting glaucoma screening programs one night a month during the summer months. We met with their director and asked to have an oral cancer program in conjunction with their clinic. We agreed to publicize each other's clinic in our posters and press releases. Sixteen clinics were jointly held. Attendance was excellent and good results were reported.

Recently, the public has been inundated with statistics concerning high blood pressure. Oral cancer screening in conjunction with screenings for blood pressure has proved valuable in several instances. Likewise, oral cancer screening in conjunction with health fairs in community centers has proved helpful.

In evaluating some programs, we were a little surprised to have some patients, after getting up from an examining chair, ask "Is that all? Aren't they going to do something 'special' to detect cancer?" The thoroughness, expertise, and depth of the oral examination by the doctor is sometimes not evident to the patient.

We have urged the doctors to utilize oral cytology more frequently. The patients seem to think that taking the cytologic smear is more meaningful than having only the oral examination. In one city, after cytologic smears were taken extensively, attendance increased dramatically.

For some unknown reason, many dentists seem apprehensive or hesitant about using oral cytology. It is difficult to understand this rationale. Oral cytology is an extremely simple examination to use, does not require special skills or training, is painless, and is readily accepted by the patient.

In evaluating the role of oral cytology, it is essential that one recognize its potential as well as its limitations. Cytology should never be considered as a substitute for a biopsy. Furthermore, all positive cytology reports must be confirmed by biopsy before treatment is planned or instituted. The clinican must know how to evaluate the cytology report and how to apply it to the specific clinical case, because the ultimate responsibility lies with the clinician who sees the patient. No laboratory is foolproof, and no laboratory test can replace good clinical judgment.

SUMMARY

Screening is a necessary approach to the detection of oral cancer and should be highly successful, based on many features of the program:

1. Oral cancer is a serious disease with a high mortality rate. Many patients who are

treated and survive have serious aesthetic and functional problems.

2. Prognosis for survival increases with early detection of small lesions that have not spread.

3. Esthetic and functional impairment is decreased by treatment of early, small lesions.

4. A good screening test is available (oral cytology), and this can immediately be followed by a simple diagnostic test (biopsy).

5. Cytology has a relatively high sensitivity and high specificity, no discomfort, and low cost.

6. Initial biopsy is diagnostic in virtually all cases.

7. Screening for oral cancer requires little special equipment and no inconvenience or embarrassment to the patient.

8. Oral cancer screening has been shown to be high in both positive and negative predictive value.

9. High-risk populations for oral cancer can be identified to some degree.

10. Treatment and rehabilitative facilities are usually available and are usually of high quality.

The problem in dealing with oral cancer is not treatment— it is lack of early diagnosis.

REFERENCES

1. Cramer, D. W.: The role of cervical cytology in the declining morbidity and mortality of cervical cancer. Cancer, *34*:2018, 1974.
2. Gardner, J. W., and Lyon, J. L.: Efficacy of cervical cytologic screening in the control of cervical cancer. Prev. Med., *6*:487, 1977.
3. Henderson, M.: Validity of screening. Cancer, *37*:573, 1976.
4. Keller, A. Z., and Terris, M.: The association of alcohol and tobacco with cancer of the mouth and pharynx. Am. J. Public Health, *55*:1578, 1965.
5. Mashberg, A., Morrissey, J. B., and Garfinkel, L.: A study of the appearance of early asymptomatic oral squamous cell carcinoma. Cancer, *32*:1436, 1973.
6. Sandler, H. C., Stahl, S. S., Cahn, L. R., et al.: Exfoliative cytology for detection of early mouth cancer. Oral Surg., *13*:994, 1960.
7. Shklar, G.: The precancerous oral lesion. Oral Surg., *20*:58, 1965.
8. Stark, A. M., and Way, S.: The screening of well women for the early detection of breast cancer, using clinical examination with thermography and mammography. Cancer, *33*:1671, 1974.
9. Strax, P.: Results of mass screening for breast cancer in 50,000 examinations. Cancer, *37*:30, 1976.

10

Tumors of salivary glands

JOHN L. GIUNTA, D.M.D., M.S.

Although salivary gland neoplasms represent only a small percentage of oral neoplasms, they are an interesting and complex array of microscopic varieties that sometimes behave unpredictably despite an otherwise relatively benign appearance. In this chapter, some of the well-recognized neoplasms will be reviewed according to classifications, with particular emphasis on the microscopic patterns. Several excellent reviews and monographs that are concerned with the classifications and histopathology of salivary gland tumors have been published. The microscopic patterns of both the extraoral (major) and intraoral (minor) salivary gland neoplasms will be presented together, because the patterns are essentially similar.

The classification follows that of the World Health Organization. In Table 10–1, a classification of salivary gland tumors, plus comments on relative incidence rate, recurrence, and survival rate, is given.

Prior to presenting the histopathology, some statistics and general features of salivary gland tumors will be reviewed. Most neoplasms of the salivary glands occur in the parotid gland; some occur only in the parotid (e.g., Warthin's tumor and acinic cell tumors). In the parotid, approximately 75 percent of the neoplasms are benign, and most of those are pleomorphic adenomas. Of the malignant neoplasms in the parotid, the most common is the mucoepidermoid tumor, followed closely by the adenoid cystic carcinoma. Interestingly, as the size of the involved gland decreases, the proportion of malignant neoplasms that occur in the gland increases. Thus, neoplasms of the sublingual gland are rare, but most of them are malignant. As for the minor salivary glands of the oral mucosa, the most common location is the palate, followed by the upper lip. The most

common neoplasm is the pleomorphic adenoma. However, the proportion of malignant neoplasms has greatly increased, with the ratio of benign to malignant being 6:4 and approaching 1:1. The most common intraoral malignant salivary neoplasm is the adenoid cystic carcinoma, followed by the mucoepidermoid tumor.

The gross features of both benign and malignant salivary neoplasms are similar, with some exceptions. Generally, the neoplasms originate as firm, smooth, rounded nodules that vary in size depending upon the length of time they have been growing. In the major glands, they are larger at the time of investigation than in the minor glands, primarily because there is less room for expansion in the oral cavity. They are usually several centimeters in greatest diameter. Slowly growing, many benign tumors reach the size of a grapefruit or even larger (Fig. 10–1). Benign and malignant tumors may be slow growing; however, the history of sudden growth, or perhaps ulceration, usually suggests malignancy. In the parotid, a history of Bell's palsy indicates invasion by a malignant tumor into the branches of the facial nerve. If the mass is fluctuant, the tumor is probably cystic. In the parotid, the tumor usually originates anterior and inferior to the ear, and the ear lobe may be everted anteriorly because of the expansive mass. In the submandibular gland, there will be a notable, asymptomatic mass or lump in the neck inferior to the inferior border of the mandible. In the oral mucosa, there may be a prominent, asymptomatic swelling of the palate or the upper lip. On the hard palate, the swelling may be mistaken for a fibroma or a dental abscess. Regardless of the site, both benign and malignant neoplasms may resemble each other clinically (Fig. 10–2), and a biopsy will

98

Table 10-1. SALIVARY GLAND TUMORS

	Relative Incidence Rate (%)		Recurrence	Survival Rate (%)
	Major	*Minor*		
Benign				
Pleomorphic adenoma	90	90	Often	100
Monomorphic adenomas				
Warthin's tumor	8			100
Oncocytoma	1			100
Other adenomas	1	10		100
Malignant				
Mucoepidermoid tumors	34	20		
Low-grade			Often	95
High-grade			High	15
Adenoid cystic carcinoma	11	41	High	12 (20 yr)
Acinic cell tumors	5			
Low-grade			Often	80 (5 yr)
High-grade			High	Poor
Other adenocarcinomas	17	31	High	Poor
Carcinoma in pleomorphic adenoma	15		High	50
Other (squamous, lymphoma, etc.)	18		High	Poor

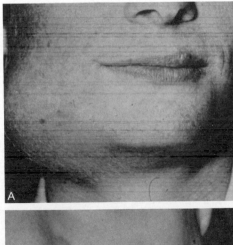
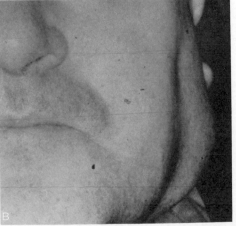

Figure 10-1. *A,* Pleomorphic adenoma of the right parotid gland in a 55-year-old female. *B,* Papillary cystadenoma lymphomatosis of the left parotid gland in a 60-year-old male.

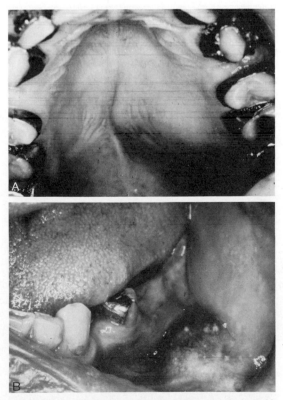

Figure 10-2. *A,* Adenocarcinoma of the palate in a 13-year-old male who was undergoing orthodontic treatment. *B,* Adenocarcinoma of the buccal mucosa in a 40-year-old female. The lesion was highly vascular.

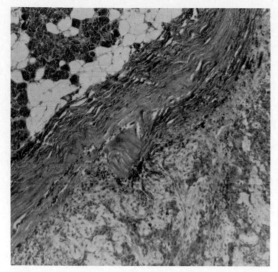

Figure 10–3. Pleomorphic adenoma of the parotid gland. A relatively thick capsule separates the normal parotid from the cellular and myxomatous tumor (lower right) (Hematoxylin and eosin, × 120).

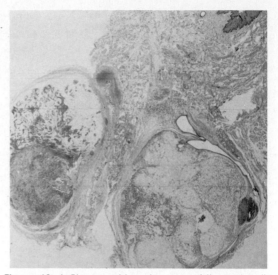

Figure 10–4. Pleomorphic adenoma of the upper lip. Oral mucosa overlies the striated muscle and two apparently separated, circumscribed, and encapsulated tumors showing variable morphology, including myxomatous areas. These tumors may be multicentric in origin (Hematoxylin and eosin, × 25).

determine the nature of the lesion and, hopefully, its ultimate classification. Because some of the malignant patterns can appear benign histologically, the behavior of the neoplasm determines its true classification. The histological findings are diverse, despite the fact that most salivary neoplasms apparently originate from adult ductal epithelium (intercalated duct epithelium). Rarely, a salivary gland tumor originates from connective tissue or is metastatic, but most are epithelial.

BENIGN EPITHELIAL TUMORS

Pleomorphic Adenoma

The benign pleomorphic adenoma is the most common of all salivary gland neoplasms and has an array of histologic features. It is characterized by an epithelial element that may or may not be composed of ductal structures, a prominent .myoepithelial element, and a prominent mesenchymal stroma, which is frequently myxomatous. Both the epithelial component and the stroma can be quite variable, thus yielding a pleomorphic pattern.

Pleomorphic adenomas are frequently encapsulated, but the thickness of the capsule is variable and at times appears nonexistent, a finding that occurs more commonly in the intraoral tumors (Figs. 10–3 through 10–5). Not infrequently, the tumor cells will be found in the capsule, a factor, in addition to the myxomatous stroma, that probably accounts

for recurrences if the resection of the tumor is minimal. Because of the slow but progressive expansion, the margins of the tumors are rounded and the adjacent normal glands and tissue become atrophied and compressed. The pleomorphic adenoma may be multinodular, yielding a picture of multiple foci histologically

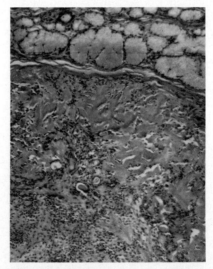

Figure 10–5. Pleomorphic adenoma of the upper lip. *Upper,* A very thin to nonexistent capsule lies between a cluster of minor, mucus-secreting salivary glands. *Lower,* The tumor showing prominent hyalinization below the capsule, a few ducts, cellular areas of myoepithelial cells, and some myxomatous stroma (Hematoxylin and eosin, × 200).

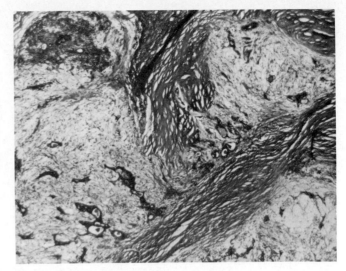

Figure 10–6. Intraoral pleomorphic adenoma. Dense connective tissue capsule surrounds the nodular, budding extensions of a primarily myxomatous tumor that contains islands of epithelium-forming ducts. Such extensions suggest multicentricity and may account for recurrences if they are not removed (Hematoxylin and eosin × 80).

(Figs. 10–4 and 10–6). Rarely, there are truly multiple foci of separate tumors.

Most helpful in the diagnosis is the finding of myxomatous areas, which are very pale staining (Figs. 10–6 and 10–7). Within this wispy stroma are single stellate-shaped or spindle-shaped nuclei with streaming cytoplasm that blend with the stroma (Fig. 10–8). These are myoepithelial cells, which are most abundant in these tumors. In the normal gland, they surround the duct-lining cell. At times, this myxomatous tissue may strongly resemble cartilage (Fig. 10–9), and in some tumors, both cartilage and bone have been found.

In addition to being myxomatous, the stroma may be hyalinized. These areas may have flattened cells of ductal epithelium that

have formed ductal structures. The ductal structures may be numerous or sparse and may be filled with an eosinophilic material.

The epithelial component is variable. There may be prominent ductal structures or only small clusters of epithelial cells. They may undergo a squamous metaplasia, and keratin may be seen. At times, there may be sheets of spindle-shaped myoepithelial cells, and these may give rise to a clear-cell variety. Although rare, normal mitoses may be seen (Fig. 10–10). At times, a ductal pattern may simulate the cylinders seen in the adenoid cystic carcinoma. Rarely, crystals or crystalloid elements may be noted.

The treatment requires adequate surgical margins beyond the capsule and the myxoma-

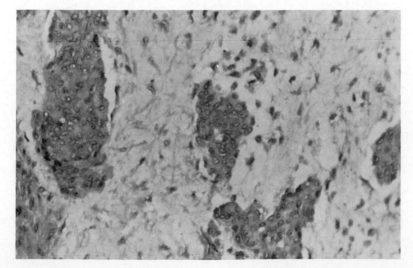

Figure 10–7. Pleomorphic adenoma of the parotid gland. Myxomatous stroma with single stellate and cartilagelike myoepithelial cells, as well as islands of probable myoepithelial cells (Hematoxylin and eosin, × 200).

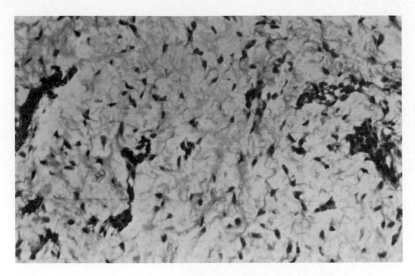

Figure 10–8. Pleomorphic adenoma of the palate. This tumor was primarily myxomatous, with spindle-shaped and stellate myoepithelial cells (Hematoxylin and eosin, × 250).

Figure 10–9. Pleomorphic adenoma of the parotid gland. Cartilage-like stroma that contains myoepithelial cells and is associated with islands of epithelium, which appears squamous (Hematoxylin and eosin, × 250).

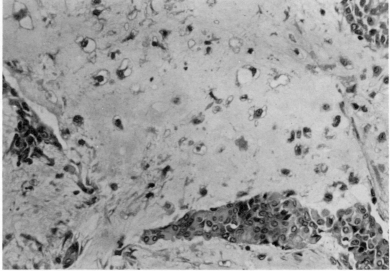

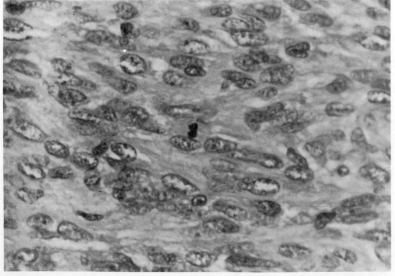

Figure 10–10. Pleomorphic adenoma of the parotid gland. A mitotic figure is in the center of densely packed myoepithelial cells. These tumors can be very cellular (Hematoxylin and eosin, × 600).

tous component. Recurrences may occur, but they probably relate to inadequate surgery at the outset. In the rare malignant counterpart, there is an adenocarcinoma or a squamous cell carcinoma that originates in a recognizable pleomorphic adenoma. The prognosis is related to the type of carcinoma and is poor.

Monomorphic Adenomas

This less common group of tumors is characterized by an epithelial pattern that is fairly uniform and a connective tissue component that is not a major feature diagnostically.

Warthin's Tumor (Papillary Cystadenoma Lymphomatosum)

This benign tumor occurs predominantly in the parotid gland and usually appears in older men as a cystic swelling anterior to the ear. These tumors may occur bilaterally. Histologically, the tumor is pathognomonic. It is characterized by papillary epithelial infoldings of ductal cells into the lumen of a cyst and the presence of organized lymphoid tissue beneath the epithelium (Fig. 10–11). The epithelium is composed of tall, columnar cells toward the lumen and shorter, cuboidal cells beneath it. The nuclei of the columnar cells are arranged in a palisading pattern in the middle of the cells. Just subjacent to these ductal (adenomatous) cells are densely packed lymphocytes, which may surround germinal centers (Fig. 10–12). One of the theories of histogenesis is that the tumor originates from ductal epithelium

within a lymph node in the parotid. The ductal cells stain eosinophilic and resemble oncocytes.

Papillary Cystadenoma (Lymphomatosum)

This tumor may be the intraoral counterpart of the Warthin's tumor. Benign, it is characterized by a similar pattern of adenomatous infoldings of a double row of ductal epithelial cells into the lumen of a cyst (Figs. 10–13 and 10–14). However, no lymph tissue with germinal centers is present. The ductal cells may or may not be oncocytic. These tumors are benign and adequate surgical margins assure nonrecurrence.

Oncocytoma (Oxyphilic Adenoma)

This uncommon tumor is composed of oncocytes, cells with prominent eosinophilic granules associated with aging. It can be found in the parotid as well as intraorally as an asymptomatic swelling.

The oncocytoma is composed of an encapsulated mass of eosinophilic staining cells with a prominent granular cytoplasm. The cells are large with a round nucleus and are grouped in rounded clusters that are surrounded by compressed capillaries or occur in sheets (Figs. 10–15 and 10–16). Occasionally, tubules or ductal structures are formed. The distinct granular appearance is due to large numbers of mitochondria. It should be remembered that oncocytic cells may be a feature of other salivary gland neoplasms. These tumors are benign and sometimes recur, but rarely are they malignant.

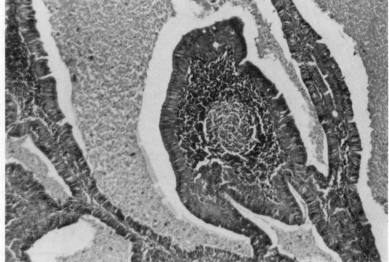

Figure 10–11. Warthin's tumor, in the parotid gland. A papillary projection of ductal cells surrounds the lymph nodal tissue and extends into the lumen, which contains fluid and cellular debris (Hematoxylin and eosin, × 80).

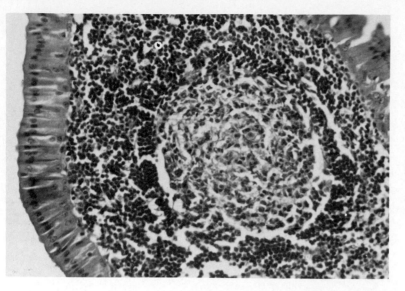

Figure 10–12. Warthin's tumor, in the parotid gland. A closer view of the tumor seen in Figure 10–11, showing the double row of outer columnar, eosinophilic cells with nuclei in a line and an inner row of cuboidal cells, which is next to the stroma with lymph tissue, including a germinal center (Hematoxylin and eosin, × 250).

Figure 10–13. Papillary cystadenoma of the palate. Two cysts with papillary, adenomatous infoldings of ductal epithelial cells are encapsulated and surrounded by lobules of mucous glands, some of which are atrophic. There is no lymphoid tissue (Hematoxylin and eosin, × 80).

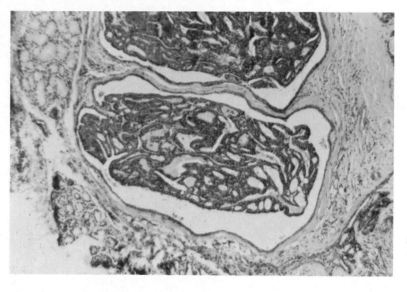

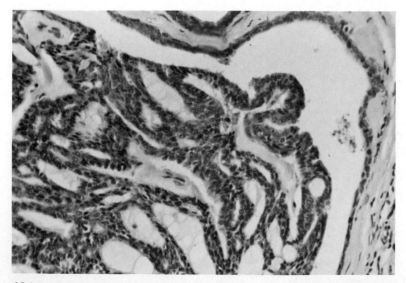

Figure 10–14. Papillary cystadenoma of the palate. High-power view of the papillary cystadenoma seen in Figure 10–13, showing projection of the double row of epithelial cells into the cyst lumen and the formation of ductal spaces with an eosinophilic coagulum (Hematoxylin and eosin, × 250).

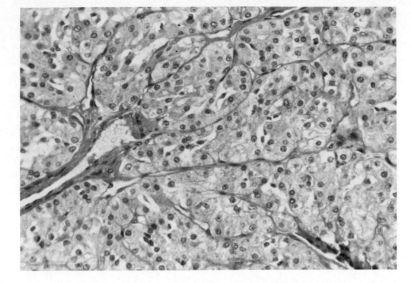

Figure 10–15. Oncocytoma in the parotid. Rounded clusters of large granular cells are surrounded by thin, often compressed capillaries. Occasional ductal outline is noted (Hematoxylin and eosin, × 250).

Basal Cell Adenoma

Although there are several other types of monomorphic adenomas that have a uniform pattern throughout, only the basal cell adenoma will be discussed, primarily because it is a clinicopathologic entity. The basal cell adenoma occurs in the parotid and in the minor salivary glands, particularly in the upper lip, where it originates as a firm nodule in the elderly. These tumors are rounded, smoothed, outlined nodules with capsules and are easily removed at surgery. Histologically, they are composed of darker-staining cells that resemble basal cells, the nuclei of which are aligned in a palisading manner. Several arrangements, such as tubular, trabecular, canalicular, and even solid sheets of cells, may be noted (Figs. 10–17 through 10–19). The presence of prominent vascular channels within the stroma between the epithelial cells is characteristic of basal cell adenomas. Benign in appearance and behavior, they do not recur after conservative removal.

MALIGNANT EPITHELIAL TUMORS

Mucoepidermoid Tumors (Mucoepidermoid Carcinoma)

The mucoepidermoid tumor is characterized by a nonencapsulated mass that is composed of mucus-secreting, epidermoid, and intermediate cells in varying proportions. The stroma

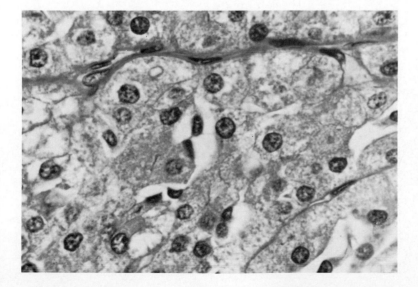

Figure 10–16. Oncocytoma in the parotid. High-power view of the oncocytoma seen in Figure 10–15, showing large cells with round central nuclei and prominent eosinophilic granular cytoplasm. Spindle-shaped nuclei are of the endothelial cells of capillaries that surround the oncocytic cells (Hematoxylin and eosin, × 600).

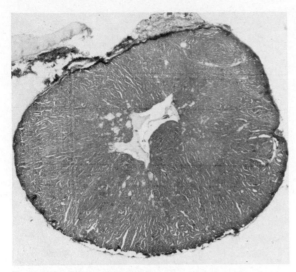

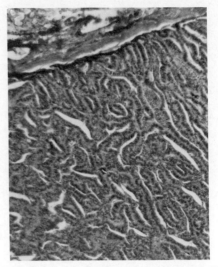

Figure 10–17. Basal cell adenoma of the upper lip. In this overview, a cross section showing a neatly, rounded mass with a thin capsule lying beneath the lip mucosa can be seen. Central cystic spaces are present (Hematoxylin and eosin, × 25).

Figure 10–18. Basal cell adenoma of the upper lip. This moderate-power view of the basal cell ademoma seen in Figure 10–17 shows slitlike spaces created by the trabecular and canalicular arrangement of the epithelial cells. The tumor capsule separates the tumor from the adjacent mucous glands (Hematoxylin and eosin, × 120).

is usually fibrous, and there are no myxoid areas or variations as in the pleomorphic adenoma. There may be numerous small or large cystic spaces with mucus (Fig. 10–20). These are usually surrounded by mucus-secreting cells, which may resemble goblet cells (Fig. 10–21). In addition, there are islands of epidermoid cells. Both intercellular bridges and foci of keratinization may be seen (Fig. 10–22). The intermediate cells are smaller and are undifferentiated cells. Whereas the proposed behavior cannot unequivocally be predicted,

histologically, there are two grades of these tumors. The high-grade tumor is supposedly more aggressive and more likely to metastasize than the low-grade tumor. The low-grade tumor generally behaves similarly to the pleomorphic adenoma and is therefore likely to recur. It is characterized by having primarily mucus-secreting cells, with cyst formation and epidermoid cells. The high-grade tumor usually has few mucus-secreting cells and a high proportion of squamous and intermediate

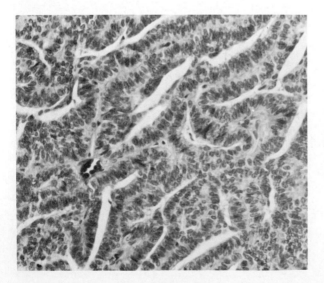

Figure 10–19. Basal cell adenoma of the upper lip. High-power view of the basal cell adenoma seen in Figure 10–17, showing palisading basaloid cells in a canalicular and trabecular pattern. Note the prominent blood vessel in the stroma *(center)* (Hematoxylin and eosin, × 250).

Figure 10–20. Low-grade mucoepidermoid tumor of the parotid gland. Small or large cystic spaces that contain mucin are surrounded by compressed mucus-secreting cells accompanied by nests of epidermoid cells in a collagenous stroma (Hematoxylin and eosin, × 80).

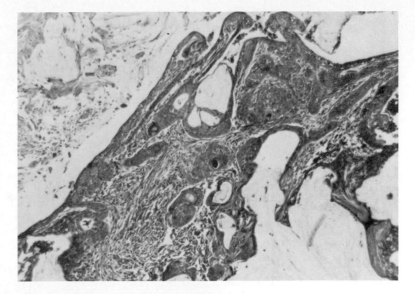

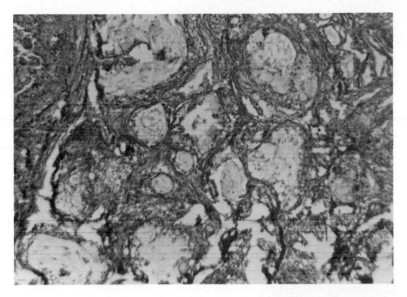

Figure 10–21. Mucoepidermoid tumor of the lower lip. In this view of the tumor, primarily mucous cells are seen, with some acinar structures and irregular small cystic spaces that contain mucin (Hematoxylin and eosin, × 120).

Figure 10–22. Low-grade mucoepidermoid tumor of the parotid gland. Higher magnification of the mucoepidermoid tumor seen in Figure 10–20, showing epidermoid cells with keratinization, mucin-filled cysts, and fibrous stroma with chronic inflammatory cells (Hematoxylin and eosin, × 250).

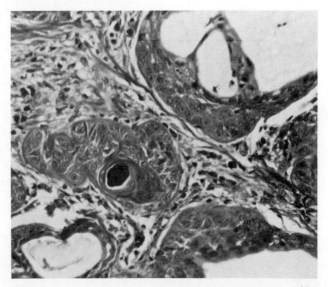

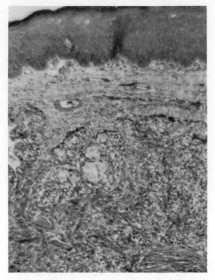

Figure 10–23. Mucoepidermoid tumor of the hard palate. The oral mucosa overlies the pushing margins of the nonencapsulated tumor, which is infiltrating the connective tissue (Hematoxylin and eosin, × 120).

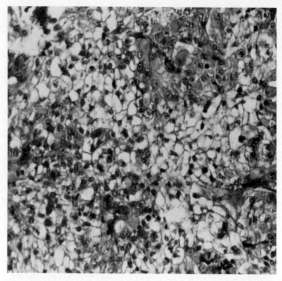

Figure 10–24. Mucoepidermoid tumor of the hard palate. This higher magnification of the mucoepidermoid tumor seen in Figure 10–23 shows mucous cells, clear cells, and darker squamous cells. Sometimes the tumor may be composed of only the hydropic cleared cells (Hematoxylin and eosin, × 250).

cells. It may be difficult to distinguish from an epidermoid carcinoma unless special stains reveal mucin with the cellular cytoplasm. Some mucoepidermoid tumors reveal notable hydropic degeneration, resulting in a tumor with cleared cells (Figs. 10–23 and 10–24). Mitotic activity may be noted, but it is not a frequent finding. As indicated previously, the prognosis is determined by clinical behavior. Treatment usually consists of surgery with adequate margins.

Adenoid Cystic Carcinoma (Cylindroma)

The adenoid cystic carcinoma is a slow-growing infiltrative lesion with rather benign-appearing cells. However, because of its behavior, which includes a high recurrence rate and a low survival rate after 15 or 20 years, the histopathology is correlated with its behavior, and it is separated from other adenocar-

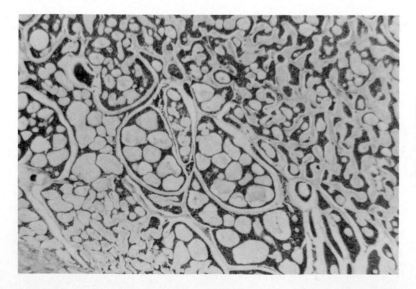

Figure 10–25. Adenoid cystic carcinoma of the submandibular gland. Deeply staining cells surround the cystic and ductal spaces. Many of the groupings are interconnected, yielding a cylindromatous and cribriform (sievelike) pattern (Hematoxylin and eosin, × 120).

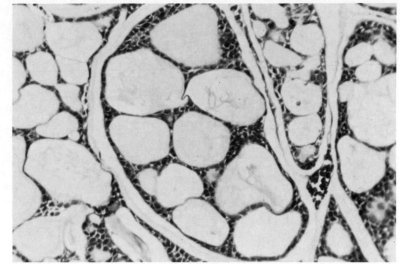

Figure 10–26. Adenoid cystic carcinoma of the submandibular gland. Higher magnification of the adenoid cystic carcinoma seen in Figure 10–25, showing a cylinder of basaloid ductal and myoepithelial cells around spaces that contain mucinous material. At the left, similar cells are forming a lacelike pattern (Hematoxylin and eosin, × 250).

cinomas (which usually have a worse prognosis) and from certain cutaneous neoplasms.

The adenoid cystic carcinoma may have many patterns. However, one pattern is characteristic. It is composed of groupings of very dark-staining nuclei with indistinct cytoplasmic boundaries. These basaloid cells include both small duct-lining cells and myoepithelial cells. They are usually arranged around spaces that form ducts, which, when packed together without stroma, yield a cribriform (sievelike) pattern (Figs. 10–25 and 10–26). Some of these formations are surrounded by a hyalinized connective tissue, yielding an appearance of cylinders with a round to oval shape (Fig. 10–27). Both of these patterns have been said to resemble "swiss cheese." The tubular struc-

tures often contain an eosinophilic coagulum.

Another pattern of adenoid cystic carcinoma is cellular, and there are trabeculae of cells without any tubular arrangement. The deeply staining cells appear monotonously uniform, and mitoses are very rare. There is a fibrous stroma that may be hyalinized and even acellular, mimicking that of a pleomorphic adenoma. Perineural infiltration is a characteristic feature that is helpful in diagnosis (Fig. 10–28). This neoplasm is nonencapsulated and extends by infiltrating and invading along perineural spaces (Fig. 10–29). Treatment consists of surgery with adequate margins. Because of possible neural extension at the time of surgery, prognosis is guarded, and after approximately 20 years, few patients survive.

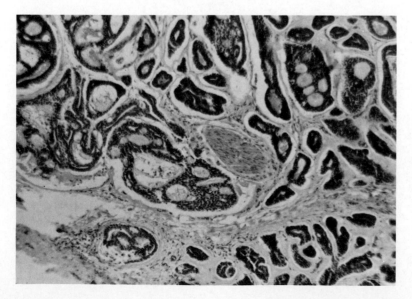

Figure 10–27. Adenoid cystic carcinoma of the palate. Ductal forms, trabeculae, and cylinders have infiltrated around the nerve in the center of the field. Stroma is collagenous and hyalinized (Hematoxylin and eosin, × 120).

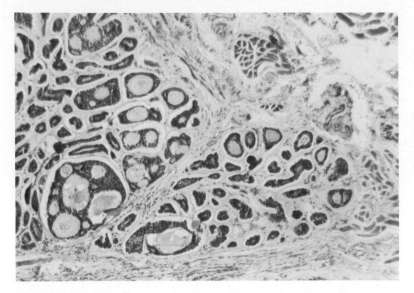

Figure 10–28. Adenoid cystic carcinoma of the palate. This view shows the infiltrative growth pattern of a nonencapsulated tumor invading striated muscle (Hematoxylin and eosin, × 120).

Acinic Cell Tumor (Acinic Cell Adenocarcinoma)

The acinic cell tumor is a rare, slow-growing, solitary, nodular, partially encapsulated lesion that occurs primarily in the parotid gland. Although the cellular morphology appears uniform and benign, the behavior may be similar to pleomorphic adenoma and mucoepidermoid tumor in that recurrences are common and occasionally tumors metastasize, with no relationship to morphology.

The acinic cell tumor is characterized by cells that resemble serous acinar cells. They have a prominent round deeply stained nucleus ("blue dot" tumor) and an abundant cytoplasm that usually contains basophilic granules (Fig. 10–30). The granularity may be absent at times, resulting in a cleared cytoplasm. By light microscopy, the granules correspond to secretory granules. There is scant stroma and rare mitotic activity, and the cells may be arranged in small groups or sheets. Cystic spaces may be seen. Treatment consists of adequate surgical excision.

Connective Tissue Tumors

Other benign and malignant tumors, epithelial and connective tissue, occur in the salivary

Figure 10–29. Collision tumor. Adenoid cystic carcinoma (above) infiltrating a pleomorphic adenoma (below) (Hematoxylin and eosin, × 120).

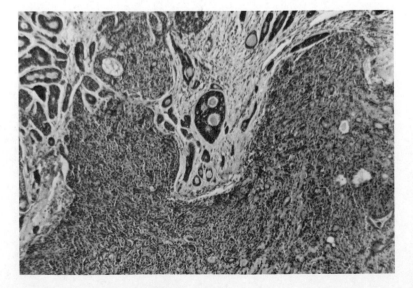

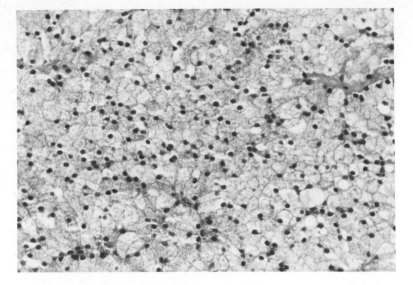

Figure 10–30. Acinic cell tumor of the parotid gland. This tumor ("blue dot" tumor) is composed of densely packed cells that resemble serous acini, with prominent round nuclei and abundant basophilic granular cytoplasm. Occasional clear cells are noted (Hematoxylin and eosin, × 250).

glands. We will briefly discuss one that is of connective tissue origin, hemangioma.

Hemangioma

This benign tumor composed of vascular tissues is the most common salivary gland tumor seen in infants and children. Clinically, there can be a slight swelling and a blue disfigurement on the skin of the face over and about the parotid gland. Whereas this can be disconcerting to parents and a point for ridicule by peers of the children, caution is to be exercised in treatment. These lesions regress spontaneously at puberty. Radiation therapy is contraindicated. Microscopically, there are numerous small blood vessels and endothelial proliferations that occur in and around the parotid gland.

Other Tumor-like Lesions

Several lesions and conditions may manifest as tumors or mimic tumors both clinically and histologically, such as benign lymphoepithelial lesion, chronic sialadenitis, lipomatosis, granulomatous inflammations, and necrotizing sialometaplasia. Necrotizing sialometaplasia will be mentioned because of the potential for error in its diagnosis.

Necrotizing Sialometaplasia

Necrotizing sialometaplasia is a benign condition that primarily affects the salivary glands of the hard palate. It originates clinically as large ulcerations that do not heal and therefore are suspected of being either malignant or granulomatous disease. Microscopically, the condition has been misdiagnosed as mucoepidermoid or epidermoid carcinoma. It is characterized by a pseudoepitheliomatous hyperplasia of the mucosal epithelium, a squamous metaplasia of ducts of the salivary glands, and an ischemic necrosis of the lobules of mucous acini. The etiology is related to a compromise of the vascular supply. The lesions spontaneously heal without further intervention in 8 to 10 weeks.

REFERENCES

1. Abrams, S., Cornyn, J., Scofield, H. H., et al.: Acinic cell carcinoma of the major salivary glands. Cancer, *18*:1145, 1965.
2. Batsakis, J. G., Wozniak, K. J., and Regezi, J. A.: Acinous cell carcinoma: histogenetic hypothesis. Oral Surg., *35*:904, 1977.
3. Busuttil, A.: Pathology of salivary gland tumors. Clin. Otolaryngol., *3*:161, 1978.
4. Chen, S.: Adenoid cystic carcinoma of minor salivary gland. Histochemical and electron microscopic studies of cystlike space. Oral Surg., *42*:606, 1976.
5. Eversole, L. R.: Mucoepidermoid carcinoma: review of 815 reported cases. Oral Surg., *28*:490, 1970.
6. Foote, F. W., and Frazell, E. L.: Tumors of the major salivary glands. Cancer, *6*:1065, 1953.
7. LiVolsi, V. A., and Perzin, K. H.: Malignant mixed tumors arising in salivary glands. 1. Carcinomas arising in benign mixed tumors: a clinicopathological study. Cancer. *39*:2209, 1977.
8. Melrose, R. J., Abrams, A. M., and Howell, F. V.:

Mucoepidermoid tumors of the intraoral minor salivary glands; a clinicopathologic study of 54 cases. J. Oral Pathol., 2:314, 1973.

9. Perzin, K. H., et al.: Adenoid cystic carcinomas arising in salivary glands: a correlation of histologic features and clinical course. Cancer, 42:265, 1978.

10. Rosenfeld, L., et al.: Malignant tumors of salivary gland origin. 37 year review of 184 cases. Ann. Surg., 163:726, 1966.

11. Skolnik, E. M., et al.: Tumors of the major salivary glands. Laryngoscope 87:843, 1977.

12. Spiro, R. H., et al.: Malignant mixed tumors of salivary origin: a clinicopathologic study. Cancer, 39:2209, 1977.

13. Spiro, R. H., et al.: Acinic cell carcinoma of salivary origin: a clinicopathologic study of 67 cases. Cancer, 41:924, 1978.

14. Thackray, A. C., and Lucas, R. B.: Tumors of the Major Salivary Glands. Atlas of Tumor Pathology. Armed Forces Inst. Pathology Fascicle No. 10, 1974.

11

Benign oral lesions in the differential diagnosis of oral cancer

DENNIS B. SOLT, D.M.D., Ph.D.

Several benign conditions may clinically resemble oral cancer. Of these conditions, inflammatory hyperplasia, ulcerations, vascular and other developmental malformations, and benign neoplasms are frequently encountered.

INFLAMMATORY HYPERPLASIA

Localized inflammatory hyperplasias probably account for most of the tumor-like masses that originate in the oral cavity. These lesions develop in response to a variety of traumatic and irritating influences to which the oral cavity is consistently subjected. Histologically, they consist of varying amounts of fibrous stroma and granulation tissue with a covering of hyperplastic stratified squamous epithelium. The hyperplasia may superficially resemble well-differentiated carcinoma on low-power microscopic survey (Fig. 11–1).

Multiple papillary lesions often develop from the mucosa of the palatal vault region that underlies a maxillary complete denture. Bite trauma may lead to inflammatory hyperplasia of the buccal mucosa or lower lip. Inflammatory hyperplasias also frequently develop in the buccal and labial sulcus in association with the flange or border of a complete denture (Fig. 11–2A and B). In this site, the hyperplastic tissue is usually fissured to conform to the denture flange, and secondary ulceration is common. Denture inflammatory hyperplasias are more likely to form when a denture is ill-fitting or unhygienic. These lesions may closely resemble neoplastic growths. Because epidermoid cancers sometimes develop in denture-bearing mucosa, the true nature of the tissue must always be established by biopsy.

HEMANGIOMA

Hemangiomas are vascular malformations that are very commonly seen in the head and neck region (Fig. 11–3). When large, they can be quite disfiguring and surgical management may be difficult, particularly for intraosseous lesions. The vascular nature of soft-tissue hemangiomas is usually appreciated clinically because of the deep red to blue color and the soft consistency of the tissue. Flat mucosal hemangiomas may resemble mucositis or erythroplasia of a neoplastic nature. Because early oral squamous cell carcinoma or carcinoma-in-situ may be manifested clinically as a red patch, the distinction between the diagnosis of hemangioma and early neoplastic disease is an important consideration.[7] The superficial capillary hemangioma will usually blanch upon digital compression of the lesion. Biopsy may be necessary to establish a definitive diagnosis.

MUCOCELE (MUCUS RETENTION PHENOMENON)

The mucocele is an extremely common oral lesion that results from blockage or severance of salivary ducts, with resultant mucous pooling and distention of glandular tissue. The overlying mucosa is usually elevated because of the retained mucus and the ensuing inflammatory response (Fig. 11–4). The lower lip is a common site of occurrence due to accidental

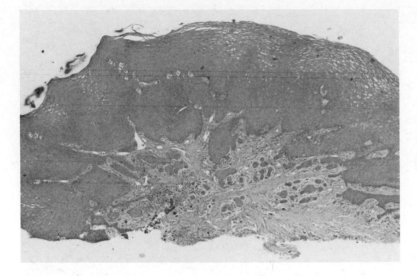

Figure 11–1. Epithelial hyperplasia and chronic inflammation of the palate, with extension of epithelial projections into the connective tissue (Hematoxylin-eosin stain, × 100).

or habitual lip biting. A history of trauma or multiple recurrence of a local tissue swelling can often be elicited from the patient. Excisional biopsy is both diagnostic and curative.

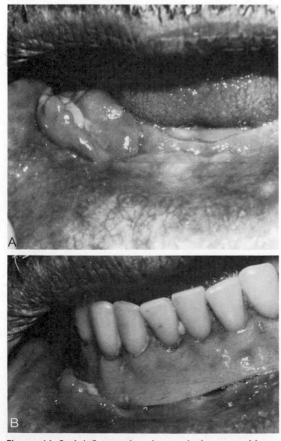

Figure 11–2. *A*, Inflammatory hyperplasia caused by a denture. *B*, Denture in position.

MEDIAN RHOMBOID GLOSSITIS

This benign condition consists of a reddish diamond-shaped or oval patch on the posterior midline region of the lingual mucosa (Fig. 11–5). The surface of the lesion is usually lobulated, and the mucosa is smooth as a result of a loss of the filiform papillae. Although the lesion has long been considered a developmental disorder, recently it has been suggested that median rhomboid glossitis may in fact be a form of localized chronic candidiasis.[9, 10] Epithelial hyperplasia and chronic inflammation are common microscopic features.

Although the posterior midline region of the tongue is an uncommon site of occurrence for squamous cell carcinoma, indurated or otherwise suspicious-appearing lesions that are encountered in this region should, of course, be biopsied.

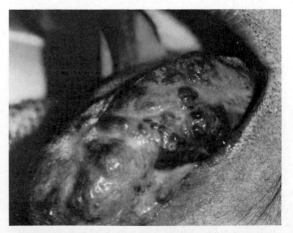

Figure 11–3. Extensive hemangioma of the tongue.

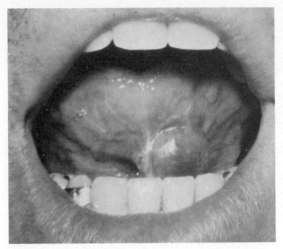

Figure 11–4. Mucocele of the ventral surface of the tongue.

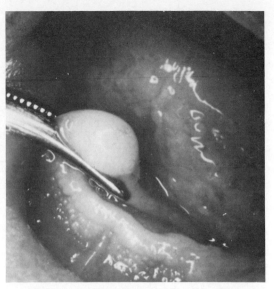

Figure 11–6. Fibroma of the alveolar ridge.

IRRITATION FIBROMA

Constant irritation may lead to proliferation of submucosal connective tissue, resulting in the formation of a firm submucosal nodule that is covered by normal-appearing mucosa (Fig. 11–6). The most commonly involved site is the buccal mucosa at the line of occlusion.

LINGUAL TONSIL

The foliate papillae on the posterolateral aspects of the tongue are soft, red, irregularly shaped masses that primarily consist of lymphoid tissue. This tissue may become enlarged

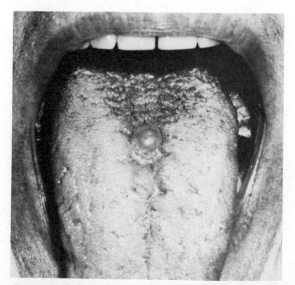

Figure 11–5. Raised area of median rhomboid glossitis.

and hyperplastic in response to chronic low-grade infection in the oral pharyngeal region. The characteristic bilateral distribution and the soft consistency of the tissue are usually sufficient signs to render an accurate clinical diagnosis of enlarged lingual tonsil. Squamous cell carcinoma rarely develops in the posterolateral border of the tongue.

GRANULAR CELL TUMOR (GRANULAR CELL MYOBLASTOMA)

The intraoral granular cell tumor usually manifests as a soft submucosal mass on the dorsal surface of the tongue. Clinically, the mucosa is elevated, but otherwise it is unremarkable in appearance. Microscopically, the lesion consists of a syncytium of large cells with granular eosinophilic cytoplasm and small nuclei (Fig. 11–7). These tumors are not encapsulated but invariably are benign in their behavior. In the squamous epithelium that covers the tumor, there is usually a striking degree of hyperplasia, with the formation of downward extensions and keratin pearls. This unusual feature should not be confused with squamous cell carcinoma.

PYOGENIC GRANULOMA

This is a soft friable mass of epithelialized granulation tissue that results from chronic irritation of the oral mucosa (Fig. 11–8). The pyogenic granuloma frequently forms on the gingiva, where dental plaque and calculus or

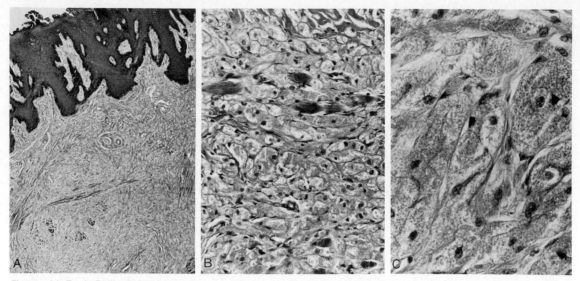

Figure 11–7. *A,* Epithelial hyperplasia overlying granular cells in granular cell myoblastoma of the tongue (Hematoxylin-eosin stain, × 100). *B,* High-power view of granular cells (× 200). *C,* High-power view showing small nuclei and granular cytoplasm (× 350).

ill-fitting partial denture clasps may act as the inciting agents. Because of their rich vascularity, these lesions may bleed readily following minor trauma. The epithelium is often ulcerated. Development of the pyogenic granuloma may be triggered by the altered hormonal environment that accompanies pregnancy or the onset of puberty. During pregnancy, these lesions may recur if the dental calculus or other causative agents were not removed at the time that the lesion was excised. Following pregnancy, they often regress spontaneously.

may range from pink to white depending upon the degree of vascularity and keratinization. The tongue and the hard and soft palates are common sites of involvement. Microscopically, the papilloma consists of finger-like projections of squamous epithelium with a delicate fibrovascular core. Although mild epithelial dysplasia is a common histologic feature, these growths are not considered to be premalignant.[1] Recent reports suggest that many cutaneous and mucosal papillomas are viral in origin.[3, 4]

PAPILLOMA

This is an exophytic cauliflower-like epithelial lesion (Figs. 11–9 and 11–10). The color

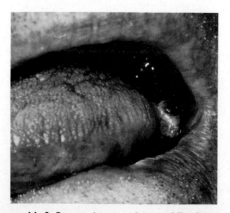

Figure 11–8. Pyogenic granuloma of the tongue.

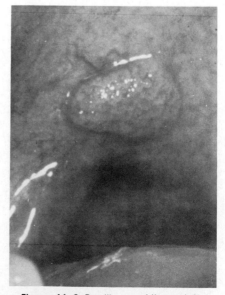

Figure 11–9. Papilloma of the palate.

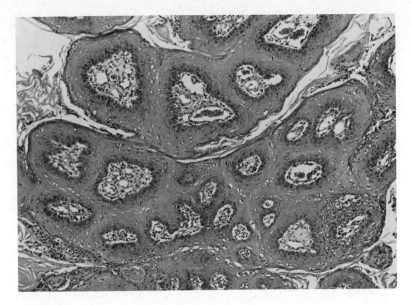

Figure 11–10. Papilloma of the palate. Note the extensive epithelial proliferation with thin cores of connective tissue (Hematoxylin-eosin stain, × 150).

TRAUMATIC ULCER

Traumatic ulcers of the oral mucosa are extremely common lesions.[7] They may result from continual trauma associated with the sharp edges of fractured or carious teeth, the jagged edges of restorations, or overextended or otherwise ill-fitting dentures. Traumatic episodes that result from sharp crusts or other firm foodstuffs, toothbrush trauma, or any number of foreign objects introduced into the oral cavity are frequent causes of oral ulcerations. These lesions are usually well circumscribed with a zone of erythema adjacent to the margin. The margins of the traumatic ulcer are not elevated as are the margins of an ulcerated oral carcinoma (Fig. 11–11). Whereas the malignant oral ulcer is usually asymptomatic, the traumatic oral ulcer is frequently accompanied by pain. Traumatic oral ulcers usually heal without scarring within 7 to 10 days. Oral ulcers that persist for more than 2 weeks should be biopsied.

NECROTIZING SIALOMETAPLASIA

Necrotizing sialometaplasia is a benign entity that has only recently been described. It is often confused clinically and histologically with squamous cell carcinoma or mucoepidermoid carcinoma.[2, 5, 8] The lesion is a non-neoplastic, self-healing inflammatory involvement of the salivary glands and usually manifests as a bilateral or unilateral ulceration of the palate. Although the pathogenesis is unclear, most of these lesions are considered infarctive in nature. Histologically, the involved salivary glands manifest acinar necrosis, mucous pooling, acute and chronic inflammation, and squamous metaplasia of the involved ducts. Although there is no cellular atypia, the squamous metaplasia is often extensive, creating a superficial resemblance to invading squamous cell carcinoma (Fig. 11–12).

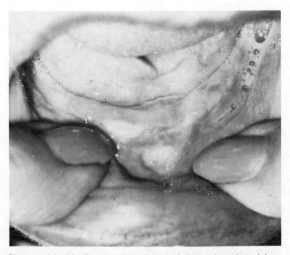

Figure 11–11. Traumatic ulcer of the alveolar ridge mucosa caused by an ill-fitting denture.

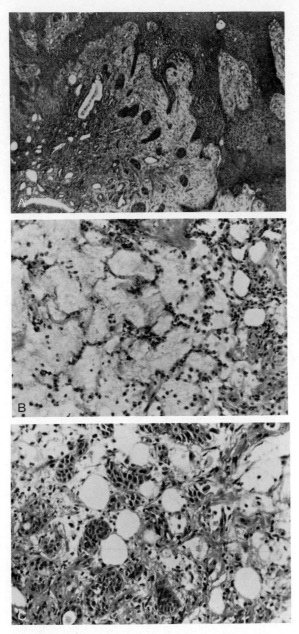

Figure 11–12. *A*, Necrotizing sialometaplasia of the palate. There is pseudoepitheliomatous hyperplasia of the mucosal epithelium that overlies the connective tissue, with spaces that are salivary ducts, some of which display a squamous metaplasia (Hematoxylin and eosin × 120). *B*, Higher-power view of *A*, showing a portion of a lobule with outlines of necrotic mucous acini and neutrophils (Hematoxylin and eosin, × 250). *C*, Higher-power view of *A*, showing squamous metaplasia of mucous ducts among some lipoid tissue and necrotic acini (right) (Hematoxylin and eosin, × 250).

REFERENCES

1. Abbey, L. M., Page, D. G., and Sawyer, D. R.: The clinical and histopathologic features of a series of 464 oral squamous cell papillomas. Oral Surg., *49*:419, 1980.
2. Abrams, A. M., Melrose, R. J., and Howell, F. V.: Necrotizing sialometaplasia: a disease simulating malignancy. Cancer, *32*:130, 1973.
3. Angevine, D. M., Norback, D. H., and Dortzbach, R. K.: Virus in papilloma. J.A.M.A., *246*:1087, 1981.
4. Jenson, A. B.: Human wart virus found in many papillomas. J.A.M.A., *224*:2041, 1980.
5. Lynch, P., Crago, C. A., and Martinez, M. G.: Necrotizing sialometaplasia: a review of the literature and report of two additional cases. Oral Surg., *47*:63, 1979.
6. Mashberg, A., Morrissey, J. B., and Garfinkel, L.: A study of the appearance of early asymptomatic oral squamous cell carcinoma. Cancer, *32*:1436, 1973.
7. McCarthy, P. L., and Shklar, G.: Traumatic lesions of oral mucosa. *In* Diseases of the Oral Mucosa, 2nd ed., Chapter 25. Philadelphia, Lea and Febiger, 1980.
8. Rye, L. A., Calhoun, N. R., and Redman, R. S.: Necrotizing sialometaplasia in a patient with Buerger's disease and Raynaud's phenomenon. Oral Surg., *49*:233, 1980.
9. Van der Waal, I., and van der Kwast, W. A. M.: Median rhomboid glossitis caused by *Candida?* Oral Surg., *47*:31, 1979.
10. Wright, B. A., and Fenwick, F.: Candidiasis and atrophic tongue lesions. Oral Surg., *51*:55, 1981.

12

Basic principles of radiotherapy

RALPH R. WEICHSELBAUM, M.D.
DAVID SHERMAN, M.D.
THOMAS J. ERVIN, M.D.

In this chapter we will attempt to explain the general principles of radiation biology and physics and to highlight their importance and applicability to the management of head and neck cancer.

RADIATION PHYSICS

The energy and penetrating power of ionizing radiation increase as photon wavelength decreases; therefore, the differences in physical characteristics are of major importance. Radiation over 500 kilovolts (Kv) is termed *supervoltage*. Clinically important advantages are seen when radiation reaches 500 Kv, because at this energy, there is reduced absorption in bone, less damage to skin at the portal entry, and reduced lateral scatter of radiation into other tissues. Supervoltage radiation is also of great importance in treating tumors that are deep in the body, because skin tolerance does not limit the dose delivered, with maximal ionization occurring below the level of the epidermis. Also, the percentage of radiation at any specific depth compared with the maximal electron build-up (usually 0.5 cm below the skin) increases as energy increases and thus produces a therapeutic advantage. Radiation between 140 and 500 Kv is termed *orthovoltage,* and superficial radiation is designated to be between 50 and 140 Kv. Orthovoltage and use of superficial machines may yield an advantage in the treatment of skin or other superficial tumors. Supervoltage radiation should be used exclusively in the curative treatment of carcinoma of the oropharynx and oral cavity. In a given dose to the soft tissues of the oral cavity, the osteocytes and vascular structures of the mandible absorb much less energy from supervoltage than from an orthovoltage beam.

Radiation may be applied close to tumors by means of hollow containers that are loaded with radioactive isotopes after placement is obtained. In the head and neck region, this is especially applicable for tumors of the antrum, sinuses, and nasal cavity. This is referred to as intracavitary irradiation. Interstitial radiation refers to the application of removable sources such as radium, cobalt-60, or iridium or of nonremovable sources such as radon or radioactive gold, which are inserted directly into the tumor. These techniques are employed in the treatment of carcinomas of the tongue, tonsil, and oral cavity, and metastatic neck nodes. A combination of the application of physical concepts as well as a natural history of malignant disease is essential for optimal therapeutic results.

Treatment planning is essential for radiotherapy. Guidelines for anatomic localization of the tumor may be necessary. In the head and neck region, this may include tomograms, computerized tomography, soft-tissue films of the neck, and xerography or contrast radiography. Treatment planning ensures that a tumor will receive an optimal dose and that the normal tissue will receive as little dose as is possible. Reproducibility of daily treatments is necessary to ensure accuracy of delivery of radiation to the tumor. This may include immobilization devices such as head straps and bite blocks as well as frequent comparisons of portal films with original planning films to ensure the reproducibility of the set-up.[3, 7, 9]

BIOLOGIC ASPECTS OF RADIATION THERAPY

Ionizing radiation interacts with molecules and causes excitation and ionization of constituent atoms. In an excited atom, electrons are shifted to different orbits and become more chemically reactive. In ionization, oribiting electrons are completely ejected from atoms, leaving free radicals that cause changes because of the breakage of the chemical bonds, thus producing biologic effects. Charged particles such as electrons or protons are directly ionizing with sufficient energy to break the chemical bonds. X-rays, gamma rays, and neutrons are indirectly ionizing, that is, they themselves do not disrupt chemical bonds but produce secondary electrons with high kinetic energy, which breaks these bonds. Neutrons interact with the nuclei of atoms of the absorbing material and impart kinetic energy to quickly recoil upon protons or other nuclear fragments, exerting a biologic effect.[3, 7, 9]

LINEAR ENERGY TRANSFER (LET)

Linear energy transfer (LET) refers to the energy that is transferred per unit length in the absorbing material. The unit that is usually used for this quantity is KeV per micron of unit density material. Differences in LET account for the fact that although various types of radiation generally produce qualitatively similar effects initially (ionization), there are marked quantitative differences as well as different biologic end effects. This is due to dissimilarity in the proximity of ionization and the influence of secondary processes (secondary electrons). Equal doses of different types of ionizing radiation do not produce equal biologic effects. It is customary to express the relative biologic effectiveness (RBE) of some test radiation compared with 250 KeV x-rays, used as the standard. Thus, the relative biologic effectiveness is the ratio of the dose of 250 KeV x-rays to the test radiation required for an equal biologic effect. The RBE varies with the biologic system and with the level of damage, which is related to the dose delivered in that system. For many cellular systems, the RBE has been known to rise with increasing LET, peaking at about 100 KeV per micron and then decreasing (Fig. 12–1). Thus, there appears to be an optimal LET (density of ionization). Sparse ionization is less efficient than densely ionizing radiation, because more than one particle must pass through the cell in order for it to be inactivated. Very densely ionizing radiation is also inefficient, because it deposits more than enough energy in a critical site; thus, the excess energy is considered to be wasted.[3, 7, 9, 20]

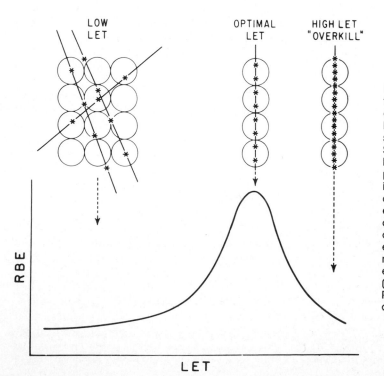

Figure 12–1. Diagrammatic representation of the concept of optimum linear energy transfer (LET). For a cell to be killed, energy must be deposited in several critical sites within the cell. Sparse ionizing radiation is inefficient, because more than one particle must pass through the cell to kill it. Dense ionizing radiation is also inefficient, because it deposits more than enough energy in critical sites within the cell, and energy is thus wasted. Radiation of optimum LET deposits just enough energy to inactivate critical targets. In mammalian cells, this is usually considered to be approximately 100 KeV/μ. (From Hall, E. J.: Radiobiology for the Radiologist, 2nd ed. New York, Harper and Row, Publishers, Inc., 1978.)

CONCEPTS OF RADIOCURABILITY AND RADIOSENSITIVITY

The term *radiosensitive* refers to the inverse of the slope of the straight line portion of the radiation survival curve (Do) when survival data are plotted in a semilogarithmic fashion. Also, this is the dose necessary to reduce the surviving fraction in the straight line portion of the curve by 0.63 to a survival level of 0.37 (Fig. 12–2). The radiobiologic definition of death is an inability to reproduce.[3, 6] Some cells may take a long time to express lethality by division, and irradiated cells may actually result in several generations of progeny and then all generations may die.[11, 15] Furthermore, until cell division occurs and lethality is expressed, cells may appear morphologically intact. The extrapolation number (ñ) is the width of the initial shoulder, and the back extrapolation at the linear portion of the survival curve to the ordinate is a measure of the ability of the cells to accumulate sublethal x-ray damage (see Fig. 12–2).[5, 7]

Radiocurability is a clinical term that refers

to whether a tumor is cured by a maximal tolerable dose of radiation. *Radioresponsive* refers to regression after radiation but not to whether a tumor is radiocurable. For example, carcinoma of the prostate is characterized by a relatively slow cell renewal system; thus, estimates of regression are meaningless because the ultimate local control rates for early prostate cancer are extremely high. The surgeon must not be misled by positive biopsies obtained at inappropriate time intervals or by a slow regression rate of the tumor. Thus, the concept of "divisional death" explains why some radiocurable tumors do not appear radioresponsive. Conversely, oat cell carcinoma of the lung regresses rapidly after delivery of relatively low doses (3000 to 3500 rads), yet up to 50 percent of these lesions fail locally even with relatively high doses (5500 to 6000 rads). Therefore, oat cell carcinoma is radioresponsive but not necessarily radiocurable.

CELL CYCLE EFFECTS

The lethal effects of radiation are cell cycle specific. The effects of radiation at different stages in the cell cycle can be studied using synchronized populations of cells. These effects may vary from cell line to cell line, although some generalizations can be made.[7, 20]

1. Cells are generally more sensitive near or at mitosis.

2. If G_1 (the pre-DNA synthetic gap) is appreciable in length, a resistant period is seen early, followed by a decline in survival toward S (the phase of DNA synthesis). The end of G_1 may be as sensitive as M (mitosis).

3. In most cell lines, resistance increases during S to a maximum in the latter part of S, and this is usually the most resistant part of the cycle.

4. In most cell lines, G_2 (the pre-mitotic gap) is as sensitive as M (Figs. 12–3 and 12–4).[7, 12, 13]

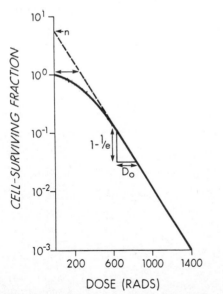

REPAIR

After the cells are irradiated, one of four events is possible.

1. No damage may have occurred in the critical target in the cell.

2. Damage may have occurred in all critical targets, and the cell may be killed.

3. A cell may have some of its critical targets damaged, and given time, these may be repaired. This is referred to as sublethal damage repair (SLDR), and the amount of sublethal damage that a cell can accumulate is expressed

Figure 12–2. Typical survival curve for mammalian cells exposed to radiation. The fraction of the surviving cells is plotted on a logarithmic scale against a linear plot of the dose, expressed in rads. The dose response curve has an initial shoulder (as measured by the extrapolation number ñ), which is the extrapolate of the slope of the survival curve and represents the ability to accumulate sublethal damage. The slope of the straight line portion of the curve is represented by Do, which indicates the radiosensitivity of the cells. (From Hall, E. J.: Radiobiology for the Radiologist, 2nd ed. New York, Harper and Row, Publishers, Inc., 1978.)

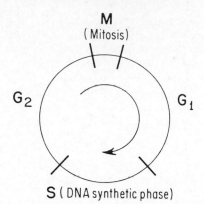

Figure 12–3. Mitotic cycle for actively growing mammalian cells. M represents mitosis, S is the phase of DNA synthesis, G_1 is the pre-DNA synthetic gap, and G_2 is the pre-mitotic gap. The "gaps" indicate periods of apparent inactivity, separating the major discernible events of the cell cycle. (M = mitosis; S = DNA synthesis phase; G_1 = pre-DNA synthetic gap; G_2 = premitotic gap). (From Hall, E. J.: Radiobiology for the Radiologist, 2nd ed. New York, Harper and Row, Publishers, Inc., 1978.)

as the extrapolation number of the survival curve (ñ).

4. Cells may repair lethal damage under certain postradiation conditions, and this is referred to as potentially lethal damage repair (PLDR).[5, 10, 17]

DETERMINANTS OF RADIOCURABILITY

It is unlikely that there is a consistent difference in the intrinsic sensitivity between normal and malignant tissue (although some radiation-sensitive and -resistant human malignant cell types have been described in vitro). However, differences in the way that cells repair sublethal or potentially lethal radiation damage may vary from tumor type to tumor type and may explain some of the variations in clinical radio-curability.[17]

Other factors may alter cellular radiosensitivity or the repair of radiation damage or

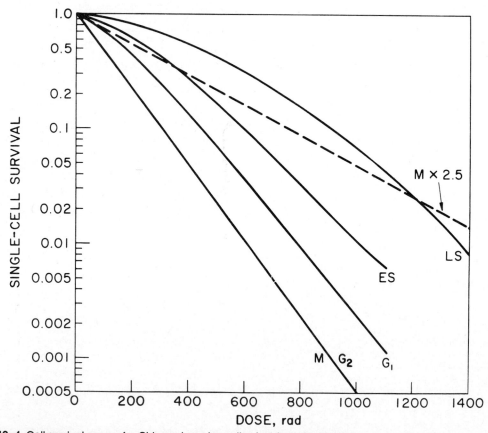

Figure 12–4. Cell survival curves for Chinese hamster cells at various stages of the cell cycle. The surviving fraction is on the ordinate and the dose, in rads, is on the abscissa. (From Sinclair, W. K.: Cyclic x-ray responses in mammalian cells in vitro. Radiat. Res., *33*:620, 1968.)

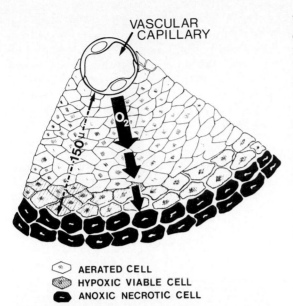

VASCULAR
CAPILLARY

○ AERATED CELL
◍ HYPOXIC VIABLE CELL
◖ ANOXIC NECROTIC CELL

Figure 12–5. The diffusion of oxygen from a capillary through tumor tissue. The distance to which oxygen can diffuse is limited by the rate at which it is metabolized by tumor cells. Cells are well oxygenated to approximately 150 μ from a capillary. At greater distances, they become hypoxic and then anoxic as the distance from the capillary is increased. Completely anoxic cells may be dead; however, hypoxic cells may form a layer between 1 and 2 cells thick, and enough of these cells may be viable and limit the radiocurability of the tumor. (From Hall, E. J.: Radiobiology for the Radiologist, 2nd ed. New York, Harper and Row, Publishers, Inc., 1968.)

both. For example, it is well known that the center of a tumor is necrotic and that there may be a significant number of hypoxic cells around the necrotic center of some tumors. It has further been shown that hypoxia makes cells more resistant to ionizing radiation, because molecular oxygen is necessary for free radical formation (Figs. 12–5 and 12–6).[14, 17] If hypoxic tumor cells are more resistant than well-aerated cells, this may alter the therapeutic ratio unfavorably (see Figs. 12–5 and 12–6).

The use of electron affinic agents specific for radioresistant hypoxic cells is an important area of research in clinical radiotherapy.[7, 14, 19] These studies have progressed from development in radiation chemistry to clinical examination. The nitroimidazole misonidazole is efficient in the killing of hypoxic tumor cells in experimental systems and is currently under clinical investigation.[1, 2] The use of high LET radiation (densely ionizing neutrons, pi mesons), which is not as dependent upon molecular oxygen for the production of free radicals as is sparsely ionizing radiation, is also currently under clinical investigation to circumvent the problem of hypoxic cells.[4]

Reoxygenation of tumors may also be an important determinant of radiocurability, because it has been presumed that the oxygen-

Figure 12–6. Survival curves for cultured hamster cells exposed to x-rays under aerated and hypoxic conditions. This data is typical of that found in the literature in which oxygen appears to be dose modifying at all levels of survival. The dose required to produce a given amount of damage is three times greater under hypoxic conditions than under aerated conditions. The ratio of these doses is known as the oxygen enhancement ratio (OER). (From Hall, E. J.: Radiobiology for the Radiologist, 2nd ed. New York, Harper and Row, Publishers, Inc., 1968.)

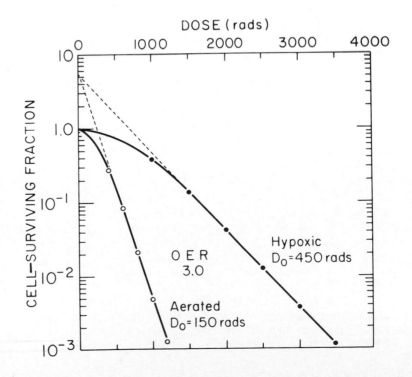

ated cells are killed and that previously hypoxic cells migrate to the periphery of a tumor, where they become better oxygenated.[16] Differential repopulation between normal and malignant tissue also may be a determinant of radiocurability, because it has been postulated that normal tissues may repopulate more efficiently than tumors. This fact re-emphasizes techniques in treatment planning and interstitial implantation in maximizing tumor dose while minimizing normal tissue dose. In the process of irradiating cancers of the oral cavity and oropharynx, changes are produced in the salivary glands, mandible, teeth, and neighboring soft tissue, and protection of these structures may enhance the therapeutic ratio as well as increase the number of tumor cells that are killed. Investigation with certain sulfhydryl compounds such as cysteine, a sulfhydryl-containing amino acid, has shown that they protect tissues against the effects of ionizing radiation, probably by reacting with free radicals that are in competition with oxygen. Thus, certain normal tissues, such as salivary glands, might be protected against the effects of radiation if selective uptake of sulfhydryl-containing compounds can be obtained.

TIME-DOSE RELATIONSHIPS IN RADIOTHERAPY

Pioneers in radiation therapy found that radiation produced a more effective therapeutic ratio when small doses were given each day as opposed to one large, single dose. The final effects of radiation in both normal and malignant tissues depend upon

1. Final overall dose.
2. Fraction size or dose of radiation per session.
3. Time over which radiation is delivered.
4. Volume of tissue that is irradiated.

Although sophisticated mathematical formulae have been developed to equate fractionation schemes, experience plays the most important role in the development of this concept.[6] It must be pointed out that the ultimate dose-limiting normal tissue effects are not usually the acute effects of radiation (mucositis, diarrhea, and so on) but the long-term effects on the vasculoconnective tissue and possibly the somatic cells, which seem to be responsible for long-term complications (radionecrosis, fibrosis, and so on).[8, 18]

These biologic concepts are valuable in the treatment of malignant disease, because in making therapeutic determinations, the clinical radiation oncologist must keep in mind not only the probability of cure but also the consequences of treatment. In certain circumstances, the consequences of radiation (or any therapeutic modality) may produce disastrous results. Also, patients might elect a therapeutic modality that produces a lower cure rate but that preserves function, that is, sexual function, voice, cosmesis, and so on. Certainly, when cure rates are equal or close to equal, nonmutilating therapy must be given preference. The end results in neoplastic disease are analyzed not only by survival but also by detailed study of failure, that is, local, regional, or distant.

TUMOR SIZE AS THE DETERMINANT OF RADIOCURABILITY: CONTROL OF SUBCLINICAL DISEASE

An important concept in clinical radiation therapy is that subclinical (microscopic) disease is controlled with lower doses than is grossly detectable cancer. The probability of local control for a variety of carcinomas increases as a function of dose. This is especially true in the head and neck region. Most patients who have subclinical disease are controlled with doses of 5000 rads. For example, patients who have carcinoma of the oral cavity and oropharynx may have an incidence rate of 40 to 80 percent of developing metastatic cancer in lymph nodes, even when the neck proved to be negative in the initial clinical examination. However, 5000 rads in 5 weeks may diminish the probability of the development of lymph node metastasis to 2 to 5 percent. This concept is supported not only by extensive clinical data but also by previously stated biologic data. For example, small tumors (microscopic) are much less likely to have hypoxic or necrotic centers. In any case, because radiation kills a fixed proportion of cells, the fewer cells that are present, the higher the probability of local control. This concept may be extended to gross clinical cancer and is supported by the fact that T1 lesions, regardless of site or histology, are more curable than T3 or T4 lesions. Smaller tumors have fewer tumor cells and a smaller hypoxic fraction than larger tumors. Also, larger tumors may be more efficient in the repair of certain types of radiation damage than their smaller counterparts.

Clinical and biologic observations have led to consideration of conservative surgery combined with moderate doses of irradiation. The advantage of such an approach is in using

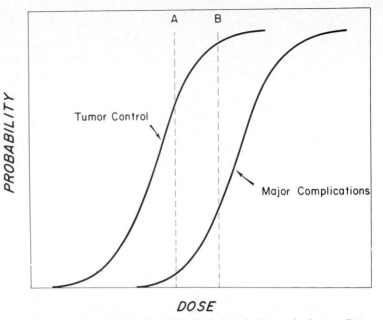

Figure 12–7. Relationship between tumor control and major complications to radiation dose. The sigmoid curve on the left shows the relationship between local control and dose. For low doses no control is seen. However, as the dose is increased, an increased likelihood of local control is seen. Balanced against tumor control are complications observed in irradiated normal tissues. The sigmoid curve on the right traces the relationship between these complications and the dose. The same type of sigmoid relationship is seen for both tumor control and complications. However, the complications curve is displaced to the right. If the curves are significantly separated, the likelihood of an uncomplicated cure is favorable. If they are in positions where they may be superimposed on one another, there is less chance for an uncomplicated cure. The choice of dose is dependent upon these factors. The optimal therapeutic ratio occurs when the complications curve is displaced as far to the right as possible and the tumor control curve is displaced as far to the left as possible. Note that both curves are extremely "steep" functions of the dose.

nonmutilating surgery with doses of radiation that are not apt to have a high likelihood of long-term complications but that are adequate to control the disease, which is reduced to cell numbers that are manageable by radiation therapy.

RADIATION DOSE AND COMPLICATIONS

Successful therapy for a tumor requires an adequate dose of radiation, but the dose that can be used is limited by the complications or radiation reactions that will occur in normal tissues adjacent to the tumor. One way of illustrating this problem is to graphically plot the probability of tumor control and the probability of major complications of the radiation against radiation dose. The curves are sigmoid, and the separation between the tumor control curve and the complication curve is usually small. Increasing the radiation dosage will increase the probability of tumor control but will also increase the likelihood of significant radiation damage to the tissues (Fig. 12–7).

REFERENCES

1. Adams, G. E.: Chemical radiosensitization of hypoxic cells. Br. Med. Bull., 29:48, 1973.
2. Adams, G. E., Dische, S., Fowler J. F., et al.: Hypoxic cell sensitizers in radiotherapy. Lancet, 1:186, 1976.
3. Buschke, P., and Parker, R.: Radiation Therapy in Cancer Management. New York and London, Grune and Stratton, Inc., 1972.
4. Catterall, M.: The treatment of advanced cancer by fast neutrons from the Medical Research Council cyclotron at the Hammersmith Hospital, London. Eur. J. Cancer, 10:343, 1974.
5. Elkind, M. M., and Sutton, H.: Radiation response of mammalian cells grown in culture. 1. Repair of x-ray damage in surviving Chinese hamster cells. Radiat. Res., 13:556, 1960.
6. Ellis, F.: Dose, time, and fractionation in clinical hypothesis. Clin. Radiol., 20:1, 1969.
7. Hall, E. J.: Radiobiology for the Radiologist, 2nd ed. Hagerstown, Maryland, Harper and Row Publishers Inc., 1978.
8. Hopwell, J. W.: The importance of vascular damage in the development of late radiation effects in normal tissue. In Meyn, R. E., and Withers, H. R. (eds.): Radiation Biology in Cancer Research. New York, Raven Press, 1980, pp. 439–448.
9. Johns, H. E., and Cunningham, J. R.: Physics of Radiology. Springfield, Illinois, Charles C Thomas, Publishers, 1969.
10. Little, J. B., Hahn, G. M., Frindel, F., et al.: Repair of potential lethal radiation damage in vitro and in vivo. Radiology, 106:689, 1973.
11. Puck, T. T., and Marcus, P. I.: Action of x-rays on mammalian cells. J. Exp. Med., 103:653, 1956.
12. Sinclair, W. K.: Cyclic x-ray responses in mammalian cells in vitro. Radiat. Res., 33:620, 1968.
13. Sinclair, W. K., and Morton, R. A.: X-ray sensitivity during the cell generation cycle of cultured Chinese hamster cells. Radiat. Res., 29:450, 1966.
14. Thomlinson, R. H., and Gray, L. H.: The histologic

structure of some human lung cancers and possible implications for radiotherapy. Br. J. Cancer, 9:539, 1955.

15. Thompson, L. H., and Suit, H. D.: Proliferation kinetics of x-irradiated mouse L-cells studied with time lapse photography. Int. J. Radiat. Biol., 15:347, 1966.

16. van Putten, L. M.: Tumor reoxygenation during fractionated radiotherapy. Studies with a transplantable osteosarcoma. Eur. J. Cancer, 4:173, 1968.

17. Weichselbaum, R. R., Nove, J., and Little, J. B.: Response of human tumor cells in vitro. In Meyn, R. E., and Withers, H. R. (eds.): Radiation Biology in Cancer Research. New York, Raven Press, 1980, pp. 345–351.

18. Withers, H. R., Peters, L. J., and Kogelnick, H. D.: The pathobiology of late effects of radiation. In Meyn, R. E., and Withers, H. R. (eds.): Radiation Biology in Cancer Research. New York, Raven Press, 1980, pp. 439–448.

19. Wright, E. A., and Howard-Flanders, P.: The influence of oxygen on the radiosensitivity of mammalian tissue. Acta Radiol., 48:26, 1957.

20. Zirkle, R. E.: The radiobiological importance of linear energy transfer. In Hollander, A. (ed.): Radiation Biology. Vol. 1, New York, McGraw-Hill, Inc., 1954, pp. 315–350.

13

Radiotherapy in carcinomas of oral cavity and oropharynx

C. C. WANG, M.D.

Carcinomas that originate in the mucous membrane of the oral cavity and oropharynx are predominantly squamous cell carcinomas of varying degrees of differentiation, ranging from carcinoma in situ to poorly differentiated carcinoma, including so-called lymphoepithelioma. The early mucosal lesion may appear as an indurated nodule or as a shallow ulcer with poorly defined margins. These areas are not well endowed with pain fibers; thus, pain is not an early symptom. Most patients present with a unilateral sore throat or canker sore in the mouth, frequently of several weeks' duration, as the only symptom of the presence of extensive disease. These tumors may be exophytic or infiltrative in nature and may extend rapidly into the underlying muscle and cause fixation with resultant difficulty in speaking or eating, and in the advanced stage may result in trismus of the jaw. Except for the lesions that arise from the tip and base of the tongue, the metastatic disease usually occurs in the homolateral cervical lymph nodes. Distant metastases below the clavicles are not common, but they do occur late in the disease.

For an adequate evaluation of the extent of the lesion, careful inspection and palpation of the primary site and neck areas are mandatory whenever possible. Indirect laryngoscopy is an extremely informative examination in evaluating the extent of the lesion as well as the mobility of the involved parts. Direct laryngoscopy and multiple biopsies to define mucosal and submucosal extension of tumor or to rule out a second primary cancer, or both, should be carried out prior to any definitive therapeutic program. Appropriate x-ray examinations, for example, soft-tissue films of the lateral oropharynx, polytomograms of the jaw, and xerograms of the base of the tongue, are indicated to assess the extent of the lesion as well as bone and muscle invasion. As part of the medical work-up, a general physical examination, chest radiographs, and a basic liver profile are necessary to assess the condition of the patient. Any electrolyte imbalance or anemia that is found should be corrected.

In evaluating and reporting the therapeutic results of any malignant disease, a commonly accepted classification must be followed. Because staging affects prognosis and treatment decisions more than any other factor, it is imperative that it be done meticulously. For oral and oropharyngeal cancer, the following TNM system was adopted by the American Joint Committee for Cancer Staging and End Results Reporting in 1978:[1]

T1—Tumor 2 cm or less in diameter.
T2—Tumor greater than 2 cm but less than or equal to 4 cm in diameter.
T3—Tumor greater than 4 cm in diameter.
T4—Massive tumor greater than 4 cm in diameter, with invasion of bone, soft tissue, and so on.
N0—No clinically positive node.
N1—Single clinically positive homolateral node less than 3 cm in diameter.
N2a—Single clinically positive homolateral node 3 to 6 cm in diameter.

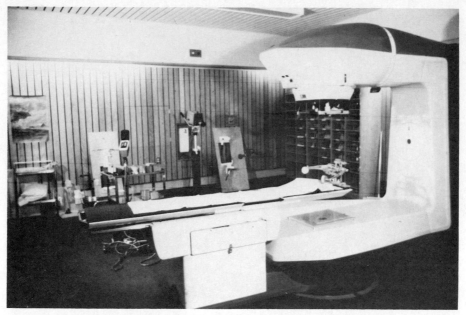

Figure 13–1. Telecobalt unit at Massachusetts General Hospital.

N2b—Multiple clinically positive homolateral nodes, none more than 6 cm in diameter.

N3a—Clinically positive homolateral nodes, one over 6 cm in diameter.

N3b—Bilateral clinically positive nodes.

N3c—Contralateral clinically positive nodes only.

M0—No distant metastases.

M1—Distant metastases present.

A variety of therapeutic measures are available for the management of localized carcinomas of the oral cavity and oropharynx, including surgical excision, radiation therapy, electrodesiccation, laser beam excision, cryotherapy, and a combination of these methods.[2, 3, 9, 15] The choice of treatment depends upon the site and size of the primary lesion, the presence or absence of metastatic disease in the neck, the general health and age of the patient, and, lastly but not the least in importance, the morbidity of the treatment program and the experience and skill of both the surgeon and the radiation therapist.

The use of radiation therapy in the management of squamous cell carcinoma of the oral cavity and oropharynx, as is true for most carcinomas of the head and neck, is based on the following principles:

1. Squamous cell carcinomas are usually radioresponsive and in the early stages are highly radiocurable.

2. The more differentiated the tumors, the less the radiation response, and the higher the radiation dose required.

3. Exophytic and well-oxygenated tumors are more radioresponsive than deeply ulcerative and infiltrative hypoxic tumors.

4. Squamous cell carcinomas, when limited to mucosa, are highly radiocurable.

5. Bone and muscle involvement by carcinoma adversely alters the radioresponsiveness of carcinomas and subsequently decreases the radiocurability.

6. Advanced cervical lymph node metastases, N2 and N3, are better treated by combined surgery and radiation therapy than by either method alone.

The radiotherapeutic modalities used for treatment of carcinomas of the oral cavity and oropharynx are primarily megavoltage radiations with energies of several million volts such as cobalt-60 radiations (Fig. 13–1) and x-rays generated from 4 to 10 meV linear accelerators (Fig. 13–2) with interplay of interstitial isotope implant. Electron beam is used for the treatment of lip cancers as well as for eccentrically situated lesions of the oral cavity, that is, buccal mucosal and gingival carcinomas, and can be collimated traveling through an intraoral cone for treatment of small tumors, T1

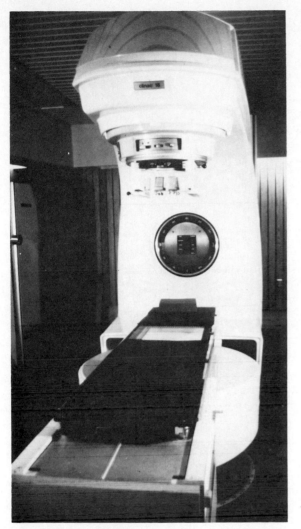

Figure 13–2. Clinac 18 linear accelerator at Massachusetts General Hospital.

and T2, of the anterior tongue or floor of the mouth in cooperative patients. Intraoral cone radiation therapy spares the jaw and salivary glands, thus reducing the magnitude of xerostomia and radiation injuries to the mandible and teeth, and is commonly used as a tool to boost the primary site to a high dosage.

The radiation dosage is determined by the tumor site, irradiated volume, number of fractions of treatment, total elapsed time of the treatment course, various techniques of delivery of radiations, tolerance of the patient, and response of the tumor. In general, a dose of 5000 to 5500 cGy* in 5 to 6 weeks is considered adequate for sterilization of a microscopic or occult disease, and a dose of 6500 to 7000 cGy in 7 weeks is considered adequate for control

*1 cGy = 1 rad

of gross squamous cell carcinoma.[10] Such a dosage is usually given initially as 5000 cGy wide-field irradiation to include the primary site and the regional nodal areas, with a further boost to the primary site by reduced portal toward completion. However, although dose response curves reveal the importance of adequate dosage for tumor control, these same curves cannot convincingly show that higher doses, over 7000 cGy, produce substantial further improvement in cure rates. Yet such large doses carry a substantially high increased risk of severe complications, such as painful fibrosis of the subcutaneous tissues of the neck, osteoradionecrosis of the mandible, orocutaneous fistulas, and severe problems related to wound healing if salvage surgery is performed for radiation failures.

Each carcinoma that arises from various sites of the head and neck has distinct clinical features, course, and prognosis, and the therapeutic approach must be individualized. With a few exceptions, radiation therapy is applicable as the first treatment for all sites whether the growth is early or late. In certain instances, surgical removal is as effective for the treatment of small, localized lesions of the oral cavity as radiation therapy. This is particularly true in old, feeble patients, in whom small lesions can be expediently excised with less discomfort than would be caused by radiation therapy. By and large, the aged and frail patients tolerate surgical excision much better than high-dose external beam therapy, interstitial implant in the mouth, or intraoral cone therapy. Radical surgery, however, with total or hemiglossectomy and partial mandibulectomy and radical neck dissection, so-called "commando procedure," is technically feasible and is generally reserved for advanced carcinomas with preoperative or postoperative radiation therapy or for recurrent tumors that have previously been treated by radiation therapy. Electrodesiccation, laser beam excision, or cryotherapy can be used as a primary method of management of superficial carcinomas of the oral cavity and oropharynx, but they are usually reserved for the treatment of leukoplakia or for the removal of small residual nidi or areas of marginal recurrence after high-dose radiation therapy.

ANATOMIC ORIGIN AND MANAGEMENT

Carcinoma of the Oral Cavity

From the standpoint of anatomic origin and method of management, oral cancer can be

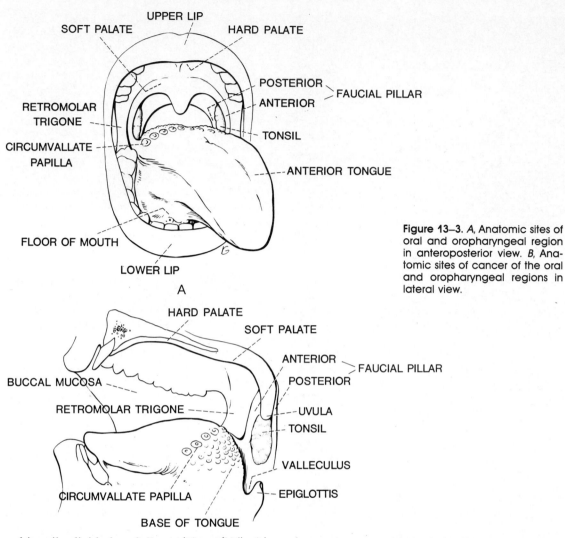

Figure 13–3. *A,* Anatomic sites of oral and oropharyngeal region in anteroposterior view. *B,* Anatomic sites of cancer of the oral and oropharyngeal regions in lateral view.

arbitrarily divided as follows (Fig. 13–3): Lip, anterior two thirds of the tongue (mobile tongue), floor of the mouth, anterior faucial pillar and retromolar trigone, buccal mucosa, gum (alveolar ridge), and palate (soft and hard). In contrast to oropharyngeal cancers, most of these lesions, ranging from 65 to 75 percent, are either well-differentiated or moderately well-differentiated carcinomas.

Lip. Squamous cell carcinoma of the lip behaves differently than other cancers of the oral cavity. These lesions occur in older males and are usually situated in the lower lip, are well differentiated, and are less than 1 cm in size. As a rule, therapy is directed toward the primary lesion if there are no palpable nodes. A small carcinoma of the lip can be removed expediently and successfully by "V" excision, and the procedure will not result in cosmetic and functional deformity. Radiation therapy is best suited for superficial cancers that involve

more than one third of the lip, tumors of the oral commissure, recurrent tumors after previous excision, or patients who refuse surgery. Surgical excision is mandatory for radiation failures, for extensive cancers that involve the mandible, or for cancer that is associated with significant loss of soft tissue, which will require major reconstruction after the lesion has been controlled by radiation therapy. Because radiation therapy or surgery has yielded extremely high cure rates for small limited cancers, that is, 3-year NED* rates of 90 percent, the selection of treatment modality must depend upon the cosmetic result that follows the procedure. Radiation therapy for superficial, small tumors, T1, consists of x-rays with superficial penetration or low-energy electrons. For extensive tumors, T2 and T3, combined external beam therapy and interstitial isotope

*NED—No evidence of disease.

implant yield excellent cure rates and cosmetic results. For the far-advanced tumors, high-energy x-rays or cobalt-60 radiations are used to include the primary site as well as the metastatic nodes.

In the follow-up of these patients after definitive therapy, as in the management of patients who have other head and neck cancers, it is desirable to have a thorough understanding of the pattern of lymphatic drainage. The upper lip drains to the parotid as well as the upper cervical nodes, whereas the lower lip drains to the submental, submandibular, and subdigastric nodes. Thus, careful examination of these nodal drainage areas should be undertaken. Bilateral drainage is not uncommon. Lymphatic drainage may involve the mandibular canal and subsequently the middle ear, though this pattern of metastasis is rare.

Anterior Two Thirds of Tongue (Mobile Tongue). Cancer of the anterior two thirds of the tongue is a common type of oral cancer and includes the lesions that arise from the mobile portion of the tongue, anterior to the circumvallate papillae. It frequently invades the underlying muscle, causing fixation of the organ, and is accompanied by a high incidence of cervical lymph node metastases.

Surgical resection is often indicated for tumors that arise from syphilitic glossitis, for recurrences or residual disease following unsuccessful radiation therapy, for lesions limited to the tip of the tongue, or for tiny lesions that are suitable for simple excision in aged, feeble patients. Small tumors, T1, that arise from the lateral border of the tongue can be removed either by partial glossectomy or by radiation therapy with equal success. If such primary

lesions are treated by surgical excision alone, the neck nodes should be carefully followed. If metastases develop postoperatively, they must be dealt with comprehensively. For superficial, medium-sized tumors, T2 with involvement of the adjacent floor of the mouth, surgical treatment must include partial glossectomy, partial mandibulectomy, and radical neck dissection. For such lesions, therefore, comprehensive radiotherapy is preferred owing to its superior cosmetic and functional results with a high cure rate. Advanced disease, T3 and T4, with deep muscular invasion often associated with cervical lymph node metastases, is unlikely to be cured by radiotherapy alone and therefore is best managed by the combined usage of radiation therapy and radical surgery, if possible.

Irradiation is performed with a megavoltage machine initially for 4500 to 5000 cGy in 6 weeks to the primary site and regional nodes, and the primary lesion is boosted either by interstitial isotope implant, such as radium needles or iridium 192, or by intraoral cone electron beam therapy to bring the total dose to a cancericidal level. Such an approach can avoid excessive xerostomia, which commonly occurred in large portal external beam irradiation alone. For advanced disease, T3 and T4, interstitial implantation is ineffective; therefore, external beam therapy is used exclusively.

Floor of Mouth. Carcinoma of the floor of the mouth frequently is situated in the anterior portion and involves the undersurface of the tongue, the adjacent gum, and the orifice of Wharton's duct.[6] Early mucosal lesions, T1 and T2, are controlled satisfactorily by a com-

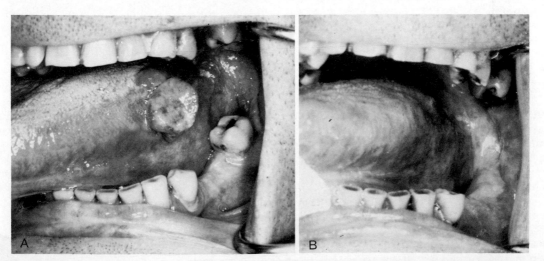

Figure 13–4. Squamous cell carcinoma of the left oral tongue. A, Pre-radiation. B, Post-radiation.

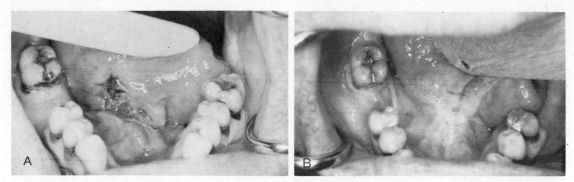

Figure 13–5. A, Squamous cell carcinoma treated by external x-rays and by interstitial implant (pre-treatment). B, Post-treatment. No evidence of disease, with excellent local control and cosmesis.

bination of megavoltage radiation therapy and interstitial implant or intraoral cone electron beam therapy, with 3-year NED rates of approximately 80 and 60 percent, respectively. If the disease becomes extensive, T3 and T4, with involvement of the gum and the mandible or if it extends deeply into the adjacent musculature, often with cervical lymph node metastases, control by radiation therapy is poor. Under such circumstances, preoperative or postoperative radiation therapy and radical surgery with removal of the primary tumor as well as the metastatic nodes in the neck are indicated if the lesions are operable.

Anterior Faucial Pillar and Retromolar Trigone. Squamous cell carcinoma that arises from this region should not be confused with carcinoma of the tonsillar fossa. This tumor may spread to the adjacent soft palate, the buccal mucosa, or the gum as well as inferiorly to the base of the tongue or the floor of the mouth. Approximately one third of the patients who have this disease have homolateral lymph node metastases at the time that the diagnosis is made. Most of these tumors are well differentiated, and the superficial lesions can be treated successfully with external beam therapy. Primary radical surgery is generally accompanied by marked facial deformity and impairment of swallowing function and often results in a high incidence of marginal recurrence.[8, 12, 14] Because these lesions tend to remain localized, salvage surgery is frequently effective if radiation therapy fails to eradicate the entire lesion. The most common sites of failure after radiotherapy are the base of the tongue and the adjacent mandible infiltrated by tumor. The residual disease, after high-dose radiotherapy, is best managed by limited resection, that is, nidusectomy. The large, infiltrative lesions, T3 and T4, with or without

pterygoid invasion are best treated by a combination of high-dose radiotherapy and composite resection.

Buccal Mucosa. Carcinomas of the buccal mucosa are relatively well-differentiated squamous cell carcinomas and are frequently associated with areas of leukoplakia. Because the mucous membranes adhere closely to the muscles of the cheek, early invasion of the masseter muscle is likely to occur and may result in trismus. Once the deeper structures and muscles are involved, there is a high incidence of cervical lymph node metastases. For the early lesions, the best results seem to have been achieved by a combination of external beam therapy and interstitial isotope implant. For advanced tumors, T3 and T4, the cure rates following radiation therapy are extremely poor. Therefore, preoperative radiation therapy and en bloc excision of the primary lesion and its regional lymph node metastases followed by plastic closure constitute the preferred treatment.

Gum (Gingival Ridge). Carcinoma of the gum usually arises in the posterior portion of the lower dental arch and is often associated with leukoplakia. Because the mucous membrane adheres directly to the periosteum of the mandible, tumor that originates on the gum may invade the underlying bone early. Most of these tumors are well differentiated. Carcinoma of the upper gum is an uncommon disease and should not be confused with tumor that originates in the maxillary antrum secondarily extending to the gum. Radiographic examination of the paranasal sinuses is helpful in differentiating these two cancers as well as in evaluating the extent of the bone involvement.

Treatment depends upon the extent of the lesion, the degree of bone involvement, and

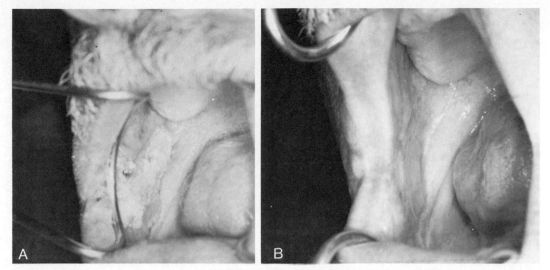

Figure 13–6. *A,* Verrucous carcinoma of the buccal mucosa (pre-radiation). *B,* Post-radiation, showing no evidence of disease after 10 years, without malignant transformation.

the status of the cervical lymph node metastases.[11] A distinction should be made between the smooth erosive pressure defect of the bone caused by slowly expanding tumor and the moth-eaten type of bone destruction caused by tumor infiltration. The former can be treated successfully by radiation therapy, whereas the latter cannot. Small, exophytic lesions, T1, without bone involvement can be treated by external beam therapy with satisfactory control of the disease. For advanced lesions with extensive bone destruction of the mandible with or without metastases, radical surgery is preferred; partial mandibulectomy and radical neck dissection have good control rates.[5] Because of the likelihood of local spread of the disease along the subperiosteal lymphatics, radiation therapy is given either before or after mandibular resection in the hope of decreasing the incidence of local recurrence and improving cure rates.

Palate. The palate may be divided into two portions, the hard and soft palates. The hard palate is the most common site of minor salivary gland malignant tumors in the oral cavity. Squamous cell carcinoma that arises from the hard palate is rare and usually ulcerative. As in the gum lesions, carcinoma of the hard palate is likely to involve the underlying bone early. Small lesions, T1, without bone involvement can be treated by external beam therapy, with satisfactory control. For the advanced lesions, combined radiotherapy and surgical removal of the primary tumor with the underlying bone constitute the treatment of choice. Malignant salivary gland tumors of the palate should be treated by excisional procedure if operable, followed by postoperative radiotherapy. Some improved cure rates have been obtained.

Most malignant tumors of the soft palate are well-differentiated squamous cell carcinomas and are ulcerative with poorly defined borders. Surgical excision of such lesions is unsatisfactory, causing impairment of swallowing and speech functions, and often results in marginal recurrences. For the early tumors, T1 and T2, very good control rates have been achieved by radiation therapy, with 3-year NED rates higher than 80 percent. In certain small mucosal tumors with well-defined borders, excellent radiotherapeutic results can be accomplished by intraoral cone electron beam therapy without radiation sequelae. Advanced tumors, T3 and T4, often associated with bilateral cervical lymph node metastases, respond poorly to radiation therapy or surgery; such lesions are considered to be rarely curable and therefore are often treated by radiation therapy with palliative intent. Occasionally, limited surgery after radiation therapy can be undertaken to remove minimal residual disease to effect a cure, but this is rare.

Carcinoma of the Oropharynx

The oropharynx includes the tonsil, the base of the tongue, and the oropharyngeal wall (Fig. 13–4). Cancers that arise from these areas are often large when first detected and tend to be infiltrative in nature.

In contrast to carcinoma of the oral cavity, oropharyngeal carcinomas are generally poorly differentiated, including a special variant, the so-called lymphoepithelioma. These lesions are characterized by a high incidence of regional lymph node metastases, irrespective of the stage of the primary lesion, ranging between 50 and 75 percent at the time that the diagnosis is made. More than half the lesions with cervical lymph node metastases from the base of the tongue are manifested with bilateral involvement. Radiation therapy for this disease consists primarily of external beam therapy, either from a cobalt-60 unit or a low-megavoltage linear accelerator. Technically, it is extremely difficult to obtain a satisfactory interstitial isotope implant in lesions situated in the base of the tongue or in the tonsillar fossa. Owing to the unusually high incidence of nodal metastases, radiotherapy must include the primary tumor as well as the regional lymphatics comprehensively, even in patients in whom clinical examination of the neck proved to be negative.

Tonsil. As previously noted, squamous cell carcinoma of the faucial tonsil is different from that which originates from the retromolar trigone and anterior tonsillar pillar. These lesions are prone to spread posteriorly to the lateral pharyngeal wall, base of the tongue inferiorly, and the soft palate superiorly. Most carcinomas of the tonsil are poorly differentiated and radiosensitive and in the early stages are highly radiocurable. Therefore, for the early lesions, radiotherapy is the treatment of choice, with 3-year NED rates higher than 80 percent. Advanced tumors of the tonsil that are often associated with tongue involvement and nodal metastases are best treated by combined therapies, such as high-dose external beam therapy through shrinking field technique to a total dose of approximately 6500 cGy, followed by sequential surgery with removal of the residual disease, commonly present in the base of the tongue or adjacent mandible. Any residual disease in the neck following high-dose radiotherapy should be treated by neck dissection.

Base of Tongue. This is the fixed portion or the posterior third of the tongue starting anatomically from the circumvallate papillae posteriorly toward the epiglotticopharyngeal folds and vallecula. In order to evaluate the extent of the disease, indirect laryngoscopy and digital palpation of the base of the tongue are mandatory as routine procedures. Xerograms of the lateral base of the tongue may delineate the depth of muscular invasion. Treatment of this disease primarily by surgery is extremely mutilating, with impairment of the speech and swallowing mechanisms. The poor surgical results are further compounded by the high incidence of marginal recurrence and bilateral cervical lymph node metastases. Therefore, management of carcinoma of the base of the tongue at the present time is by high-dose external beam therapy. Any residual disease following radiation therapy, however, should be treated by limited excision. Unfortunately, most primary cancers of the base of the tongue are situated so that appropriate surgery would have to be extremely mutilating, including excision of the entire tongue and total laryngectomy, for there to be any potential for cure. For small, T1 and T2, exophytic lesions, the 3-year NED rate can be as high as 70 and 50 percent, respectively, following radiotherapy.

Oropharyngeal Wall. The oropharyngeal wall includes the lateral and posterior walls and the posterior tonsillar pillar. Primary lesions that arise from the posterior tonsillar pillar alone are extremely rare. Squamous cell carcinomas that arise from these sites tend to be ulcerative, and their exact extensions upward and downward are difficult to determine. Therefore, lateral soft-tissue xerograms of the posterior pharynx are essential to assess the extent of the tumor. Because of the strategic location, surgery is unlikely to be successful due to difficulty in obtaining clear resection margins, with a resultant high frequency of local recurrences. These tumors are better treated by external beam therapy, which must include the entire pharynx from the nasopharyngeal vault down to the pyriform sinus. Because of the proximity of the tumor to the spinal cord, care must be taken to avoid excessive irradiation and subsequent damage to the spinal cord. Because of the high sensitivity of the oropharyngeal mucosa, patients generally experience rather severe painful radiation reaction with impairment of their nutritional status. Therefore, radiotherapy must be carried out with caution. Any residual disease limited to the lateral pharyngeal wall after a course of radiation therapy occasionally may be treated by pharyngectomy, although cure rates are usually poor.

COMBINED RADIATION THERAPY AND SURGERY FOR ORAL AND OROPHARYNGEAL CANCER

The cure rates for early carcinomas of the oral cavity and oropharynx, T1 and T2, are quite good. However, the radiotherapeutic results for advanced tumors, T3 and T4, are less than satisfactory whether treated by radiation therapy or by surgery alone. In these extensive lesions, failures of surgical treatment are usually the result of marginal recurrences, and failures of radiation therapy are primarily due to inability to control either the radioresistant nidus at the primary site or the nodal disease. Because of this, a program of combined radiation therapy and surgery has frequently been undertaken. The planned use of combined radiation therapy and surgery permits surgical resection of gross disease, even when the resection margins are "dirty" or inadequate by previous standards, followed by irradiation for subclinical or occult disease. Such an approach allows effective palliation and even occasional cure of many patients who are not otherwise salvageable or who are faced with functionally and cosmetically crippling alternatives. Two conceptual approaches to combined radiotherapy and surgery have emerged, preoperative and postoperative radiation therapy.

Preoperative Radiation Therapy

The aims of preoperative radiotherapy are to prevent marginal recurrences, control subclinical disease in the primary site or in the nodes, and convert technically inoperable tumors into operable ones. Theoretically, preoperative radiation therapy that is performed with the cancer cells in their maximum stage of oxygenation has a possible advantage over irradiation in the postoperative hypoxic condition. This form of combined approach has been found to decrease both local recurrence and the incidence of distant metastases.

The disadvantages of preoperative radiation therapy are that the exact extent of the tumor is obscure at the time of surgery, there is a delay in the surgery, and there is increased risk of postoperative complications. The dosage employed in this conventional preoperative radiotherapy program is subcancericidal, consisting of 4500 cGy in 1 month. This is followed in 1 month by radical surgery that encompasses all possible areas of disease, as if radiation therapy had not been given. The program is applicable to medium-sized or advanced tumors that have poor radiotherapeutic or surgical cure rates, including tumors of the oral cavity such as the tongue, floor of the mouth, gum, and oropharynx, and commonly is not associated with significant postoperative functional and cosmetic morbidity.

The radiation dosage used in preoperative radiotherapy or so-called "sequential postradiation resection" is cancericidal, that is, 6000 to 6500 cGy in 6 to 7 weeks, and is delivered homogeneously to the primary site as well as to the first-echelon lymph nodes. The treatment portal must be progressively reduced after 5000 cGy has been administered. Contrary to the conventional moderate-dose preoperative program, radiation therapy is followed by limited surgical resection, and only the residual nidus of the primary lesion, mostly in the muscles or bones, is excised, on the assumption that the peripheral, superficial disease has been controlled by high-dose radiation therapy. This approach is intended to avoid excessive functional and cosmetic mutilation by radical surgery and has been found useful in advanced lesions that arise from the retromolar trigone and faucial tonsil with involvement of the adjacent soft palate and the base of the tongue or gum. Following high-dose preoperative radiation therapy, radical surgery with intent to remove all involved areas according to the original extent of the tumor will most likely result in a high rate of postoperative complications and therefore is not advised.

Postoperative Radiation Therapy

The advantages of postoperative radiation therapy are that a higher dosage of radiation can be delivered and the clinician has a better understanding of the known sites of residual disease and the extent of pathologic involvement. Therefore, the aim of postoperative radiation therapy is to eradicate residual cancer at the resection margin and subclinical disease implanted in the wound or in the neck nodes. The procedure is usually carried out approximately 3 to 4 weeks after surgery, when the wound is healed. Generally, a dose of 5500 cGy in 6 weeks should not be exceeded if the surgery is radical in extent. On the other hand, if the surgery is primarily a debulking procedure, high-dose radiotherapy for gross residual disease must be given, that is, 6500 cGy in 7 weeks through shrinking field technique to the area of known disease.

The question as to whether radiation therapy should be used preoperatively or postoperatively has been the subject of much discussion.[13] Although the local control of the primary lesions and the survival rate of patients have not revealed any major differences between these two approaches, in certain sites with exophytic tumors, such as the larynx, tonsil, and tongue, good tumor response following preoperative irradiation has encouraged additional radiation to a curative level, thus eliminating the need for a mutilating surgical procedure. Therefore, the decision should be made on an individual basis, according to personal preference and experience. At our institution, preoperative radiotherapy is often preferred.

Treatment of metastatic nodes in the neck is as important as therapy of the primary site in the oral cavity and oropharynx. Except for early carcinomas of the lip, floor of the mouth, buccal mucosa, and retromolar trigone, patients who have N0 disease should receive elective neck treatment. For patients who have N1 disease, a modified radical neck dissection is an adequate procedure. However, the patients who have N2 and N3 disease should receive combined therapies, that is, radical neck dissection for removal of metastatic nodes and bilateral neck irradiation to prevent recurrent disease in the resected neck and contralateral cervical metastasis. A dosage of 4500 to 5000 cGy in 5 weeks is planned.

COMPLICATIONS OF RADIATION THERAPY

Minor side effects such as xerostomia, loss of taste, and dental caries may occur following curative radiation therapy. Major complications include soft-tissue ulceration, orocutaneous fistulas, and osteoradionecrosis of the mandible.[4, 7] Osteoradionecrosis may be affected by the proximity of the growth, recent dental extractions, and the health and integrity of the mucous membrane of the gum as well as by radiation dosage. Osteoradionecrosis may also occur in the edentulous jaw from excessively high dose of radiations. Once it develops, removal of the devitalized, infected bone by surgery, including sequestrectomy or partial mandibulectomy, may be indicated. Although carious teeth should be removed prior to irradiation for hygienic reasons, good, well-repaired teeth either within or without the treatment portals need not be sacrificed if the radiation dosage is kept within the limits of the tolerance of the mandible. Radiation-induced dental caries can be avoided by observing meticulous dental care with fluoride treatment during and after radiation therapy.

Although such radiation complications of varying extent are considered to be undesirable, they should be accepted as risks in the treatment of malignant tumors of the oral cavity and oropharynx; however, they may be minimized by observing careful radiotherapeutic and surgical techniques.

SUMMARY

Squamous cell carcinomas of the oral cavity and oropharynx are potentially curable malignant tumors (Table 13–1). When the tumor is diagnosed and treated in the early stages, T1 and T2, the cure rates either by surgery or by radiation therapy are high. The choice of therapeutic modalities for such lesions is complex and depends upon the site of origin; size of the tumor; presence or absence of nodal metastases; age, physical, medical, and social status of the patient; reliability of the patient to return for a prolonged course of radiation therapy; skill and expertise of the physicians involved; and relative morbidity and cosmesis of the two forms of treatment rather than any differences in 5-year survival rates. In general, for early T1 lesions of the oral tongue and floor of the mouth, if the deformity resulting from surgery is minimal, perhaps related to freedom from radiation sequelae, surgery is preferred. If surgical resection involves major morbidity, such as deformity that alters cosmesis or the function of speech and swallowing mechanisms, radiation therapy is the treatment of choice. For medium-sized tumors, superficial T2, of the oral tongue, floor of the mouth, and oropharynx, radiation therapy is the treatment of choice. It not only provides satisfactory control of the disease but also affords preservation of normal function and anatomic parts. Surgery is reserved for radiation failures. Extensive disease, T3 and T4, often associated

Table 13–1. THREE-YEAR NED RATES FOLLOWING RADIATION THERAPY ALONE* (updated 1978)

	T1	T2	T3 and T4
Floor of mouth	35/43— 81%	37/71—52%	4/48— 8%
Oral tongue	19/30— 63%	25/61—41%	8/70—11%
Retromolar trigone	7/12— 58%	28/59—47%	10/53—19%
Soft palate	18/18—100%	23/36—64%	4/29—14%
Tonsil	11/13— 85%	61/102—60%	17/86—20%
Base of tongue	25/30— 83%	26/48—54%	13/88—11%

*Excluding surgical salvage patients.

with bone and muscle involvement and cervical lymph node metastases, is rarely curable by either radiotherapy or surgery alone; therefore, a combined approach using radiation therapy and surgery is the procedure of choice. If the lesions are obviously incurable by any means, palliative radiation therapy may offer symptomatic relief.

Metastatic disease to the cervical nodes should be treated aggressively by combined therapies if the primary lesion is controlled. The fact that 30 to 40 percent of patients who have T2 and T3 lesions with a clinically negative neck will have evidence of metastatic nodal disease on microscopic examination of the dissected neck specimens or on subsequent follow-up of untreated neck, so-called "occult" or "subclinical" disease. With the exception of small mucosal tumors, modern management of carcinoma of the oral cavity and oropharynx by surgery or irradiation must include comprehensive management of the cervical nodes by either elective neck irradiation or neck dissection as part of the overall therapeutic program. Post-treatment rehabilitation with the use of an internal prosthesis or oral surgery to aid in postoperative reconstruction should be offered to patients in the overall management of this disease. Cooperation between the various physicians involved is what ultimately benefits patients who are afflicted with this disease.

REFERENCES

1. American Joint Committee: Manual for Staging of Cancer, 2nd ed. Philadelphia, J. B. Lippincott Co., 1978.
2. Ash, C. L.: Oral cancer: a twenty-five year study. Am. J. Roentgenol., 87:417, 1962.
3. Ballantyne, A. J., and Fletcher, G. H.: Management of residual or recurrent cancer following radiation therapy for squamous cell carcinoma of the oropharynx. Am. J. Roentgenol., 93:29, 1965.
4. Bedwinek, J. M., Chavoski, L. J., Fletcher, G. H., et al.: Osteonecrosis of the oral cavity and naso- and oropharynx. Radiology, 119:665, 1976.
5. Cady, B., and Catlin, D.: Epidermoid carcinoma of the gum: a 20-year survey. Cancer, 23:551, 1968.
6. Campos, J. L., Lampe, I., and Fayos, J. V.: Radio-
therapy of carcinoma of the floor of the mouth. Radiology, 99:677, 1971.
7. Cheng, V. S. T., and Wang, C. C.: Osteoradionecrosis of the mandible resulting from external megavoltage radiation therapy. Radiology, 112:685, 1974.
8. Fayos, J. V., and Lampe, I.: Radiation therapy of carcinoma of the tonsillar region. Am. J. Roentgenol., 111:85, 1971.
9. Fayos, J. V., and Lampe, I.: Treatment of squamous cell carcinoma of the oral cavity. Am. J. Surg., 124:493, 1972.
10. Fletcher, G. H.: Elective irradiation of subclinical disease in cancers of the head and neck. Cancer, 29:1450, 1972.
11. Lampe, I.: Radiation therapy of cancer of the buccal mucosa and lower gingiva. Am. J. Roentgenol., 73:628, 1955.
12. Perez, C. A., Lee, F. A., Ackerman, L. V., et al.: Nonrandomized comparison of preoperative irradiation and surgery vs. irradiation alone in the management of carcinoma of the tonsil. Am. J. Roentgenol., 126:248, 1976.
13. Powers, W. E., and Palmer, L. A.: Biologic basis of preoperative radiation treatment. Am. J. Roentgenol., 102:176, 1968.
14. Wang, C. C.: Management and prognosis of squamous cell carcinoma of the tonsillar region. Radiology, 104:667, 1972.
15. Wang, C. C.: Radiation therapy in the management of oral malignant disease. Otolaryngol. Clin. North Am., 12:73, 1979.

General Text References

Ackerman, L. V., and del Regato, J. A.: Cancer, 5th ed. St. Louis, The C. V. Mosby Co., 1977.
Buschke, F., and Parker, R. G.: Radiation Therapy in Cancer Management. New York, Grune and Stratton, Inc. 1972.
Casarett, A. P.: Radiation Biology. Englewood Cliffs, NJ, Prentice-Hall, Inc., 1968.
Fletcher, G. H.: Textbook of Radiotherapy, 3rd ed. Philadelphia, Lea and Febiger, 1980.
Hall, E. J.: Radiobiology for the Radiologist, 2nd ed. New York, Harper and Row Publishers, Inc., 1978.
MacComb, W. D., and Fletcher, G. H.: Cancer of the Head and Neck. Baltimore, The Williams and Wilkins Co., 1967.
Moss, W. T., Brand, W. N., and Battifora, H.: Radiation Oncology, 5th ed. St. Louis, The C. V. Mosby Co., 1979.
Rubin, P., and Casarrett, G. W.: Clinical Radiation Pathology, Vols. 1 and 2. Philadelphia, W. B. Saunders Company, 1968.
Wang, C. C.: Radiation Therapy for Head and Neck Neoplasms: Indications, Techniques and Results. Littleton, John Wright-PSG, Inc., 1983.

14

Dental management for cancer patients receiving head and neck radiation

DEBORAH LUCKS, D.D.S.
STEPHEN T. SONIS, D.M.D., D.M.Sc.

As cancer therapy is becoming more successful and survival rates are significantly prolonged, the noninstitutional dentist will see more patients who have been treated for cancer. Dentists will be confronted with the task of making treatment decisions about patients who have received radiation therapy to the head and neck. It will be important that dentists understand the effects of cancericidal therapy on the normal oral tissues and the influence that such treatment has on dental treatment.

Radiation therapy is commonly used to treat squamous cell carcinomas of the head and neck. It may also be used to treat regional malignant lymphomas. Patients who are treated for Hodgkin's disease often receive radiation treatment that includes the mandible and submandibular and sublingual salivary glands.

Side effects of head and neck radiation therapy include mucositis, xerostomia, loss of taste, loss of elasticity of the skin of the neck, osteoradionecrosis, and fibrosis of the temporomandibular joint. The type and severity of radiation side effects depend upon the tissues in the radiation field, the amount of radiation given, and the course of treatment.

Profound xerostomia and the risk of osteoradionecrosis are the two side effects that are of most concern to the dentist.

Salivary glands in the radiation field usually undergo irreversible and severe functional

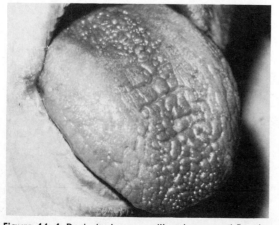

Figure 14–1. Red, dry tongue with edema and fissuring in a patient who has xerostomia. There is also some angular cheilosis.

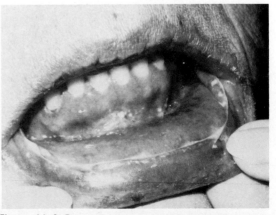

Figure 14–2. Dry oral mucous membrane with surface accumulation of nondesquamated cells in a patient who has xerostomia.

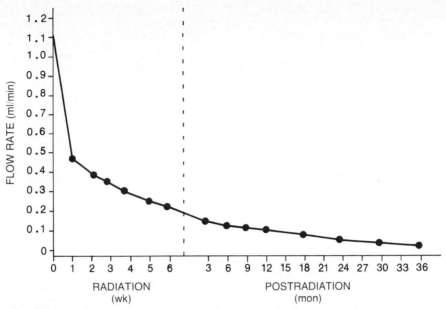

Figure 14–3. Graphic illustration of diminished salivary flow rate in 42 cancer patients during and following radiation. (From Dreizen, S., Brown, D., Daly, T. E., and Drane, J. B.: J. Dent. Res., *56:*99, 1977.)

changes. Saliva may become thick and ropy or may be reduced severely. Serous elements of the salivary glands are the most radiosensitive. Thus, the patient who receives head and neck irradiation loses most of the serous component of saliva. When the mucous glands are also affected, the patient may have almost total loss of salivary gland function (Figs. 14–1 through 14–3).

A significant consequence of xerostomia is radiation caries, which usually appears in the cervical region or the incisal edges of teeth a few months following treatment. Left untreated, caries and decalcification may become so severe that the structural integrity of the teeth is destroyed until the clinical crowns snap off (Fig. 14–4).

The causes of radiation caries are multifold and include loss of the buffering capacity of saliva, elimination of mechanical flushing by saliva, and reduction of salivary IgA. Salivary electrolytes are lacking and thus do not prevent demineralization of the teeth. There is also a shift of the oral flora to a more cariogenic bacterial population, that is, a shift to increase concentrations of *Streptococcus mutans,* lactobacillus, and yeast.[2, 4, 5, 11]

A second potential side effect of radiation therapy is osteoradionecrosis. Reported incidence in the literature varies from 2 to 22 percent (Table 14–1). As a result of radiation, the blood supply to bone is decreased, leading to a reduction in osseous vitality and resistance to infection, as well as impaired healing potential. The mandible, because of its naturally limited blood supply, is at greater risk than the maxilla. The more radiation that the patient receives, the greater the risk of osteoradionecrosis. However, the problem is generally unusual in patients who receive less than 6000 rads (Table 14–2).

Osteoradionecrosis may occur spontaneously or may be caused by an invasive surgical procedure such as a tooth extraction (Table 14–3). Trauma, such as that caused by an ill-fitting dental prosthesis, may result in ulcera-

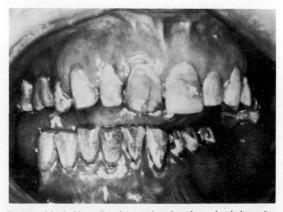

Figure 14–4. Xerostomia and extensive dental caries following radiation therapy.

Table 14–1. INCIDENCE OF OSTEORADIONECROSIS OF JAWS IN PATIENTS IRRADIATED FOR ORAL AND HEAD AND NECK CANCER

Investigators	Year	Center	No. Patients Irradiated	No. Cases Osteoradio-necrosis	Percentage
Watson and Scarborough[18]	1939	Memorial Hospital, NY	1891	235	13
Wildermuth and Cantril[20]	1953	Swedish Hospital, WA	104	6	6
Meyer[12]	1958	Westfield, MA	491	26	5
Dodson[9]	1962	Geisenberger, VA	108	10	9
Beumer, Silverman, Benak[3]	1972	University of California, CA	278	10	4
Carl, Schaaf, Sako[6]	1973	Roswell Park, NY	47	2	4
Bedwinek, et al.[1]	1976	M.D. Anderson, TX	381	54	14
Morrish, et al.[13]	1981	University of California, CA	100	22	22

tion and subsequent osteoradionecrosis. Clinically, osteoradionecrosis may appear as an open, sometimes painful, occasionally foul-smelling wound with underlying necrotic bone. Sequestration may be evident. Interestingly, not all lesions of osteoradionecrosis are infected. Most areas of osteoradionecrosis heal spontaneously, but slowly, following scrupulous and constant débridement and hygiene.

Great care must be taken with the patient who has received radiation to the jaws. It is important that the dentist contact the radiotherapist to establish the field of radiation, the location of the tumor, and the type and amount of radiation administered. When a patient is being irradiated and none of the major salivary glands is in the field, the degree of xerostomia is reduced, as is the risk of radiation caries. Inclusion of the mandible or maxilla in the field of radiation heightens the risk of osteoradionecrosis. Patients who have tumors with periosteal involvement or tumors that are close to bone are at a greater risk of developing osteoradionecrosis than are patients who have soft-tissue tumors. The proximity of the necessary radiation field to the bone is the prob-

able cause for this observation. Moreover, radioactive implants are more likely to cause osteoradionecrosis than is conventional radiotherapy.[9, 10] Generally, the risk of osteoradionecrosis is directly proportional to the amount of local radiation which the patient receives (see Table 14–2).

PREVENTIVE TREATMENT FOR PATIENTS ABOUT TO UNDERGO RADIATION THERAPY

When a patient is scheduled to begin head and neck radiotherapy, the dentist should be consulted to examine the patient and to recommend proper dental treatment. Preradiation dental evaluation should include a clinical examination and full-mouth radiographs.[8, 16] Teeth that show periodontal or pulpal infection should be extracted. A thorough dental prophylaxis should be performed. The patient should receive instruction in preventive home care. It is important for the patient to understand the relationship among poor hygiene, radiation, and caries. The patient's restorative needs should be treated. Generally, the most conservative restoration possible is the one of choice. Amalgam restorations are preferable to cast restorations. Removable prostheses may be more desirable than fixed bridges, because home care is easier and the likelihood of recurrent caries is diminished. Because the prognosis for these patients may be unpredictable, it may be unwise to become involved with extensive, expensive, and time-consuming fixed bridges.

A daily fluoride regimen should be prescribed; results of studies have consistently revealed its effectiveness in reducing the frequency of radiation-induced caries. The most

Table 14–2. INCIDENCE OF RADIONECROSIS ACCORDING TO THE RADIATION DOSE TO THE BONE

Rads	Incidence of Osteonecrosis Dentulous Patients	Edentulous Patients
<6500	0/36 (0%)	0/3 (0%)
6500–7500	8/29 (27.6%)	1/15 (6.6%)
>7500	11/13 (84.6%)	2/4 (50%)
Total	19/78 (24.4%)	3/22 (13.6%)

(From Morrish, R. B., Chan, E., Silverman, S., et al.: Osteonecrosis in patients irradiated for head and neck carcinoma. Cancer, 47:1980, 1981.)

Table 14–3. ASSOCIATION OF DENTAL EXTRACTIONS AND OSTEONECROSIS IN 78 IRRADIATED DENTULOUS PATIENTS

	Incidence of Osteonecrosis	Radiation Dose in Rads: Range (average)	Average Time of Onset of Osteonecrosis After Treatment (in months)
No extractions	5/41 (12.2%)	6940–9280 (7871)	29
Before radiotherapy	3/19 (15.8%)	7580–9610 (8500)	41
After radiotherapy	11/18 (61.1%)	6700–8100 (7346)	20
TOTAL	19/78 (24.4%)	6700–9610 (7666)*	22

*Radiation in dentulous patients who did not have osteonecrosis ranged between 4950 and 9700 rads (average 6450 rads).

(From Morrish, R. B., Chan, E., Silverman, S., et al.: Osteonecrosis in patients irradiated for head and neck carcinoma. Cancer, *47*:1980, 1981.)

effective and convenient way to administer fluoride to the patient is through the use of fluoride gels, which the patient uses on a daily basis, placed in customized trays (see Chapter 13).[10, 19]

Trays can be constructed simply by using a thick flexible mouth guard material on a vacuum (Omnivac) machine. Alternatively, a laboratory can be used. It is important that the margins of the tray extend onto the gingiva above the crowns of the teeth. The tray edges should be trimmed smoothly so as not to be an irritant to the oral mucosa.

The patient is instructed to place 5 to 10 drops of an acidulated phosphate fluoride gel (e.g., Thera-flur) into each tray and to spread the gel around so that it is thoroughly dispensed inside the tray. The patient should then place the trays over the teeth and bite lightly for 6 minutes. The trays are then removed, and both the trays and the mouth are rinsed.

The patient should take nothing by mouth for 30 minutes. This regimen should be followed daily. Caries is prevented when compliance is good (Table 14–4).

If the patient has mucositis, a nonacidulated fluoride gel may be substituted, because it is less irritating to mucosa than is the acidulated gel. However, its anticaries activity is not as effective.

If the trays cannot be tolerated, a fluoride rinse (such as Phos-Flur or Phos-Flur N) may be substituted as a 1-minute rinse. The acidulated fluoride rinse has a greater anticaries activity, but the neutral rinse is indicated when the patient has mucositis.

The patient should discontinue daily fluoride usage only when the xerostomia has subsided, which may not occur for months after the completion of radiotherapy. In some cases, it is necessary to continue fluoride use indefinitely.

Table 14–4. COMPARISON OF RESULTS IN THE UNCOOPERATIVE, NONCOMPLIANT PATIENTS, WHO EITHER DID NOT USE OR ONLY SPORADICALLY USED THE 0.4 PERCENT SnF₂ GEL WITH THOSE IN COOPERATIVE PATIENTS WHO USED THE GEL ON A DAILY BASIS

			Caries Activity	
Use of 0.4% SnF₂ Gel	No. of Patients	Teeth Present	Crowns Amputated	Additional Carious Surfaces
None	5	72	54	36
Sporadic	4	75	3	39
Noncooperative total	9	147	57	75
Daily Cooperative total	6	139	0	1
Group total	15*	286	57	76

*Seven deceased patients and two others who failed to return for examination were lost to follow-up.

(From Wescott, W. B., Starcke, E. N., and Shannon, I. L.: Chemical protection against postirradiation dental caries. Oral Surg., *40*:709, 1975.)

Fluoride may also be used in an attempt to remineralize teeth in which radiation caries has begun. Shannon and colleagues had great success with VALube, a fluoridated artificial saliva.[17] If the teeth show evidence of demineralization, the fluoride gel should be used for 15 minutes t.i.d. with rinses interspersed with a fluoridated rinse of 1 percent fluoride.

SPECIAL CONSIDERATIONS IN THE TREATMENT OF CANCER PATIENTS

Oral Surgery

The major consideration in performing oral surgical procedures in the patient who will or who has received radiation therapy is the avoidance of osteoradionecrosis. Ideally, all extractions should be performed at least two weeks prior to the start of radiation therapy to allow for sufficient healing. If necessary, radiotherapy should be delayed until there is epithelium covering the extraction socket, leaving no exposed bone.[4]

Before extractions are contemplated, a complete medical history should be taken and all necessary information should be discussed with the medical oncologist, the radiotherapist or both.

If the patient has also been treated with chemotherapy, there is a chance of myelosuppression (see Chapter 17). The degree of myelosuppression should be determined with appropriate laboratory tests. Patients should have antibiotic coverage on the day of and for 1 week following extractions.

Care should be taken to perform extractions as atraumatically as possible with alveoloplasty and primary wound closure. Hemostatic agents should not be allowed in the socket, because they may become a nidus for infection.

If the patient has a fair to good prognosis and if the jaw bones are directly in the radiation portal, all teeth with questionable prognosis should be extracted in the preradiation phase to avoid the need for extractions after radiation and the associated increased risk of osteoradionecrosis. Although there is a risk of osteoradionecrosis due to extraction in the preradiation phase, there is even greater risk after radiation due to diminished blood supply, delayed healing, and decreased blood supply.[14]

In the patient who has already received radiation, a less aggressive approach is needed. It is best to ignore all asymptomatic teeth. If a tooth becomes infected or painful after radiation, the most conservative treatment should be attempted. If a tooth must be extracted, it should be done with antibiotic prophylaxis. A convenient form is oral penicillin (2 g 1 hour preoperatively and 500 mg q.i.d. × 10 days). The extraction should be as atraumatic as possible. Any rough bone should be eliminated, and the wound should be irrigated thoroughly. Primary closure is desirable. The patient should have a closely monitored postoperative course. Endodontic therapy may be more desirable than extraction, although its long-term effectiveness may be questionable in patients who have cancer.

Endodontics

The effects of megavoltage radiation on the dental pulp have not yet been resolved. However, if a patient develops pulpitis, root canal treatment should be considered. Antibiotic coverage is advisable. Care should be taken not to push the necrotic debris beyond the tooth apex.

Because of the decreased bone vitality, periapical radiolucencies may not resolve.

Pulpotomy is not advisable because of the inherent risk of infection.

Periodontics

Periodontal surgery is contraindicated in patients who have received radiation therapy to the head and neck. Conservative periodontal maintenance is important. Scaling, root planing, and curettage should be done as often as necessary, with proper antibiotic coverage.

Operative Dentistry

Restorative procedures should be as conservative as possible in the patient who has received radiation therapy. The clinician should be as atraumatic as possible with the gingival margin when using rubber dam clamps and matrix bands. If the clinician believes that the gingiva or the underlying bone has been traumatized during caries removal or gingival retraction for amalgam condensation, the patient should be given a course of antibiotics and oral lavage with 3 percent hydrogen peroxide USP diluted with two parts warm water to one part peroxide, or with saline.

Prosthodontics

As a result of surgical resection or extractions, removable prostheses are frequently required for the patient who has head and neck cancer. In constructing a denture, one must try to minimize the possibility of chronic irritation. A soft liner material may be helpful for the first 2 to 3 months.

When the dentist has the occasion to rehabilitate a patient who has been treated with radiotherapy, the following facts should be taken into consideration. The oral tissues are compromised and atrophied, with delayed healing, and the host resistance is lowered. The dental prosthesis should be as nonirritating to the oral mucosa as possible.

If removable dentures are to be constructed, careful follow-up must be enforced. There must be a 24-hour, 48-hour, 1-week, 1-month, and then every 3-month follow-up until the denture has been trouble-free for 1 year; then a follow-up every 6 months is indicated.

Care must be taken to prevent any denture sores from forming, because a mucosal ulceration could easily result in a nonhealing atrophied mucosa with exposed bone, leading to osteoradionecrosis.[7]

The patient must be instructed to remove the dentures if he or she feels a sore spot or even if a red spot is noticed. If there is any doubt whether such instructions can be communicated to and understood by the patient, a removable prosthesis should not be recommended.

Some clinicians believe that dentures for irradiated patients should be fabricated from a soft, flexible denture material. To date, the softer denture materials have been found to be too porous, therefore harboring bacteria, leading to an increased risk of osteoradionecrosis.

Audi-flex has been mentioned as an alternative denture material. This is a material used in the construction of hearing aids.

Trismus

When the patient is suffering from trismus as a sequela to head and neck irradiation, a stent may be constructed to reduce the trismus (see Chapter 21). Trismus can be minimized by a jaw exercise program.

Above all, the dentist should take care to maintain the oral health of the patient and to do no harm.

When the dentist is an integral part of the head and neck cancer team and when preventive dentistry is utilized, minimal complications and greater comfort to the patient may result. Esthetics and function can be maintained with a reduction in time-consuming and costly post-therapy dental rehabilitation.[8]

REFERENCES

1. Bedwinek, J., Shukoosky, L. J., Fletcher, G. H., et al.: Osteonecrosis in patients treated with definitive radiotherapy for squamous cell carcinomas of the oral cavity and naso- and oropharynx. Radiology, *119*:665, 1976.
2. Ben-Aryeh, H., Gutman, D., Spargel, R., et al.: Effects of irradiation on saliva in cancer patients. Int. J. Oral Surg., *4*:205, 1975.
3. Beumer, J., Silverman, S., and Benak, S.: Hard- and soft-tissue necrosis following radiation therapy for oral cancer. J. Prosthet. Dent., *27*:640, 1972.
4. Brown, L. R., Dreizen, S., Handler, S., et al.: The effect of radiation induced xerostomia on human oral microflora. J. Dent. Res., *54*:740, 1975.
5. Brown, L. R., Dreizen, S., Rider, L. J., et al.: The effect of radiation induced xerostomia on saliva and serum lysozyme and immunoglobulin levels. Oral Surg., *41*:83, 1976.
6. Carl, W., Schaaf, N. G., and Sako, K.: Oral surgery and the patient who has had radiation therapy for head and neck cancer. Oral Surg., *36*:651, 1973.
7. Curtis, T. A., Griffith, M. R., and Firtell, D. N.: Complete denture prosthodontics for the radiation patient. J. Prosthet. Dent., *36*:66, 1976.
8. Daly, T. E.: Dentistry for the irradiated head and neck cancer patient. Cancer Bull., *29*:74, 1979.
9. Dodson, W. S.: Irradiation osteomyelitis of the jaws. J. Oral Surg., *20*:467, 1962.
10. Dreizen, S., Brown, D., Daly, T. E., et al.: Prevention of xerostomia related dental caries in irradiated cancer patients. J. Dent. Res., *56*:99, 1977.
11. Dreizen, S., Brown, L. R., Handler, S., et al.: Radiation induced xerostomia in cancer patients—effect on salivary and serum electrolytes. Cancer, *38*:273, 1976.
12. Meyer, I.: Osteoradionecrosis of the Jaws. Chicago, Year Book Medical Publishers, Inc., 1958.
13. Morrish, R. B., Chan, E., Silverman, S., et al.: Osteonecrosis in patients irradiated for head and neck carcinoma. Cancer, *47*:1980, 1981.
14. Murray, C. G., Daly, T. E., and Zimmerman, S. O.: The relationship between dental disease and radiation necrosis of the mandible. Oral Surg., *49*:99, 1980.
15. Murray, C. G., Herson, J., Daly, T., et al.: Radiation necrosis of the mandible: a ten year study. Part 1, Factors influencing the onset of necrosis. Part II, Dental factors, onset, duration, and management of necrosis. Int. J. Radiat. Oncol. Biol. Phys., *6*:543, 1980.
16. Regezi, J. A., Courtney, R. M., and Kerr, D. A.: Dental management of patients irradiated for oral cancer. Cancer, *38*:994, 1976.
17. Shannon, I. L., Trodahl, J. N., and Stareke, E. N.: Remineralization of enamel by a saliva substitute designed for use by irradiated patients. Cancer, *41*:1746, 1978.
18. Watson, W. L., and Scarborough, J. E.: Osteoradionecrosis in intraoral cancer. Am. J. Roentgenol., *40*:524, 1939.
19. Wescott, W. B., Starcke, E. N., and Shannon, I. L.: Chemical protection against postirradiation dental caries. Oral Surg., *40*:709, 1975.
20. Wildermuth, O., and Cantril, S. T.: Radiation necrosis of the mandible. Radiology, *61*:771, 1953.

15

Surgical therapy of malignant tumors— basic principles

RICHARD E. WILSON, M.D.

The surgeon who treats malignant disease must confront a variety of factors. First, it must be understood that there is currently a resurgence of surgical interest in cancer. For the past 5 or 6 decades, cancer management was almost totally relegated to the surgeon. Only in about the last 20 years, with the advances in chemotherapy, the development of therapeutic radiology, and the potential for immune therapy as a form of management of malignant disease, has there been tremendous growth in these disciplines. The NIH Clinical Cancer Center was developed as a chemotherapy center, because there was no chemotherapy center (to speak of) in the United States. Its main objective was to convert clinical pharmacology into clinical practice in chemotherapy. With all these disciplines taking a more active role in the development of new approaches, surgery became an accepted "old hat," without any "new look." Recently, there has been a rekindling of interest of surgeons who specialize in cancer, so-called surgical oncologists, to develop this field of special expertise. I need not go into the politics of medicine and surgery, but it should be understood that surgical oncology is developing itself in many ways; it is moving in the direction of separate credentialing, separate training programs and fellowships, and a more active role in the leadership of cancer management.

Seven aspects of surgical management may be listed as the basic principles for cancer treatment. First, one must understand the *natural history* of the disease. Second, one must have expertise in the *specific anatomy*. For dentists, this is primarily the oral cavity and its environs, but for cancer surgeons, it involves many areas of the body and there is

further subspecialization. In making decisions about management, *staging* must be carried out prior to therapy. It is absolutely necessary to understand the potential for *multimodality therapy* and to start with that as a concept rather than administer one treatment and then, when you have gone as far as you can with that, try another treatment and, after a while, a third treatment. The approach to oral cancer is an excellent demonstration of this. The combination of chemotherapy, surgery, and radiation in the treatment process is more likely to achieve better results than in starting with one form of therapy and, when cancer recurs, to use another. Obviously it is most important that the surgeon use the *technical skills* that he or she has developed. Likewise, *postoperative management* is critical, and of particular importance for oral cancer is *rehabilitation*. I am happy to report that over the years head and neck surgeons and oral oncologists have been leaders in prosthetics and rehabilitation for their patients, partly because the head and face are so visible. There is even a greater need for rehabilitation to proceed hand-in-hand with treatment. The final area is *long-term follow-up*. These are the seven pillars upon which surgeons should base all cancer management.

NATURAL HISTORY

To understand the history of malignant disease, one has to think more about epidemiology. What are the factors responsible for the development of malignancy? Who is responsible for the treatment of cancer? One person who helps in the treatment of cancer is the public health officer, the person who develops screening programs in the community, the local expert who tries to reduce the incidence and severity of the disease, a medical goal for which everyone must strive. Epidemiology is a fascinating field. It is similar to a detective story in that more new things come to light for each malignancy. Population studies are very interesting. Why is breast cancer one fifth as common in Japan as in the United States? Why is colon cancer almost unheard of in India? Why is liver cancer a major cause of death in the Far East? We may see one case of primary liver cancer each year at our institution in Boston, but in Singapore, it is a common cause of death. These are not just minor differences; they are major alterations. Identification of the causes of these natural occurrences may contribute to new approaches to the prevention and treatment of cancer. It is clear that it is much harder to treat cancer after it has developed, and all the money that has been spent in trying to treat late malignancy and in developing programs for this stage of disease is not as easy to justify as is the search for cancer prevention. The efficiency probably lies in identifying early disease and in treating for cure, because, in my opinion, every cancer is curable if it can be found and resected or somehow primarily treated at a stage before it has spread. There is a natural progression of disease from premalignant to invasion to distant spread, and there is always a phase in which it might be most curable. Our entire effort must be directed toward understanding this approach.

As a corollary, it is important to recognize patients who are in high-risk groups and to watch them carefully for any signs of early disease. It is impossible to screen or to study 250 million people in this country for every disease. First, many people will not cooperate, and second, it is economically unfeasible. No screening study is valid for the entire population. The cost of finding one case of breast cancer by studying all women who come to the hospital without any reason for screening is well in excess of $10,000, and breast cancer is the most common cancer in women. Oral cancer is rare compared with other malignancies; thus, screening is even less plausible for this type of cancer. As soon as the clinician begins to focus on those factors that are found to be important from the epidemiology and natural history of the disease, he or she can begin to select patients, for example, those who have a family history of breast cancer, had late menopause, never had children, are

obese, and so on, and the screening process can be reduced to include those who are more likely to have positive findings. If one screens any woman who has lumps in her breast, one would increase the screening percentage even further; thus, one might triple and quadruple the value of screening when this process is added.

If one studies only smokers for their oral pathology, one will be selecting a high-risk group. A very small portion of people who do not smoke get cancer compared with those who do. That factor alone greatly increases the screening efficiency. The Dana-Farber Cancer Institute screening manual is an important source, because in it, the screening procedures for many of the common cancers are explained. Today, there are important screening programs in this country for breast cancer, oral cancer, thyroid cancer, and colon cancer, to mention a few. All screening programs generate controversy as to their cost effectiveness, and it has not yet been proved that early stages of malignancies can be found by screening.

In understanding the natural history of a cancer, it is important to understand the routes of spread, because they are a part of the workup and examination. One must look not only at the primary site but also at the areas to which the disease may have extended. Likewise, it is important to understand the patterns of recurrence so that when managing a patient in follow-up, the physician will know specifically what to investigate. One must have some feeling for the time course of recurrence, so that one can appropriately schedule the patient to return for re-evaluation. In managing patients, it is critical for both the patient and the family to know and for the doctor to understand the survival data. What do you tell a patient who has a carcinoma in the floor of the mouth? What are his chances of being alive in 2 years or 5 years? What are the factors that affect that survival? All this information is important in understanding and treating a patient who has a malignant disease.

KNOWLEDGE OF SPECIFIC ANATOMY

One must know where to look for the disease. For instance, in the mouth, there are certain areas in which patients are more likely to develop cancer. If one knows that cancer is more likely to develop in the floor of the mouth, the side of the tongue, the tonsillar area, and certain regions in the alveolar ridge than in other areas, one should concentrate on examining there. In the rectum and the colon, 50 percent of cancers in the large bowel are within reach of the sigmoidoscope; thus, not all patients require a barium enema examination. Because the cost is always important in the effectiveness of an investigation, the following relatively inexpensive procedures are those that are usually carried out: obtaining a stool for guaiac testing, performing a rectal examination, and carrying out a sigmoidoscopy. There is no way that everyone would be able to have a barium enema examination once a year, despite the fact that colorectal cancer is the most common malignancy found in Americans. Approximately 110 thousand new cases of colorectal cancer are discovered each year in this country.

One must understand the anatomy of the local region in which the cancer is manifested. It is important to know the blood supply, nerves, muscles, and organs involved so that one can design the operation and plan the treatment to give the least deficit of function. The quality of life is the most significant factor in the management of cancer. It is very important to understand what structures are around the tumor and how they work.

The lymphatic drainage is critical, because most carcinomas initially spread by embolization into the lymphatic channels, which drain the tissue fluid that surrounds the cells. The basic biologic property of cancer is that it does not have any growth barriers. It reproduces rapidly and overgrows normal cells. Tumor cells easily get into the lymphatics and enter the bloodstream both by direct invasion and through the lymphatics. Within the lymph nodes and all along the thoracic duct, there are direct communications between the lymphatics and the veins. There are small one-way valves that prevent blood from going into the lymphatics but do not keep lymph from going into the bloodstream. All the lymphatic drainage empties into the venous system either through the thoracic duct or by one of the channels that drains the head and neck region. Thus, eventually there is no separation of lymphatic drainage from the bloodstream. We believe that most patients who have cancer have circulating tumor cells most of the time. This does not mean that they implant, which is one of the many mysteries about them. What makes cells that are circulating actually stick and grow? Why do they grow in some places? Why do certain tumors have a propensity to metastasize to certain organs even though the

spread is hematogenous? Why does lung cancer go to the brain? Why does renal cell carcinoma go to the lungs? There are many interesting questions, and if we could put all the pieces of the puzzle together, we would be better able to treat malignant disease.

Particularly important in oral cancer is an awareness of potential functional deficits. Often, patients who are missing half their colon do not know it. Their bowels move normally, and they can eat everything that they want. They may have had a major operation and a large specimen may have been removed, but they are not bothered by either. However, if a patient is missing half his tongue, he knows it and is affected by it. Planning treatment to minimize functional deficits without reducing the efficiency of cancer control takes study, experience, and skill.

STAGING OF THE MALIGNANCY

Staging refers to the natural history of the disease, where it goes, how it spreads, and where it tends to recur. Basically, staging leads to decisions for management before the operation. This is called *clinical staging* or clinical diagnostic staging. There are two kinds of staging, clinical staging and histologic or *pathologic staging*. The latter is retrospective staging after treatment. When the staging system is understood by the examiner, the patient can be evaluated more effectively. The examiner will be better able to note those clinical features that are important.

Unfortunately, staging is not equally accurate for all cancers. Those which are more superficial, such as the oral cancers, have very good staging systems. The radiotherapists, the general surgeons, and the ear, nose, and throat surgeons each had their own staging systems. Only recently have physicians from different disciplines formed the American Joint Committee for Cancer, which represents all the major societies and subspecialties. They have produced a staging manual, which was newly published in 1983 and is a valuable asset for students.

We have tried to convert most staging schemes to the TNM system (Tumor, Nodes, Metastases). For all cancers for which this is possible on a preoperative basis, there is a good classification. Head and neck cancer and breast cancer are among those that have the best schemes. Colon cancer cannot be classified preoperatively. Instead, staging is intraoperative and postoperative. In thyroid and lung cancer, clinical staging is more appropriate but is not as accurate as it is for head and neck or breast lesions. We keep trying to upgrade staging systems, because staging actually gives a prognosis preoperatively. It also helps to select therapies for particular patients. It is a data base that must be retrospectively adjusted in the light of histology. In other words, if it is found that all patients who had primary oral cancer with five or more lymph nodes in the lower neck died, a different strategy must be adopted for treating that group of patients. The end results of treatment must be examined and the staging system must be redefined accordingly.

Many new techniques are now available for identifying spread and helping with tumor staging. Staging is no longer only dependent upon physical examination. Computerized tomographic scans, angiograms, lymph angiograms, ultrasonography, and endoscopy are used. All these approaches are used in defining the true stage of disease, but sometimes surgical staging is still required. Laparotomies are often performed to stage Hodgkin's disease, because even with all these studies, it often cannot be determined whether the retroperitoneal lymph nodes or the spleen is actually involved with Hodgkin's disease. The treatment is so precise, depending upon the stage, that if the spleen is involved, one kind of treatment is used. If the liver is involved, another type of treatment is used. The more options available for treating cancer, the more accurate the staging must be. If no treatment is effective for a given malignancy, it does not matter whether the patient has a localized cancer or a widespread cancer. In this situation, staging becomes less important and mostly serves to document the observations. But as soon as one becomes more proficient with treatment, the more dependent one is on accurate staging.

Many years ago, if a patient had end-stage heart disease, there was nothing that could be done about it; he or she would die of cardiac failure. Then Dr. Harken began performing mitral valve repair, and it suddenly became important to define whether a patient had mitral stenosis or mitral insufficiency. Dr. Harken could do a valvuloplasty for stenosis but not for insufficiency; thus, it became critical to define which type of lesion a patient had. Still, it did not matter whether patients had coronary disease, because nothing could be done about that. Today, it is critical to know how much coronary artery disease a patient has, which

vessels are involved, how narrow they are, what the valve sizes are, which valves are involved, and what the status of the myocardium is. All these factors affect the type of therapy selected and are valuable data.

MULTIMODAL CAPABILITIES OF TREATMENT

The more specific the therapy, the more important it is to identify the problem. One must not start out assuming that a technique for evaluation is accurate until it has been matched with previous standards. For example, one can assume that a computerized tomographic scan is valid, but one still must match it with intraoperative experience. This is most important for surgical oncologists, because this is what separates them from other surgeons who treat cancer. Surgical oncologists must have training not only in surgery but also in chemotherapy and radiotherapy and must be familiar with immunology. The concept is that they can deal with other disciplines, both in their language and in their viewpoint. A physician who treats cancer patients must understand the many capabilities of treatment. Preoperative consultation is very important, because the chemotherapist and radiotherapist must see the lesion to be able to work with the surgeon in planning optimal therapy. After a radical neck dissection or some other major operation has been performed, they can reconstruct in their minds what things look like, how big the lesion was, whether there were possible nodes, and so on.

Cooperation among disciplines is important for the education of both the staff and residents. The best way to avoid disagreements that may develop between the disciplines is to accept the fact that everyone has something to offer and that the patient will benefit by having representatives from more than one surgical discipline look at the problem. In addition, Tumor Boards or specialty clinics such as eye clinics or head and neck clinics, where all patients with given anatomic lesions are reviewed, are valuable. Tumor Boards and Clinics have been valuable developments in most hospitals. In some institutions, Tumor Boards review problem patients; others insist that all patients should be presented prior to treatment. This is impractical for most general hospitals.

Current trials with careful randomization that compare different modes of therapy provide important information. Eventually, they can help us to properly select different kinds of treatment. Prospective, randomized studies are the best means of making advances, because bias in patient selection can be eliminated. In order to do this, we must know the end results of previous studies. This information serves as a foundation for newer investigations. Most therapeutic protocols (phase III studies) are based on previous studies. In Phase I studies, tolerance to the therapeutic procedure is assessed. In Phase II studies, one gains some idea of the effectiveness of treatment. In Phase III trials, one type of treatment is compared with another of known benefit.

TECHNICAL SKILLS

People must have the required training and experience to carry out operative procedures. The diseases and clinical problems are so varied that one must have a wide range of knowledge and know where to find information about specific anatomic parts and special techniques. Consultation among physicians in various disciplines is also valuable.

Preoperative preparation is critical, for both the psychologic and physical well-being of the patient. The bowel must be cleansed, certain medications may have to be given, the heart must be functioning properly, and blood pressure must be checked. Preparation may take hours or even a week prior to surgery. The patient may need to have intraoperative studies done, such as frozen sections or arteriography. The natural history of the disease must be known. For example, one must know which nodes to biopsy in a pancreatic carcinoma. Such information will reveal whether a given tumor is resectable. If it is resectable, an intraoperative evaluation is still the most accurate method of indicating prognosis and determining whether the patient will benefit from adjuvant therapy. Finally, there are certain basic principles in cancer surgery of which one must be aware and should utilize. The operating surgeon must not cut into the mass of the cancer. Such a maneuver will shed tumor cells that may implant in adjacent tissue. Gentle tissue handling is essential. It is now known that cancer cells frequently circulate in the blood and lymphatics and that they do not have to be expressed into the vessels by compressing or cutting the tumor. We try to plan our operations so that we do not cut across the tumor, and we try to include the draining lymphatic channels whenever possible. The surgeon must consider both resection and re-

pair of tissues and must have an understanding of nerve supply and its functional aspects, particularly in extremity surgery.

POSTOPERATIVE MANAGEMENT

Although initial surgery is the most important event in the treatment of cancer, postoperative management and rehabilitation are also critical. A surgical oncologist must perform well-planned surgery and be an expert in metabolic alterations after surgery. These changes include fluid and electrolyte balance, hormone fluxes, and energy requirements.

Because cancer often affects older people, hypertension, diabetes, cardiac disease, and other conditions with which older people are afflicted must be treated. The oncologic surgeon consults other physicians such as cardiologists and diabetologists in caring for his patient. The surgeon may be in charge of the overall management of the cancer patient, but he has to depend upon consultants.

Cancer is a problem that involves one's entire family. Both the patient and the family must be educated; it is essential that the family of a cancer patient be a part of the management. The positive aspect of the situation must be emphasized, but physicians should never lie to patients. With knowledge about the disease, physicians can present honest statements to the patient about treatment and prognosis.

Interested and knowledgeable lay groups may help the doctor to educate patients and assist in their rehabilitation. The surgeon must participate in his patient's recovery, but the assistance of others is vital.

LONG-TERM FOLLOW-UP

Tumor registries are important, because they provide the physician and the hospital the opportunity to learn from previous experience. Without this information, progress is impossible. For the patient, there is always a risk of local recurrence; therefore, thorough follow-up examinations are useful. Patients who have certain types of cancer are more likely to develop a second primary tumor of the same type. A patient who has one type of cancer is also at a higher risk of developing some other type of cancer. Likewise, new cancers may result from the treatment of an earlier cancer, particularly with radiation treatments or chemotherapy. Long-term follow-up is also necessary for patients who receive adjuvant therapy after primary surgery. Identification of recurrence at an early stage allows the best results for salvage. The smaller the tumor burden, the better the response to treatment.

CONCLUSIONS

The management of patients who have malignant disease is both complex and difficult. It is dependent upon a series of basic principles of therapy, which have briefly been outlined here. Adherence to these principles will result in better management of cancer patients and will increase the opportunity for them to achieve a better quality of life.

SUMMARY

Basic Principles of Surgical Therapy For Cancer

Understanding Natural History of the Disease
Epidemiology
High-risk groups
Screening
Route of spread
Patterns of recurrence
Survival data

Knowledge of Specific Anatomy Involved
Usual sites for presentation
Structures involved with primary site
Blood and nerve supply to area
Lymphatic drainage
Potential functional deficits

Adequate Staging of the Malignancy (i.e., Clinical Staging)
Knowledge of staging systems for specific malignancy
Diagram for preoperative staging
TNM system where possible (systems are always improving)
Understand types of presentation of tumor
Utilize all techniques to identify spread pre- and intraoperatively

Appreciation of Multimodal Capabilities in Treatment
Training in chemotherapy, radiotherapy, and immunology (formal and by experience)
Preoperative consultation
Use of Tumor Boards and Specialty Clinics
Knowledge of end results of treatment by single and combined modalities
Participation in clinical trials

Technical Skills to Perform the Planned Procedure
Required training and experience
Special knowledge and review if necessary
Preoperative preparation
Special intraoperative studies, when appropriate (e.g., frozen section, arteriography)
Observing general principles of cancer surgery

Adequate Postoperative Management for Rehabilitation
Knowledge of surgical metabolism (e.g., postoperative fluid and electrolyte balance in elderly people)
Utilize consulting services
Educate patient and family
Make use of appropriate lay groups

Long-Term Follow-up and Search for Other Malignancies
Local and distant recurrence
Adjuvant therapy where indicated
Importance of natural history and disease relationships
Treat relapses aggressively for best palliation

REFERENCES

1. Beahrs, O. H., and Myers, M. H. (eds.): Manual for Staging of Cancer, 2nd ed. Philadelphia, J. B. Lippincott Co., 1983.
2. Copeland, E. M., III (ed.): Surgical Oncology. New York, John Wiley & Sons, Inc. 1983.
3. DeVita, V. T., Jr., Hellman, S., and Rosenberg, S. A. (eds.): Cancer: Principles and Practice of Oncology. Philadelphia, J. B. Lippincott Co., 1982.
4. Pilch, Y. H.: Surgical Oncology. New York, McGraw-Hill, Inc., 1984.
5. Wilson, R. E.: Surgical Problems in Immuno-Depressed Patients, Vol. 30 in the series Major Problems in Clinical Surgery. Philadelphia, W. B. Saunders Company, 1984.

16

Surgical therapy of oral cancer

JOSEPH E. MURRAY, M.D.

Oral cancer includes head and neck cancers that are restricted to the following structures of the oral cavity: tongue, floor of the mouth, gingiva, buccal mucosa, palate, and lips. Skin cancer, odontogenic tumors, and lymphomas are specifically excluded from the scope of the guidelines that the National Cancer Institute formulated for the head and neck cancer control network program. The head and neck tumors to be considered are primarily squamous cell carcinomas. Their epidemiology and biology exclude endocrine tumors, sarcomas, and central nervous system diseases. Approximately 40 percent of all head and neck cancers occur in the oral cavity, and 15 percent occur in the oropharynx and hypopharynx. Thus, more than 50 percent of all head and neck cancers are within the realm of examination of the oral area or hypopharynx.

The male to female incidence is over 3:1, and the age and specific incidence increases markedly after 50 years of age.

The characteristics of diagnosed patients suggest the predisposing factors of heavy consumption of alcohol and tobacco use. Some studies have suggested an associated exposure to wood and metal dust, ingestion of hot drinks and spicy foods, and neglect of oral hygiene.

HISTOPATHOLOGY

Most head and neck cancers are squamous cell carcinomas and thus may be preceded by various precancerous lesions. Early lesions may be entirely epithelial, in which case the term *carcinoma-in-situ* is applied. An invasive carcinoma will be either well differentiated, moderately well differentiated, poorly differentiated, or undifferentiated. Pathologists may have difficulty determining whether a poorly differentiated or anaplastic tumor originated in squamous or glandular epithelium. Verrucous carcinomas are clinically manifested as a warty outgrowth, and such tumors progress slowly. The term *leukoplakia* means a clinically observed white patch. Microscopically, it might be hyperkeratosis or an early invasive carcinoma; on the other hand, it may represent a fungus infection or other benign oral disease.

The clinical course of cancer of the mucous membranes of the head and neck is moderately predictable from a biological viewpoint. Squamous cell carcinoma of the mucous membrane is usually preceded by a whitish plaque, leukoplakia, or velvety red plaque, erythroplakia. The symptoms of erythroplakia are more ominous than those of leukoplakia, which often does not develop into cancer.

A primary tumor may be either exophytic or infiltrative, and ulcerations are common. The symptoms produced vary from obstruction to the oral passageway or the airway, secondary infection, ulceration, involvement of the cranial nerves, pain, or bleeding.

Regional metastases to the cervical lymph nodes occur progressively, and their anatomic location is often determined by the site of the primary tumor. Most patients die from direct extension or from local metastases of the disease. Distant metastases occur infrequently and may occur to the lung, liver, or bone. The 5-year survival rate of cancer of the various locations are: lip, 86 percent; tongue, 33 percent; floor of the mouth, 45 percent; and other oral lesions, 44 percent. These are overall survival rates and, of course, vary with the size of the primary lesion and the presence or absence of regional or distant nodes. In the absence of regional adenopathy, the survival rate of cancer of the lip approaches 89 percent; tongue, 52 percent; floor of the mouth, 65 percent; and other oral lesions, 61 percent.

TREATMENT

Intraoral cancer is treated by three major modalities: surgical excision, radiation therapy, or chemotherapy, either singly or in combination. The final decision about the type of treatment to be used will be made according to the anatomic site of the tumor, the staging of classification (TNM), and the histopathology. The final decision will be influenced by medical factors such as age of the patient, systemic disease, and coexisting tumors. Nonmedical factors such as patient refusal and special occupation must also be considered.

Surgical Excision

In most cases in which it is feasible, it is best to separate the entire tumor from the patient's body by surgical removal. The advantage of surgical excision is promptness of treatment and completion within a short period of time. The excised specimen is available for microscopic evaluation of the margins. The major disadvantages of surgical excision are tissue loss and the required removal of adjacent functioning structures.

Cryosurgery, that is, freezing the tissues in situ, may be considered a form of surgical technique whereby the frozen tissue becomes necrotic and sloughs. Healing depends upon secondary scar formation. Electrocoagulation, that is, the destruction of the tumor by heat and electrocautery, might also be considered in the same way as cryosurgery, in situ destruction of tissue to allow for secondary healing.

Radiation Therapy

Radiation therapy, like surgical excision, can be effective locally. The dose required to sterilize a given neoplasm depends upon the microanatomy, size, and location of the tumor. The advantage of radiation therapy is its ability to treat a larger volume than may conveniently be removed surgically. The disadvantages relate to the prolonged treatments (often spanning weeks), radiation injury to normal tissue traversed by the beam, and depression of salivary gland function and resultant radiation caries, osteomyelitis, and soft-tissue necrosis. Later, atrophic changes in the mucosa also occur, and there is long-term potential for the development of new cancerous lesions.

Chemotherapy

The third method of treatment, chemotherapy, may be applied systemically or regionally. Chemotherapeutic agents may attack widespread disease and may augment the local effects of surgery and radiation therapy. To date, most chemotherapeutic programs have been palliative or adjunctive. There is no doubt, however, that with improved chemotherapy its use will increase both in extent and importance. Recently, the increasing use of multiple agents in combination chemotherapy has produced dramatic decreases in tumor bulk and therefore its effects seem promising.

The treatment for any patient must be evaluated in terms of all three methods, that is, surgical excision, radiation therapy, and chemotherapy. A combined treatment of cancer depends upon many factors. Of the three major treatment disciplines, surgery and radiation therapy have a high probability of controlling the tumor locally, although the probability decreases with increasing tumor bulk. Systemic chemotherapy has a lower probability of control, primarily because the therapeutic ratio is limited by the exposure of the normal cell renewal systems of bone marrow and the gastrointestinal tract to the antitumor agents. In cases in which local or regional persistence of a neoplasm is the only significant clinical problem, a combination of surgery and radiation therapy has been shown to be of value. A combination of surgical resection and x-ray therapy, however can produce dual morbidity, so their combined usage requires considerable thought and experience.

REHABILITATION

The general principle of rehabilitation is to control the cancer and minimize the functional and cosmetic impairment. Therefore, the prosthodontist, speech pathologist, and dentist are needed to help with voice impairment and eating. It is best to perform any necessary surgical reconstruction at the time of surgical excision. The common psychological problems of patients who have head and neck cancer include anxiety about recurrence, depression related to the change in body image, mourning of the loss of their face and body, with associated withdrawal from society, and finally, loss of self-esteem and self-worth, including a fear of rejection because of their disfigurement. Therefore, the treatment of these lesions requires that one have a thorough knowledge of the biology of the tumor and the surgical potential, that one knows the reconstructive techniques that are available, and that the patient will get the necessary emotional support.

CASE HISTORIES

The remainder of this chapter is devoted to illustrative case presentations of how surgical resection can be used in the management of cancer patients. It must be emphasized, however, that the critical factor is selecting the best treatment, either singly or in combination, applicable to the individual patient.

The selection of the required surgical procedures depends upon the size of the tumor, its location, its aggressiveness or biologic potential, its extension to adjacent and underlying tissues, and the presence or absence of metastases to regional lymph nodes. Surgical excisions may be used singly or may be combined with presurgical or postsurgical therapeutic radiation. The surgical approach may consist of any of the following procedures, ranging from simple excision and primary closure to complex surgical removal of the tumor and appropriate reconstruction.

1. Excision of tumor with adequate margin.

2. Excision of tumor with an adequate margin and apposition of mucosal surfaces with local pedicles (see Figure 16–1).

3. Surgical removal of tumor with adjacent tissues or with mandibulectomy and neck dissection for removal of all regional lymph nodes (see Figure 16–2 and 16–4).

4. Surgical removal of tumor with all adjacent soft tissue and bone but without neck dissection (see Figure 16–3).

5. Resection of tumor followed by reconstructive surgery to replace mandible by a rib graft (see Figure 16–5 and 16–6).

6. Reconstruction by skin grafting and maxillofacial prosthodontics to replace extensive loss of intraoral tissue and bone that cannot be replaced by bone grafts (see Figure 16–7).

Figure 16–1. *A*, An exophytic, ulcerated squamous cell carcinoma of the lower lip in a 55-year-old male. He has been a pipe smoker and has had this lesion approximately 4 months. Note the vertical scar to the right of the midline of the lower lip, indicating the site of a previous resection of a tumor of unknown histology. There are no positive nodes; the lesion is classified as T2N0M0.

Figure 16–1. *B*, Intraoperative photo of the surgical excision required to treat this lesion. Operation is performed under local anesthesia. Note the mucosa of the lower lip that is held by the forceps. This mucosa will be advanced anteriorly and sutured to the intact skin of the lower lip. Also note the V-excision of the previous scar, mentioned in *A*.

Figure 16–1. *C*, Patient after the operation has been completed, with the mucosa advanced to the skin and sutured primarily. This operation is commonly referred to as a "lip shave." The excised specimen is shown directly below the suture line.

Figure 16–1. *D*, Patient 2 years later. The well-healed scar does not show any evidence of recurrent disease. There is some loss of tissue as indicated by the exposed lower teeth.

Figure 16–1. *E*, Patient 4 years postoperatively, with a leukoplakic patch on the buccal mucosa, just behind the right commissure. Because it was ulcerated and enlarging, it was totally excised. The microscopic report showed multifocal squamous carcinoma with adequate margins of resection.

Figure 16–1. *F*, Patient 2 years following resection of the buccal mucosa. Note the thinning of the vermilion border of the right upper lip.

Figure 16–1. *G*, The opening of the mouth is adequate for speech and mastication. The patient was followed regularly at yearly intervals for 15 years. He never developed regional nodes, although other leukoplakic spots on areas of the buccal mucosa did develop, none of which showed tumor on microscopic evaluation. The course of cancer of the lower lip in this patient is typical. There is a field of cancerization, possibly associated with smoking and other environmental carcinogens. Patients who have cancer of the lip rarely develop regional node metastases (less than 10 percent), and when they occur, they are almost always first palpated in the submental or submandibular area. If they develop, regional dissection is the method of choice. Currently, prophylactic x-ray therapy to the bilateral upper necks has been advocated by some groups.

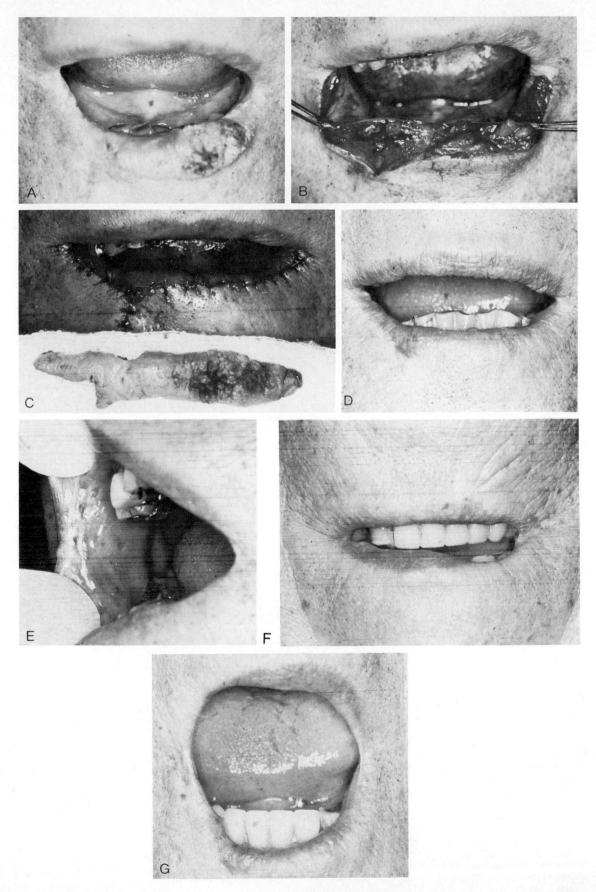

Figure 16–2. *A,* Squamous cell carcinoma of the floor of the mouth on the right side between the alveolar ridge and the side of the tongue. It measures approximately 3 cm × 2 cm, is moderately painful, and has been present for approximately 2 months. Microscopic examination showed squamous carcinoma. There are no palpable nodes in the neck. The patient is a nonsmoking female, with only minimal to moderate use of alcohol. The lesion is classified as a T3N0M0. The T3 classification is because the lesion extends over two adjacent structures, i.e., primarily the floor of the mouth, extending onto the alveolar ridge and onto the base of the tongue. The lower lip is retracted inferiorly, and the buccal mucosa is retracted to the patient's right. A stretched commissure of the lip can be seen at the left side of the photograph.

Figure 16–2. *B,* Treatment included resection of the side of the tongue, the complete lesion, and all the adjacent mandible, from the canine area to the mandible in continuity with a right radical neck dissection. The neck dissection was performed in the absence of palpable nodes because of the likelihood of cervical metastases from this type of lesion (greater than 40 percent) and because adequate surgical resection required dissection of the neck area to obtain adequate exposure. The postoperative study showed positive microscopic neck nodes in 3 of the 38 lymph nodes. Thus, the patient is classified as having clinically negative and microscopically positive neck.

Figure 16–2. *C,* Intraoperative photograph showing that the cheek has been opened like the page of a book and turned to the patient's right. The lip has been split in the midline. The neck dissection has been completed. A traction suture is placed on the side of the tongue (note the suture line extending up toward the tip of the nose). For closure, this side of the tongue will be sutured to the buccal mucosa.

Figure 16–2. *D* and *E,* Patient's appearance and function 2 years after surgical excision. Note that the neck has been irradiated as shown by the induration and discoloration. Note the skin incision *(D)* that extends from the midline of the symphysis of the chin to the midline of the lower lip. Because this patient had a T3 lesion with positive nodes, x-ray therapy was given in conjunction with the surgical resection. Note the excellent function: the patient does not drool, can open and close her mouth, has more than adequate use of the tongue, and has maintained her nutrition. This patient died 3 years following treatment with distant metastases to the cranium. This unusual site of metastases may have been related to the destruction of the lymphatics by the surgical operation or to the radiation therapy or both. The usual site of distant metastases of head and neck cancer is the lungs or liver or both.

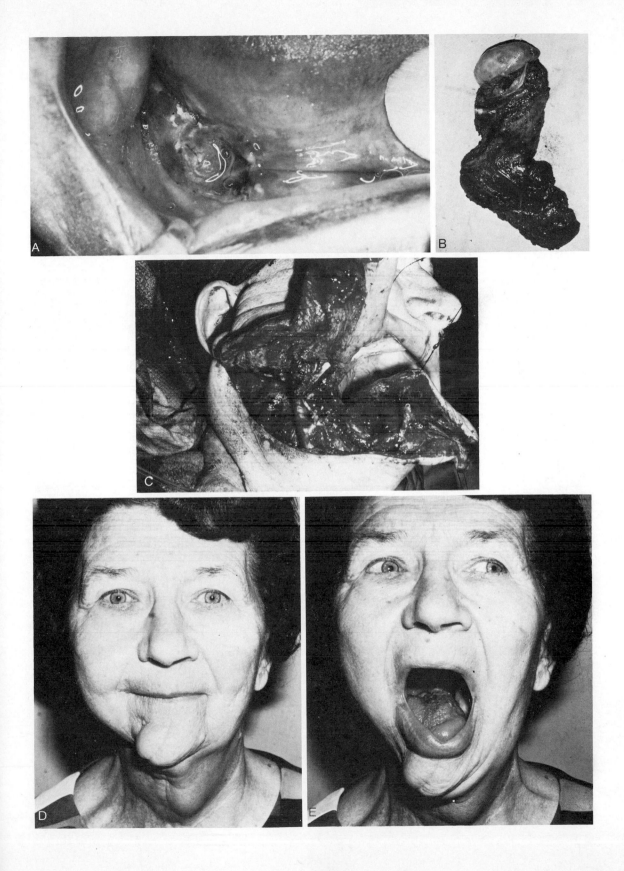

Figure 16–3. *A,* Looking into the mouth of a 52-year-old male who has had a history of squamous cell carcinoma of the left floor of the mouth that was treated with a full course of x-ray therapy one year previously. His chief complaint is a painful ulcer that is limiting his eating and sleeping. There is a strong history of alcohol intake and a moderate smoking history. The exquisite tenderness is characteristic of x-ray osteoradionecrosis of bone. The only treatment possible is resection of all the irradiated tissue. The purpose of the operation is primarily to get rid of the pain and secondarily to strive for cure of the recurrent cancer. There are no palpable nodes in the neck.

Figure 16–3. *B,* Intraoperative photograph showing the tongue and the left body of the mandible after the cheek flap has been moved to the left. Note the stitch on the tip of the tongue; the upper lip and the tip of the nose are visible in the upper middle part of the photograph. The entire body of the mandible from the symphysis back to the angle is exposed, and the recurrent tumor is seen as a small nubbin on the floor of the mouth by the side of the tongue (in the middle of the photograph).

Figure 16–3. *C,* Intraoperative photograph after resection of a block of mandible with the floor of the mouth and the side of the tongue. This was an adequate resection and included the entire recurrent tumor and the irradiated tissues.

Figure 16–3. *D,* A postoperative photograph one year later. Note the depression along the area to the left of the chin where the mandible was removed. Healing has occurred per primum in spite of the fact that the tissue had been heavily irradiated. Neither this patient nor the patient in Figure 16–2 had bone grafting, although replacement of the missing bone with either iliac or costal bone could have been done if the patients had desired it for functional or for cosmetic reasons.

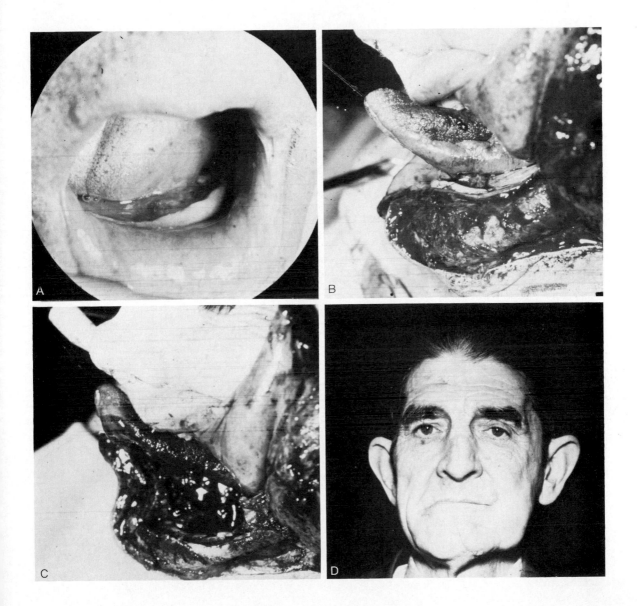

Figure 16–4. *A,* Location of a squamous carcinoma in the left tonsillar fossa. Note that it involves the left portion of the soft palate, the tonsillar fossa, the side of the tongue, and the retromolar space. There are no palpable nodes, and the lesion measures approximately 3 cm in diameter. On bimanual palpation, it has bulk that extends onto the medial aspect of the angle of the mandible.

Figure 16–4. *B,* Preoperative intraoral photograph showing the tumor in *A.* The retractor is on the dorsum of the tongue, and one can see the outline of the tumor near the middle of the photograph.

Figure 16–4. *C,* Operative specimen following radical neck dissection to remove all the draining lymph nodes on the left side of the neck, the excision of the body and ramus of the mandible, and the entire tumor. The tumor outlined in ink is facing us in the upper portion of the photograph to the left of the discolored tooth. There were no palpable nodes in the neck either pre- or postoperatively. This patient is thus classified as having a T3N0M0 lesion that was clinically and microscopically negative.

Figure 16–4. *D,* Intraoperative photograph showing the elevated large cheek flap. Note the orientation of the upper jaw with the maxilla and the palate exposed. The tongue is drawn forward in the lower left of the photograph and is dragged over the symphysis of the mandible. The huge defect is closed by sewing the side of the tongue to a buccal mucosal pedicle flap that is elevated during the same operation.

Figure 16–4. *E,* Patient several years later. He had not desired to have the mandibular deformity corrected. He could open his mouth widely and maintained his nutritional state. He died of a myocardial infarction 8 years after the resection without any sign of recurrent tumor. This type of tumor with positive nodes would have approximately a 5-year, 33-percent survival expectancy. With negative nodes, there is a 75 percent chance of a 5-year-survival period.

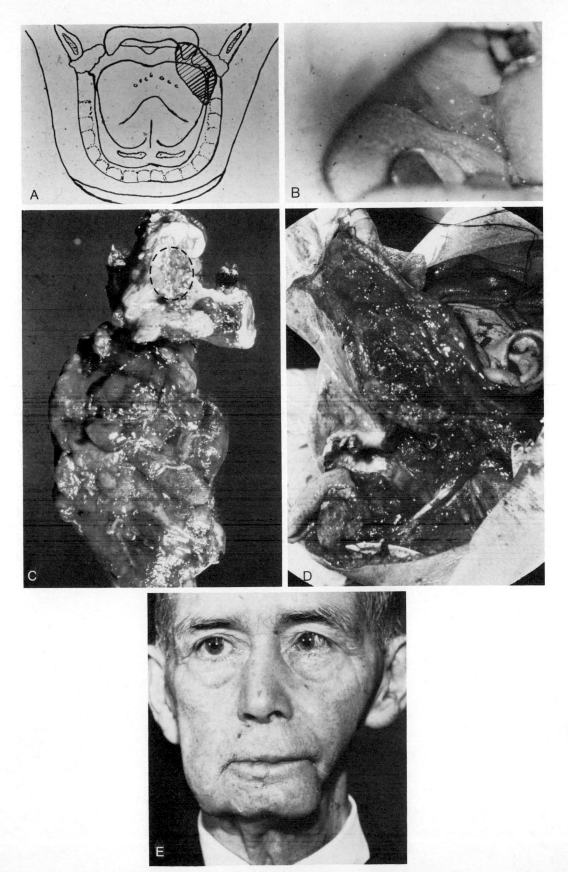

Figure 16–5. *A,* Intraoperative photograph of a resected squamous carcinoma of the left alveolar ridge. The surgical specimen is shown in lower part of photo. The patient complained of pain in the left temporal region and the simultaneous appearance of an ulcerated area in the left premolar region. He has no significant history of tobacco or alcohol usage, and his dental hygiene is satisfactory. There are no palpable nodes in this young, active businessman. The mandibular defect has been replaced by an iliac bone graft as shown in the upper portion of the figure.

Figure 16–5. *B,* The iliac bone graft wired solidly into position, replacing the missing mandible.

Figure 16–5. *C, D,* and *E,* Patient 2 years postoperatively, with normal function. The submandibular scar can be seen on the left lateral view *(E).* This was a T3N0M0 tumor treated in a one-stage procedure, with resection and immediate reconstruction. X-ray therapy was not indicated in this patient because of the proximity of the tumor to the bone. Chemotherapy was not required because of the total resection with adequate margins and the absence of nodes.

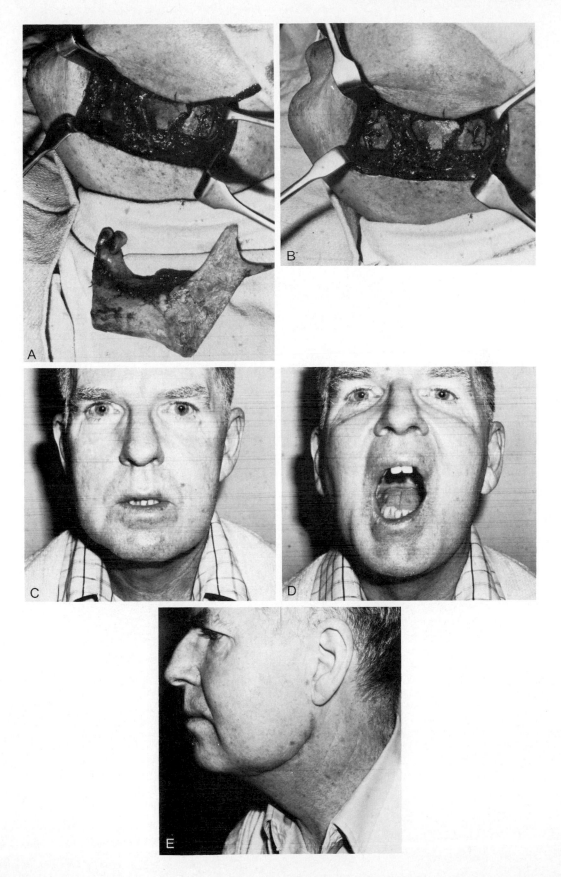

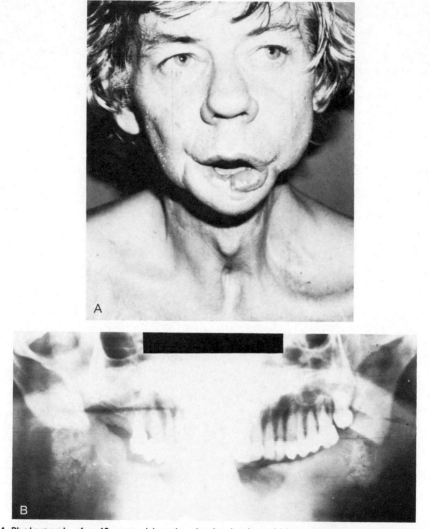

Figure 16–6. *A,* Photograph of a 48-year-old male who had a long history of chronic alcohol ingestion. He had had previous resection of squamous carcinoma of the anterior floor of the mouth, with neck dissection and pedicle flap coverage, at another institution. He presented with draining sinuses, which were possibly recurrent tumors, as well as drooling and the inability to eat satisfactorily.

Figure 16–6. *B,* Panoramic x-ray of the mandible, showing the extent of the resection required to control the lesion. One can see the resected rami just above the angles bilaterally. Following this resection, the external drainage healed and the patient was suitable for mandibular bone graft reconstruction. There was no evidence of tumor in the specimen.

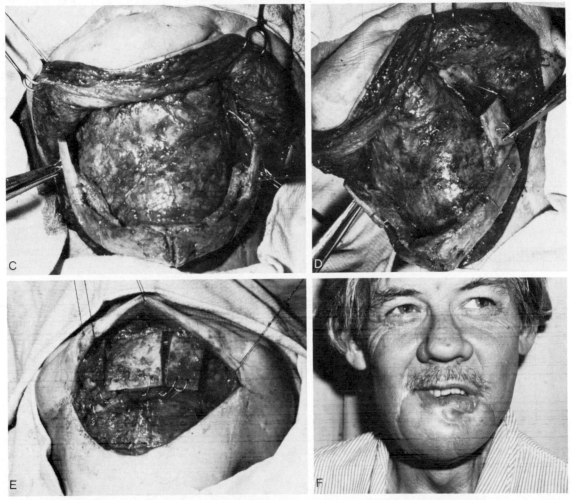

Figure 16–6. *C* and *D*, Total mandibular reconstruction, using fabricated iliac and costal bone. The new mandible is made by a combination of ribs and iliac fabricated to form a total mandible. *C*, The mandible is fitted into the right and left sides. We are looking at the patient head on; his lips and the oral cavity are at the top, middle portion of the photograph. *D*, The left side of the patient's neck. One can see the wires being placed in the left condyle and attached to the left condyle of the mandible.

Figure 16–6. *E*, One year following the initial bone graft, additional onlay bone graft was placed on the symphysis area to give support to the lower lip. One can see the osteotomized pieces of iliac bone wired onto the previously placed symphysis bone graft.

Figure 16–6. *F*, Patient one year following second bone grafting procedure. Note that he can control his saliva, he has a much more prominent chin point, and the overall reconstruction is satisfactory. Further revisions of the lower lip could have been performed if the patient had requested them. This is an example of reconstruction following surgical cure of a carcinoma of the floor of the mouth. Obviously, simultaneous correction of the deformity at the time of the curative resection of the tumor is preferable; however, in certain circumstances delayed reconstruction can be effective.

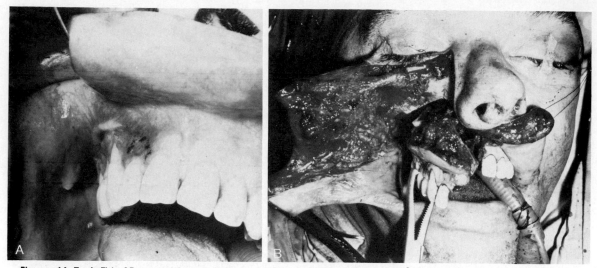

Figure 16–7. *A,* This 35-year-old male had a chronic ulcerating lesion of the right gingival, buccal sulcus for several months. The lesion extends through the alveolar bone and is visible on the palate (see the specimen in the lower portion of *C,* showing the palatal side with the ulcer directly behind both premolar teeth). Note the orifice of Stenson's duct in the right buccal mucosa. The upper lip is retracted superiorly, and one can see the fibrosity of the nostrils. This is a T3N0M0 tumor and as such can best be treated by surgical resection. X-ray therapy is not indicated because of the young age of the patient and because of the invasion of bone by the tumor.

Figure 16–7. *B,* Intraoperative photograph showing the resected portion of maxilla being held by bone forceps. The right cheek has been opened, as the page of a book, to the patient's right. In the lower portion of the cheek flap, the Stenson's duct is still present in its normal position. The osteotomy has gone through the maxilla and the maxillary antrum, removing the entire floor of the right antrum, leaving only the roof of the antrum, which is, of course, the floor of the right orbit. The infraorbital vessels on the right have been deliberately sacrificed and are included in the specimen.

Figure 16–7. *C,* Specimen is shown from the palatal side (upside down). In the maxillary area, we are looking directly into the exposed maxillary sinus.

Figure 16–7. *D,* A skin graft has been sutured to the area of the buccal flap that will be exposed intraorally. Note that the endotracheal tube is now resting superior to the dorsum of the tongue and inferior to the soft palate. The maxillary sinus is still obvious. This skin graft is held in place with an appropriate packing.

Figure 16–7. *E,* Intraoperative photograph several years later showing the well-healed skin graft and the lining of the maxillary sinus.

Figure 16–7. *F,* Postoperative view of the patient, with the prosthesis in place, shows that the scars in the right upper lip and along the side of the nose and the right lower eyelid are practically invisible. Three years following resection of the primary tumor, he developed a mass in the right midjugular area. This was considered a metastatic tumor and, as such, was treated, without microscopic biopsy, by a total neck dissection. The specimen showed 2 positive nodes out of 39 nodes. The patient has been free from disease during the past 9 years. This patient illustrates the need for prosthetic restoration in order to achieve optimal functional return. He also illustrates the vagaries of metastatic spread and the requirement of following patients indefinitely.

Figure 16–7. *G,* Maxillary prosthesis, available immediately following the surgical resection. A temporary prosthesis was used initially, and after several months and complete healing, a permanent prosthesis was constructed. Note that the clasps are attached to the normal teeth on the left side of the maxilla. The large ball of prosthetic material fits into the exposed antrum and gives solidity to the fixation of the prosthesis. The patient is able to eat and speak normally and to carry on his life as a salesman.

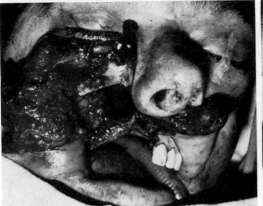

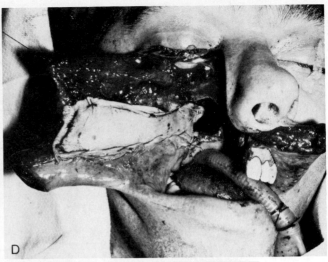

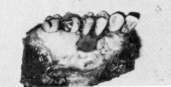

C

D

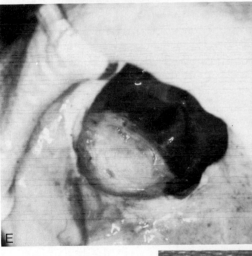

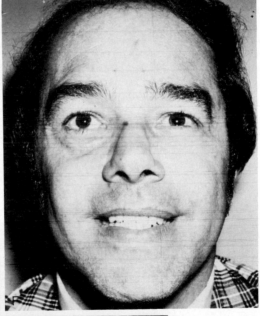

E

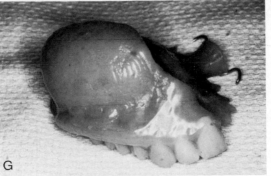

G

17

Basic principles of chemotherapy

DANIEL D. KARP, M.D.
THOMAS J. ERVIN, M.D.
EMIL FREI, III, M.D.

Since the original report by Goodman and associates in 1946 on the efficacy of nitrogen mustard in the treatment of lymphoma and Hodgkin's disease, the chemotherapy of cancer has progressed steadily and substantially.[26] Two years later, Farber reported temporary remissions in acute childhood leukemia produced by aminopterin.[21] This analog of the vitamin folic acid was later slightly modified to amethopterin (methotrexate) and is now an important agent in the chemotherapy armamentarium. During the 1950's, progress in biochemistry and molecular biology resulted in the fundamental understanding of the structure and function of DNA and the elucidation of the four key building blocks, adenine and guanine (purines) plus cytosine and thymidine (pyrimidines), which are assembled into long, double helical chains to produce the genetic and metabolic information required by all cells to divide. By making small changes or substitutions in these fundamental molecules, a new generation of agents, *the base and nucleoside antimetabolites,* was developed to initiate further gains in antitumor therapy. Another major step was taken with the alteration of the nitrogen mustard molecule to produce cyclophosphamide, which could be used in a variety of tumors both by mouth as well as by vein.

Beginning in the 1960's, taking advantage of the principles of infectious disease, in which it was established that multiple antibiotics could minimize the problems of drug resistance in treating serious infections, combination chemotherapy was initiated and resulted in major gains, so that for the first time, it became possible to produce high rates of response and *cures* in previously uniformly fatal illnesses such as disseminated Hodgkin's disease[15] and

acute leukemia.[35, 43] In the last decade, with the addition of the anthracycline family of drugs (Adriamycin and daunorubicin) and more recently the very useful *cis*-platinum, drug activity has been strengthened for a variety of tumors. Currently, there are approximately 30 agents that have been approved by the FDA for use against cancer as well as new and promising drugs in various stages of development and clinical evaluation. Survival rates are improving and despite an increase in incidence of cancer in the United States, cancer mortality rates for people younger than 45 years of age are diminishing.[19] Recent estimates indicate that 40,000 people were *cured* by chemotherapy in 1981,[23] and the list of diseases for which effective chemotherapy exists continues to grow (Table 17–1).

CHEMOTHERAPY SELECTIVITY

For a long time, it has been the goal of basic scientists and cancer chemotherapists to identify and exploit significant differences in the biology of the cancer cell in order to develop drugs and combinations of drugs that are more destructive to tumors than to normal host tissues. It has been more than 50 years since the original observations by Warburg that cancer cells have an increased production of lactic acid through accelerated glucose metabolism.[41] Recent experiments with rat hepatomas have shown several changes in key enzyme levels that occur as a cell is transformed from a normal liver cell to a malignant cell.[42] There is even a gradation of abnormalities as the tumor changes from being less malignant to more malignant. Clearly, cancer cells operate under different metabolic control (or lack of control)

166

Table 17-1. CANCER RESPONSES TO CHEMOTHERAPY

Cancers Curable by Chemotherapy	Cancers Probably Curable by Chemotherapy
Hodgkin's disease	Limited small cell CA lung
Acute lymphocytic leukemia	Acute myelogenous leukemia
Testicular cancer	Breast cancer, adjuvant setting
Diffuse histiocytic lymphoma	Osteogenic sarcoma, adjuvant setting
Gestational choriocarcinoma	
Wilms' tumor	
Ewing's sarcoma	
Embryonal rhabdomyosarcoma	
Burkitt's lymphoma	
Cancers in Which Life Prolonged by Chemotherapy	**Cancers Poorly Responsive to Chemotherapy**
Squamous cell carcinoma of head and neck	Renal
Ovarian carcinoma	Colorectal
Cervix (squamous cell carcinoma)	Pancreas
Soft-tissue sarcomas	Gastric
Chronic leukemias	Melanoma
Non-Hodgkin's lymphomas	

than do normal cells. Although chemotherapy is relatively selective and curative against Hodgkin's disease, choriocarcinoma, and testicular cancer, many other tumors such as squamous cell carcinoma of the head and neck have been less sensitive. Because cancer drugs are toxic to both normal and cancerous cells, successful chemotherapy requires both the exploitation of subtle differences such as cancer cell growth kinetics and careful attention to the pharmacology of the drugs.

Using the experimental L1210 murine leukemia model, Skipper established many of the principles that form the basis of modern cancer chemotherapy.[40] They have shown that drugs kill by first order kinetics, that is, that a given dose of drug will kill a constant fraction of cells, *not* a constant number regardless of the number of cells present at the time of therapy. This means that it would require the same amount of therapy to reduce a 1-kg tumor from 10^{12} to 10^{10} cells as it would to shrink a microscopic tumor that contains 10^5 cells down to 10^3 cells. A nodule 1 cm in diameter contains approximately 10^9 cells and is at the lower limit of clinical detectability. Skipper has also shown that the survival rate of an animal is inversely related to the number of cells inoculated or remaining after chemotherapy and that a single cancer cell capable of clonal multiplication will eventually kill the host animal. Consequently, chemotherapy must be continued for a long time after the tumor has become clinically undetectable and the patient has gone into remission if cures are to be accomplished.

If cancer cells simply "grew" much faster than normal tissue constituents, a cytokinetic attack would be easier. In the early stages of the growth of experimental tumors, cells grow in an exponential manner. As the size of the tumor increases, however, the time that is required for it to double its volume also increases. This happens for several reasons:

1. The number of cells that participate in division, the growth fraction, decreases. This is the most important factor.

2. The time for cell division becomes prolonged.

3. There is an increase in cellular losses due to the decreased vascular supply, loss of nutritional components, and local accumulation of metabolic waste products.

Tumor growth, therefore, follows a Gompertzian curve that is characterized by an initial rapid growth rate, followed by a slowing of the growth rate as the tumor burden increases (Fig. 17–1).[32] Many normal tissues such as bone marrow, gastrointestinal mucosa, and hair follicles actually grow faster than solid tumors. Therefore, agents that destroy rapidly growing cells will have these three areas as major sites of toxicity. Such toxicity must be taken into account in devising active and tolerable treatment programs. As a result, many solid tumors may have a very low proliferative thrust, with less than 5 percent of the total cell population engaging in active cell replication (Fig. 17–2), whereas a high proportion of cells in the bone marrow or gastrointestinal tract may be in the process of dividing. This makes the selection of therapy against certain types of tumors especially difficult and requires careful insight into cell kinetics and drug dosage for improved results of treatment.

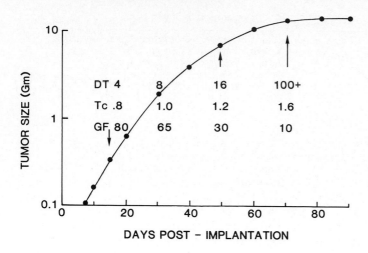

Figure 17–1. Tumor growth rate.

DOSE-RESPONSE RELATIONSHIPS

There is extensive experimental evidence that indicates a clear relationship between the dose of chemotherapy given and the antitumor effect. When the optimal dose of the folic acid antagonist methotrexate is reduced by half in the L1210 leukemia model, there is only a 25 percent antitumor effect.[25] On the other hand, when the optimal dose of medication is increased, animal survival rates decrease because of increased toxicity to normal tissues. The existence of a steep dose-response curve for many of the chemotherapeutic agents supports the generalization that patients receive the maximum amount of medication that is consistent with acceptable reversible toxicity. When more conservative dose schedules are maintained or when chemotherapy is designed to minimize the side effects of the drugs, the

response rates in general have suffered substantially. Recently, Bonadonna and Valagussa studied the use of combination chemotherapy in women who had undergone mastectomy for breast cancer.[11] It has been well established that patients in whom there has been metastatic spread to the axillary lymph nodes are at high risk for recurrent disease. The chemotherapy given in the adjuvant situation is designed to prevent tumor recurrence. Those patients who received less than 75 percent of the prescribed dose of cyclophosphamide, methotrexate, and fluorouracil (CMF) had a markedly decreased relapse-free survival. Using Adriamycin for adjuvant treatment of the malignant bone tumor, osteogenic sarcoma, Cortes and Holland[14] showed major benefits at doses greater than 75 mg/m². For those who received less than 75 percent of that dose, however, the success rate

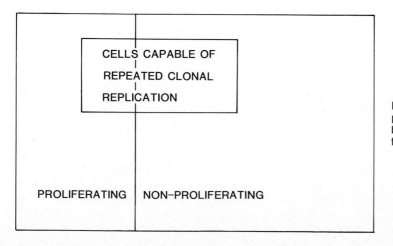

Figure 17–2. Potential tumor cell compartments within a tumor, indicating both proliferative and nonproliferative cell populations.

was markedly reduced. Although these two studies were retrospective, the dose rate is one of the most important factors that influences success and ultimately the curative potential for cancer chemotherapy.[22]

CELL KINETICS AND THE CELL CYCLE

Cells that are multiplying either to produce tissue growth or to replace cellular losses synthesize DNA and go through a series of phases known as the cell cycle. The cell cycle is defined as the interval between mitoses (the intermitotic or generation time).[3] A broader definition would include these cellular and biochemical aspects that regulate and maintain cell growth. Both tumors and normal cells consist of three populations:

1. Continually dividing cells that are actively going through the cell cycle.

2. Cells that leave the cell cycle and differentiate into mature end-stage cells. Examples of these are the polymorphonuclear white blood cell or the mature keratinized squamous cell. These end-stage cells must be replaced by the offspring of existing "stem" cells.

3. Cells that leave the cell cycle to become dormant, resting cells. These cells can be recruited into growth and re-enter the cycle if necessary.[13]

The growth of any tissue depends upon the length of the cell cycle time, the fraction of cells undergoing active growth in cell cycle activity, and the rate of spontaneous cell loss due to cellular maturation or cell death. The phases of the cell cycle are labeled M, G1, S, and G2 (Fig. 17–3).

CANCER CHEMOTHERAPEUTIC AGENTS

There are several classes of cancer chemotherapeutic agents[12] including antimetabolites, alkylating agents, antitumor antibiotics, antimitotic agents, hormones, and miscellaneous compounds. These agents, their toxicities, and the tumors for which they have established usefulness are outlined in Table 17–2. In this section, the general features of these agents will be discussed, highlighting those agents that have particular usefulness against cancers of the oral cavity and oropharynx. In Figure 17–4, the major site of action of these drugs is shown.

Antimetabolites

For the most part, antimetabolites are drugs that bear a strong chemical resemblance to the normal metabolites or cofactors required for nucleic acid synthesis. They enter normal syn-

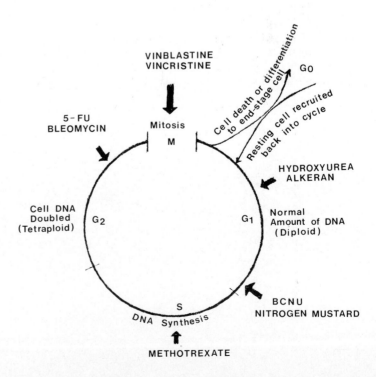

Figure 17–3. The cell cycle and sites of action of selected drug activity.

Table 17–2. GUIDE TO CURRENT CHEMOTHERAPY DRUGS

Type	Family	Drugs	Route of Administration	Mechanism of Action	Malignancies Treated
Alkylating agents	Nitrogen mustards	Mechlorethamine (HN$_2$)	IV	Alkylation of DNA primarily by linking guanine base pairs, inhibiting DNA replication. Phase–nonspecific.	Hodgkin's disease, lymphoma
		Cyclophosphamide (cyclo)	IV, PO		Acute and chronic lymphocytic leukemia, breast, lung, Hodgkin's disease myeloma, lymphoma, sarcoma, cervix, Ewing's sarcoma
		Chlorambucil	PO		Chronic lymph-leukemia, ovary, Hodgkin's disease, lymphoma
		Melphalan (L-PAM)	PO		Breast, myeloma, ovary, testis
	Nitrosoureas	Carmustine (BCNU)	IV	Alkylation and carbamylation. Phase–nonspecific.	Brain tumors, colon, gastric, lymphoma
		Lomustine (CCNU)	PO		Brain, lung, colon, Hodgkin's disease
		Semustine (MeCCNU)	PO		Brain, colon, gastric melanoma, Hodgkin's disease
	Triazenes	Dacarbazine (DTIC)	IV	Inhibition of purine, RNA and protein synthesis. Moderate alkylation. Prolongs G$_1$ and G$_2$.	Hodgkin's disease, melanoma, sarcoma
Anti-metabolites	Folic acid analogs	Methotrexate (MTX)	IV, PO	Inhibits dihydrofoliate reductase, restricting available active foliate needed for DNA and RNA synthesis. S phase–specific.	Acute lymphocytic leukemia, head and neck cancer, breast, lung, choriocarcinoma, mycosis fungoides, testis, cervix

	Drug	Route	Mechanism	Indications
Pyrimidine analogs	Fluorouracil (5-FU)	IV, topical	Blocks thymidylic acid synthesis and is incorporated into RNA. S phase–specific.	Breast, colon, gastric, hepatoma, ovary, pancreas, cervix, skin (topically)
	Cytosine Arabinoside (ARA-C)	IV, SC	Incorporation into DNA with early chain termination. S phase–specific. Blocks progression from G_1 to S.	Acute leukemia
Purine analogs	Mercaptopurine (6-MP)	PO	Inhibits adenine and guanine synthesis. S phase-specific.	Acute leukemia, chronic granulocytic leukemia
	6-Thioguanine (6-TG)	PO	Substitutes for guanine, causing defective nucleotides. S phase-specific.	Acute leukemia
Naturally occurring agents				
Vinca Alkyloids	Vinblastine (VLB)	IV	Mitotic arrest by inhibition of microtubule assembly. M phase-specific.	Breast, testis, Hodgkin's disease, lymphoma
	Vincristine (VCR)	IV		Acute lymphocytic leukemia, breast, Hodgkin's disease, lung
Anthra-cyclines	Adriamycin (ADR)	IV	DNA intercalation; free radical formation. Phase–nonspecific, but greater efficacy in S phase.	Acute leukemia, bladder, breast, lung, endometrial Ewing's sarcoma, Hodgkin's disease, lymphoma sarcoma, prostate, head and neck, thyroid, testis
	Daunorubicin (DNR)	IV		Acute leukemia
Antibiotics	Actinomycin-D (ACT-D)	IV	DNA intercalation: cycle nonspecific.	Choriocarcinoma, sarcoma, testis, Wilms' tumor
	Bleomycin (BLEO)	IV, SC, intracavitary	DNA scission and inhibition of repair. G_2 phase–specific.	Hodgkin's disease, lymphoma, penile cancer, head and neck, testis, cervix

Table continued on following page

Table 17–2. GUIDE TO CURRENT CHEMOTHERAPY DRUGS (*Continued*)

Type	Family	Drugs	Route of Administration	Mechanism of Action	Malignancies Treated
Miscellaneous agents	Platinum coordination complexes	Cisplatin (cis DDP)	IV	Alkylation and DNA cross-linking by binding to guanine residue. Phase–nonspecific, but G_1 most sensitive.	Bladder, head and neck cancer, lung, ovary, testis, cervix
	Substituted urea	Hydroxyurea (HU)	PO	Inhibits DNA synthesis. S phase–specific.	Acute leukemia, chronic granulocytic leukemia
	Methyl hydrazine	Procarbazine		Free radical formation, similar to radiation cycle. Phase–nonspecific.	Brain tumors, Hodgkin's disease, lymphoma
Hormones	Adrenal steroids	Prednisone	IV, PO	Inhibition of lymphoid proliferation, binds with steroid receptors.	Lymphoma, lymphocytic leukemia, breast, myeloma
		Estrogens	IV, PO	Binds to hormone receptors	Breast, prostate

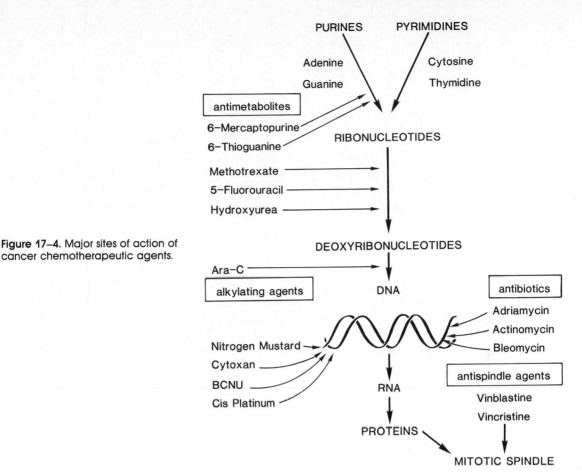

Figure 17–4. Major sites of action of cancer chemotherapeutic agents.

thetic pathways and by their incorporation produce false building blocks. Alternatively, they may compete for normal enzyme binding sites and may inhibit key synthetic processes. These drugs generally will produce both bone marrow and gastrointestinal toxicity.

Methotrexate. This drug is an analog of folic acid and has extremely high binding affinity for the enzyme dihydrofolate reductase, which is responsible for activating folic acid, which is essential for DNA synthesis. Its side effects can successfully be prevented by 5-formyl-tetrahydrofolic acid (leucovorin) when given within 24 hours of the administration of the drug.[7] Methotrexate is excreted by the kidney and may cause kidney damage when given in high doses.[8] As a single agent, it can be used as treatment for squamous cell carcinoma of the head and neck and will produce frequent but short-lived responses in 50 percent of the patients.[28]

5-Fluorouracil (5-FU). This fluorinated pyrimidine inhibits thymidylic acid synthetase and is incorporated into RNA. This drug is given intravenously and may cause mucositis, dizziness, and ataxia.[29] It has widespread use, especially against breast cancer and tumors of gastrointestinal origin.[33]

Cytosine Arabinoside (ARA-C). This antimetabolite is produced by making a substitution on the sugar moiety of the cytosine nucleoside. ARA-C is incorporated into DNA, slowing DNA synthesis, antagonizing DNA polymerase, and producing early chain termination.[31] It is rapidly inactivated by the liver and other organs by deamination. It is used primarily in cases of acute leukemia. It can be given either subcutaneously or intravenously, but its very short plasma survival requires that it be given over prolonged periods of time or in large intermittent doses.

Alkylating Agents

These drugs achieve their effects by damaging DNA. They substitute alkyl groups on the nucleophilic sites of many organic compounds. In particular, they bind to adjacent guanine residues of the DNA helix causing DNA cross-linking. This class of agents is non–cell-cycle specific. Their major toxicity is bone marrow suppression resulting in cumulative decreases in bone marrow stem cells with prolonged treatment.

Cyclophosphamide. A derivative of nitrogen mustard was originally devised to make use of the observation that many tumors contained increased phosphoramidase activity. It was hoped that the cleavage of the cyclophosphamide molecule by tumor enzymes would release the mustard compound, thereby producing selective tumor toxicity. This was proved not to be the case. Nevertheless, cyclophosphamide is active against a broad spectrum of tumors. This drug is inactive until metabolized by the liver microsomal enzyme system and then is excreted by the kidneys. If cyclophosphamide metabolites remain in the bladder for a prolonged period of time, bladder irritation (sterile cystitis) may occur. Therefore, patients must maintain a high volume of urine flow while receiving this drug.

Bis-Chloronitrosourea (BCNU). This is one of three commonly used nitrosourea compounds.[16] This fat soluble agent is administered intravenously and is active against several neoplasms. Because of its lipid solubility, it will cross the blood brain barrier and is effective in brain tumors.[17]

Antibiotics

Antibiotics are produced in large part by Streptomyces fungi and have diverse chemical structures and activity. As with most antibiotics, allergic or anaphylactoid reactions may occur.

Adriamycin and Daunorubicin. These four-ringed anthracyclines are similar in chemical structures to certain dyes and as such have a red-orange color and a natural fluorescence. They intercalate between nucleotides in the DNA helix and, therefore, interfere with DNA replication.[5] They also seem to act by generating oxygen free radicals.[2, 3] The anthracyclines are non–cell-cycle specific but have increased activity against rapidly dividing cells. They are among the most active of the cancer chemotherapeutic agents with a broad range of efficacy. Toxicity to both the gastrointestinal tract and the bone marrow is the limiting factor in drug dosage. These drugs are given by vein and must be infused with care, because skin or subcutaneous necrosis may occur with extravasation.

Bleomycin. This drug is composed of a family of compounds that were discovered in Japan. It is notable for pulmonary fibrosis and for an absence of bone marrow suppression.[9] It also causes harmless skin pigmentation and rare instances of severe allergic anaphylactoid reactions. This drug may be given subcutaneously or by vein and will often cause transient fever during its administration. Pulmonary toxicity is more frequent in elderly patients, in patients who have severe existing pulmonary disease, and in patients who are receiving a cumulative dose of more than 300 units.[6] Pulmonary toxicity may be exacerbated by inspired oxygen concentrations greater than 25 percent for any prolonged period. Therefore, during surgery, patients who have received substantial doses of bleomycin will need special attention to their oxygen demands during anesthesia.

Antimitotic Agents

These *Vinca rosea* plant derivatives are large complex alkaloids that inhibit the formation of the mitotic spindle apparatus, which is critical for cellular mitosis. Their pharmacology has been reviewed extensively.[30]

Vinblastine. This agent is an intravenous preparation whose major toxicity is bone marrow suppression. It will cause severe skin irritation if it is injected outside the vein. This drug is especially useful in treating lymphomas and testis cancer, in addition to head and neck cancer.

Vincristine. This drug differs very little structurally from vinblastine but has a minimum of bone marrow toxicity. Its major side effects are damage to the peripheral nerves with numbness and tingling (paresthesia) of the distal extremities after several doses of the drug have been given. Because of its absence of bone marrow toxicity, it has been used with great success in combination with other marrow toxic drugs to treat a variety of common tumors such as lymphoma, leukemia, breast cancer, and lung cancer.

Miscellaneous Agents

***Cis*-diaminedichloroplatinum (II).** This compound is administered intravenously and is especially useful in testis cancer, ovarian cancer, and squamous cell carcinoma of the head and neck.[34] It has alkylating properties, but unlike many other alkylating agents, its bone marrow toxicity is not severe.[44] Its major side effect is nausea and vomiting during the administration of the drug, often resulting in the need for aggressive antiemetic therapy for patient comfort. Because of its platinum constituent, it may cause kidney damage similar to heavy metal poisoning. Care must be taken to ensure high rates of urine flow to keep the concentration of drug low in the kidney tubules.[44]

TOXICITY OF CHEMOTHERAPY

Gastrointestinal. Gastrointestinal discomfort and mucosal irritation are dose limiting and are predictable for many drugs, particularly the antimetaboles such as ARA-C, fluorouracil, and methotrexate. The anthracyclines and actinomycin will produce severe oral ulceration when there has been previous radiation to the head and neck area, the so-called "radiation recall" phenomenon. Nausea and vomiting are usually well controlled by the administration of antiemetics.[36] Cis-platinum, Adriamycin, actinomycin D, and cyclophosphamide may all cause severe nausea and vomiting. Newer antiemetics such as metoclopramide and tetrahydrocannabinol have been developed and seem promising in controlling this side effect.[37] Diarrhea may result from agents such as 5-fluorouracil and ARA-C, and vincristine may cause constipation.

Bone Marrow. Bone marrow toxicity (myelosuppression) is commonly seen with the alkylating agents, many of the antitumor antibiotics, and the antimetabolites. Most effective chemotherapy programs will result in a reversible lowering of both the white blood count and platelet count, which may result in fever, infection, or bleeding complications. The blood counts of patients must be monitored frequently during the administration of chemotherapy so that drug dosages can be modified appropriately and complications can be avoided. In addition, the nadir of the blood counts serves as a reference point for the adequacy of chemotherapy. If drugs that are known to be myelosuppressive are given and if the blood counts do not fall to a certain level, it may be assumed that the dose of medication was suboptimal. By carefully monitoring blood counts, both the adequacy of chemotherapy and the safety of treatment can be assured.

Alopecia. Cyclophosphamide and the anthracycline agents are most frequently associated with alopecia, although other alkylating agents and antimetabolites may, to varying degrees, cause hair loss. It is almost always a reversible process. In attempts to prevent hair loss, scalp tourniquets and ice caps to decrease blood flow and drug delivery to the hair follicles have been tried but have been of limited value.

Cardiac Toxicity. When given over a prolonged period of time, the anthracycline agents will cause damage to the heart muscle. Patients who receive more than 450 mg/m^2 total dose of Adriamycin in intermittent doses are at increased risk for cardiac compromise.[27]

Pulmonary Toxicity. Bleomycin, which will produce harmless darkening of the skin in half the patients in whom it is used, will also produce pulmonary fibrosis in many patients who receive more than 200 mg/m^2.[39] The lung damage is cumulative and may be particularly hazardous in those patients who have preexisting emphysema or chronic bronchitis. Methotrexate may rarely cause "allergic" pulmonary infiltrates, which resolve quickly with discontinuation of the drug.

Genitourinary. Drugs may directly injure the kidney tubules and impair kidney function. Methotrexate is excreted by the kidneys and when given in conventional doses is quite safe. When given in very high doses, however, it may crystallize in the renal tubule with resulting renal dysfunction unless great care is given to fluid administration and adequate urinary output is maintained. Cis-platinum acts in the same way as other heavy metals in causing kidney tubule damage. It must be given with large amounts of saline intravenously to dilute the drug in the renal tubule and to prevent toxicity.

Bladder irritation will be produced by cyclophosphamide metabolites if the drug is allowed to remain exposed to the bladder lining for prolonged periods of time. By maintaining high rates of urine flow, this toxicity may be prevented.

STRATEGIES FOR CHEMOTHERAPY

Based upon cytokinetic principles and other factors, it is apparent that tumors that are small and, therefore, rapidly doubling should be most sensitive to chemotherapy,[10] and for most solid tumors, it is imperative that one not wait until the tumor has become bulky with a low growth fraction if any gains are to be made. The theoretic effect of drug scheduling on antitumor response is diagrammed in Figure 17–5. It is important that there be a continuous downward trend in the tumor

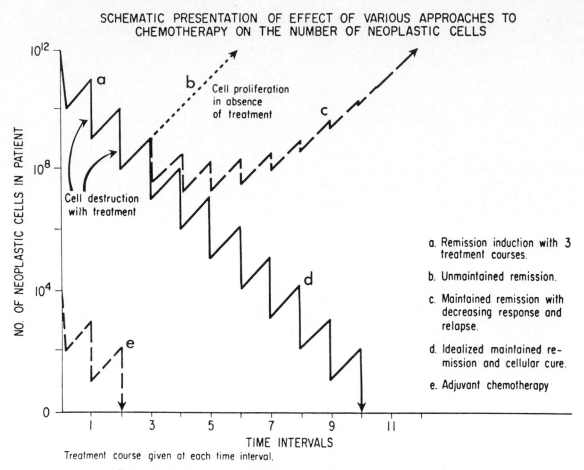

SCHEMATIC PRESENTATION OF EFFECT OF VARIOUS APPROACHES TO CHEMOTHERAPY ON THE NUMBER OF NEOPLASTIC CELLS

Cell proliferation in absence of treatment

Cell destruction with treatment

a. Remission induction with 3 treatment courses.

b. Unmaintained remission.

c. Maintained remission with decreasing response and relapse.

d. Idealized maintained remission and cellular cure.

e. Adjuvant chemotherapy

NO. OF NEOPLASTIC CELLS IN PATIENT

TIME INTERVALS

Treatment course given at each time interval.

Figure 17–5. Theoretic effect of drug scheduling on antitumor response.

growth pattern, a so-called "saw tooth downward pattern." The effectiveness of chemotherapy depends upon both tight scheduling and the delivery of optimal doses of drug. When effective drugs are given, response and survival rates may be adversely affected. Any strategy that allows drugs to be given in larger concentration (as in direct perfusion into a tumor) or at more frequent intervals (such as using drugs whose action can be reversed, for example, methotrexate) may contribute to higher rates of tumor regression.

Whenever possible, one should use a combination of drugs that is active against a given tumor but whose mechanism of action and resulting toxicity is different in order to deliver full drug doses with side effects that are tolerable for the patient. A characteristic example is the combination chemotherapy of Hodgkin's disease.[18] With a combination of drugs that includes nitrogen mustard, vincristine, prednisone, and procarbazine, it is possible to obtain a 50 percent cure rate, even in cases of

advanced Hodgkin's disease. All these drugs have different mechanisms of action and differing side effects that are spread among various organ systems to allow better tolerance by the host. Another example is the combination platinum, bleomycin, and methotrexate that is used in head and neck cancer.[20] The major toxicity of platinum results in kidney damage, bleomycin causes damage to the skin and lungs, and methotrexate is toxic to the gastrointestinal tract and bone marrow. However, when followed by leukovorin rescue, methotrexate has minimal cross toxicity with the other agents. When given in a coordinated manner, these drugs will produce high response rates.

The use of combinations of agents has other advantages.[10] In the same way that bacteria can become resistant to antibiotics, cancer cells can develop resistance to chemotherapeutic agents, whereas normal tissues, rarely, if ever, become tolerant to the toxicity of the drugs. This means that by using multiple agents simultaneously or switching to new active agents after several effective cycles of drug administration, it may be possible to minimize the emergence of resistant clones of cells. Pharmacologic approaches to improving drug action and safety are important. Thus, with methotrexate, optimizing plasma concentration time ($C \times T$) may allow for tumor kill while avoiding side effects.

On the other hand, there are a variety of factors that limit drug selectivity or that compromise chemotherapy success. Certain tumor types are especially resistant to conventional approaches. To date, malignant melanoma and renal cancer have been particularly difficult in this regard. Pre-existing comorbid conditions such as kidney or liver disease or chronic lung or cardiac conditions are significant limitations in the delivery of certain drugs, and it is important to choose agents that do not produce additional toxicity. One such example is bleomycin, which may result in pulmonary scarring if used in patients with severely impaired pulmonary function. Patients who have had previous pulmonary disease will be much less able to tolerate this drug than those who have not had pulmonary compromise. Factors of drug absorption and excretion are of critical importance in devising effective therapy. Certain agents, such as 5-fluorouracil, are inconsistently absorbed from the gastrointestinal tract, and for this reason, intravenous chemotherapy is essential to achieve reproducible effects.[1] Other drugs, such as cyclophosphamide, must be metabolized to their active form, and if liver damage exists, drug metabolism may severely be impaired, with resulting decreased antitumor effects. Alternatively, lack of metabolism of other agents, such as Adriamycin will increase plasma concentrations of active drug metabolite, will decrease the excretion of active drug, and will increase patient toxicity. Finally, many drug interactions may occur that will potentiate the side effects of a given chemotherapeutic agent, for example, the concomitant use of allopurinol, a drug used to treat gout and lower uric acid, and the antimetabolite 6-mercaptopurine. Allopurinol will decrease the breakdown of 6-mercaptopurine, thereby allowing an increased effect from the drug as well as an increase in the bone marrow toxicity of the patient.

PROSPECTS FOR THE FUTURE

Current research is directed toward making better use of existing cancer chemotherapy agents in addition to developing new or specific drugs. Improved dosage monitoring with direct drug levels will be an important advance for many agents. New devices such as implantable pumps will allow continuous infusions of drugs, which will result in constant exposure of effective agents against tumors that have low growth fractions.[1] Finally, new insights into the biology of cancer cells as well as improved ability to grow tumors in tissue culture will aid in the development of predictive tests similar to those already available for antibiotics to determine which agents or combinations of agents may be most effective against a given tumor. These specialized assay systems hold great promise for the improvement of chemotherapy.[25]

REFERENCES

1. Ansfield, F., Klotz, J., Nealon, T., et al.: A phase III study comparing the clinical utility of four regimens of 5-fluorouracil: a preliminary report. Cancer, *39*:34, 1977.
2. Bachur, N. R.: Anthracycline antibiotics, pharmacology, and metabolism. Cancer Treat. Rep., *43*:817, 1979.
3. Bachur, N. R., Gordon, S. L., and Gee, M. V.: A general mechanism for microsomal activation of quinone anticancer agents to free radicals. Cancer Res., *38*:1745, 1978.
4. Baserga, R.: The cell cycle. N. Engl. J. Med., *304*:453, 1981.
5. Benjamin, R. S., Riggs, C. E., and Bachur, N. R.: Pharmacokinetics and metabolism with Adriamycin in man. Clin. Pharmacol. Ther., *14*:592, 1973.
6. Bennett, J. M., and Reich, S. D.: Bleomycin. Ann. Intern. Med., *90*:945, 1979.
7. Bertino, J. R.: "Rescue" techniques in cancer chemotherapy. Use of leucovorin and other rescue agents after methotrexate treatment. Semin. Oncol., *4*:203, 1977.
8. Bertino, J. R.: Toward improved selectivity in cancer chemotherapy. Cancer Res., *39*:293, 1979.
9. Blum, R. H., Carter, S. K., and Agre, K.: A clinical review of bleomycin, a new antineoplastic agent. Cancer, *31*:903, 1973.
10. Blum, R. H., and Frei, E., III: Combination chemotherapy. *In* Methods in Cancer Research, Vol. XVII, Chapter 6. New York, Academic Press, Inc., 1979, p. 215.
11. Bonadonna, G., and Valagussa, P.: Dose response effect of adjuvant chemotherapy in breast cancer. N. Engl. J. Med., *304*:10, 1981.
12. Calabresi, P., and Parks, R. E.: Chemotherapy of neoplastic disease. *In* Gilman, A. G., Goodman, L. S., and Gilman, A. (eds.): The Pharmacological Basis of Therapeutics, 6th ed. New York, Macmillan, Inc., 1980.
13. Carter, S. K., and Livingston, R.: Principles of cancer chemotherapy. *In* Carter, S. K., Glatstein, E., and Livingston, R. (eds.): Principles of Cancer Treatment. New York, McGraw-Hill, Inc., 1981, p. 15.
14. Cortes, E., and Holland, J. F.: Adjuvant treatment of primary osteogenic sarcoma. *In* Bonadonna, G.,

Mathe, G., and Salmon, G. (eds.): Recent Results in Cancer Research, Vol. 68. New York, Springer-Verlag New York, Inc., 1979, p. 16.

15. DeVita, V. T., Jr.: The consequences of chemotherapy of Hodgkin's disease. Cancer, 47:1, 1981.

16. DeVita, V. T., Carbone, P. P., Owens, A. H., Jr., et al.: Clinical trials with BCNU. Cancer Res., 25:1876, 1965.

17. DeVita, V. T., Denham, C., Davidson, J. D., et al.: The physiological disposition of the carcinostatic BCNU in man and animals. Clin. Pharmacol. Ther., 8:566, 1967.

18. DeVita, V. T., Jr., Serpick, A. A., and Carbone, P. P.: Combination chemotherapy in the treatment of advanced Hodgkin's disease. Ann. Intern. Med., 73:891, 1970.

19. DeVita, V. T., Jr.: Personal communication.

20. Ervin, T. J., Weichselbaum, R. R., Miller, D., et al.: Treatment of advanced squamous cell carcinoma of the head and neck with cis-platinum, bleomycin, and methotrexate (P-B-M). Cancer Treat. Rep., 65:787, 1981.

21. Farber, S., Diamond, L. K., Mercer, R. D., et al.: Temporary remissions in acute leukemia in children produced by folic antagonist amethopteroylglutamic acid (aminopterin). N. Engl. J. Med., 238:787, 1948.

22. Frei, E., III, and Canellos, G. P.: Dose: a critical factor in cancer chemotherapy. Am. J. Med., 69:585, 1980.

23. Frei, E., III: The national cancer chemotherapy program. Science, 217:600, 1982.

24. Garnick, M. B., Weiss, G., Steele, G., et al.: A phase I trial of long term continuous Adriamycin administration. Proc. Am. Soc. Clin. Oncol., 22:106, 1981.

25. Goldin, A., Vendetti, J. M., and Mantel, N.: Preclinical screening and evaluation of agents for the chemotherapy of cancer: a review. Cancer Res., 21:1334, 1961.

26. Goodman, L. S., Wintrobe, M. M., Dameshek, W., et al.: Nitrogen mustard therapy: use of methyl bis (beta-chloroethyl) amino hydrochloride for Hodgkin's disease, lymphosarcoma, leukemia, and certain allied and miscellaneous disorders. J.A.M.A., 132:126, 1946.

27. Henderson, I. C., and Frei, E., III: Adriamycin cardiotoxicity. Am. Heart J., 99:671, 1980.

28. Hong, W. K.: Chemotherapy for advanced head and neck carcinoma. Clin. Cancer Briefs, 3:3, 1982.

29. Horton, J., Olson, K. B., Sullivan, J., et al.: 5-Fluorouracil in cancer: an improved regimen. Ann. Intern. Med., 73:897, 1970.

30. Johnson, I. S., Armstrong, J. G., Gorman, M., et al.: The vinca alkaloids: a new class of oncolytic agents. Cancer Res., 23:1390, 1963.

31. Kufe, D. W., Major, P. T., Egan, E. M., et al.: Correlation of cytotoxicity with incorporation of ARA-C into DNA. J. Biol. Chem., 255:8997, 1980.

32. McCredie, J. A., Inch, W. R., Kruuv, J., et al.: The rate of tumor growth in animals. Growth, 29:331, 1965.

33. Moore, G. E., Bross, I. D., Ausmans, R., et al.: Effects of 5-fluorouracil in 389 patients with cancer. Cancer Chemother. Rep., 52:641, 1968.

34. Prestayko, A. W., Crooke, S. T., and Carter, S. K. (eds.): Cisplatin: Current Status and New Developments. New York, Academic Press, Inc., 1980.

35. Sallan, S. E., Camitta, B. M., Cassady, J. R., et al.: Intermittent combination chemotherapy with adriamycin for childhood acute lymphoblastic leukemia: clinical results. Blood, 51:425, 1978.

36. Sallan, S. E., and Cronin, C. M.: Antiemetics. In Greenblatt, D., and Miller, R. (eds.): Handbook of Drug Therapy. New York, American Elsevier Publishers, Inc., 1979, p. 1060.

37. Sallan, S. E., Cronin, C. M., Zelen, M., et al.: Antiemetics in patients receiving chemotherapy for cancer. N. Engl. J. Med., 302:134, 1980.

38. Salmon, S. E., Hamburger, A. W., Soehnlen, B., et al.: Quantitation of differential sensitivity of human tumor stem cells to anticancer agents. N. Engl. J. Med., 298:1321, 1978.

39. Samuels, M. L., Johnson, D. E., Holoye, P. Y., et al.: Large dose bleomycin therapy and pulmonary toxicity. J.A.M.A., 235:1, 1976.

40. Skipper, H. E., and Schabel, F. M., Jr.: Quantitative and cytokinetic studies in experimental tumor systems. In Holland, J. F., and Frei, E., III (eds.): Cancer Medicine. Philadelphia, Lea and Febiger, 1982, p. 663.

41. Warburg, O.: On respiratory impairment in cancer cells. Science, 124:269, 1956.

42. Weber, G.: Enzymology of cancer cells. N. Engl. J. Med., 296:541, 1976.

43. Weinstein, H. J., Mayer, R. J., Rosenthal, D. S., et al.: Treatment of acute myelogenous leukemia in children and adults. N. Engl. J. Med., 303:473, 1980.

44. Zwelling, L. A., and Kohn, K. W.: Effects of cisplatin on DNA and the possible relationships to cytotoxicity and mutagenicity in mammalian cells. In Prestayko, A. W., Crooke, S. T., and Carter, S. K. (eds.): Cisplatin: Current Status and New Developments. New York, Academic Press, Inc., 1980.

18

Chemotherapy for advanced oral cancer

THOMAS J. ERVIN, M.D.
DANIEL D. KARP, M.D.
RALPH R. WEICHSELBAUM, M.D.

Squamous cell carcinoma arising in the oral cavity continues to be an important oncologic problem. The 1980 Amercian Cancer Society statistics predicted that there would be 15,000 new cases of oral cancer diagnosed in 1982. These statistics also predicted that there would be 9,000 deaths from squamous cell carcinoma of the oral cavity.[4] Even for patients who are cured of their disease, serious problems such as cosmetic defects from surgery or radiotherapy, psychological disturbance, and loss of vital processes, including salivation, mastication, and speech, exist and must be dealt with.

Within the past 10 years, there has been a rapid proliferation of investigation related to head and neck cancer, particularly to squamous cell carcinoma. For untreated patients, a multidisciplinary approach, including surgery, radiotherapy, and chemotherapy, has been developed. Although the usefulness of such combined modality treatment, including chemotherapy, has not been firmly established, in some institutions it has become standard treatment for previously untreated patients in whom disease is in an advanced stage.[23] Recently published reviews that concern this topic include Glick and Taylor[17] and Ervin and colleagues.[13, 15] The role of chemotherapy in the multidisciplinary treatment of advanced head and neck cancer may be very important. As shown in Table 18–1, each therapeutic discipline has its own defined potential antitumor effect, with the role of chemotherapy being important in the achievement of both local and distant control of tumor growth.

The potential role of chemotherapy as the initial treatment in the curative therapy of head and neck cancer patients who have advanced disease can be outlined in more detail. In Table 18–2, the positive and negative features of the addition of chemotherapy to standard treatment are outlined. In discussing the potential advantages of chemotherapy, several points can be emphasized.

Until recently, local tumor control has been a problem in head and neck cancer. Patients who have advanced lesions have not been helped by standard radiotherapy or surgery; the tumor has regrown in the primary treatment field. In fact, 70 percent of patients who have had relapses following standard treatment had only locoregional disease at autospy.[7, 36] By virtue of additional tumor cell kill, chemotherapy may enhance radiotherapy by decreasing the hypoxic fraction of cells that are within the tumor (such hypoxic cells are resistant to radiation) by acting as a radiosensitizer. Similarly, reduction of tumor size by chemotherapy may allow for more complete surgical resection or for better reconstructive results.

Table 18–1. THE MULTIDISCIPLINARY APPROACH TO ADVANCED HEAD AND NECK CANCER

Discipline	Potential Antitumor Effect
Surgery	Removal of bulk disease Removal of "hypoxic fraction"
Radiotherapy	Removal of bulk disease Removal of microscopic metastasis—*local*
Chemotherapy	Cytoreduction of tumor prior to definitive local treatment Removal of microscopic metastases—*distant* and *local*

Table 18–2. CHEMOTHERAPY PRIOR TO SURGERY OR RADIATION

Potential Advantages
 Decrease in locoregional tumor size resulting in:
  Increased control of primary tumor.
  Decreased local treatment.
 Increased effect on systemic micrometastases.
 Avoidance of possible adverse effects of surgery or radiotherapy on chemotherapy.
  Immunosuppression.
  Hypercoagulability.
  Altered vascular access.
 Determine the chemoresponsiveness of the tumor.
 Greater dose of chemotherapy achievable.
Potential Disadvantages
 Tumor growth.
 Selection of tumor cells inherently resistant to radiotherapy.
 Selection of tumor cells that disseminate distantly, producing distant micrometastases.
 Compromise of subsequent radiotherapy or surgery.

Traditionally, the control of distant metastases has not been a factor in the treatment of head and neck cancer. However, in patients who live longer because they have been treated with more successful and sophisticated methods of palliating local recurrences, the clinically apparent distant metastasis rate has risen dramatically. This should not be surprising because squamous cell carcinoma that arises in the upper aerodigestive tract has many properties, both morphologic and cytokinetic, similar to lung cancer, a disease that is often diagnosed at a later clinical stage and that is noted for its high incidence of distant metastasis. Goldie and Goldman[18] have developed a mathematical model that suggests that early therapy should be focused on systemic metastases. Their hypothesis supports the idea that within two or three tumor doubling times (as little as three months or the time necessary to treat head and neck cancer with local treatment) the probability of the spontaneous emergence of tumor cells that are resistant to chemotherapy becomes very high. This occurrence would, of course, exclude the possibility of cure, because systemic micrometastases are treatable only with chemotherapy. The practical implication of such a theory is that systemic treatment, that is, chemotherapy, should be administered early in the treatment of head

and neck cancer in patients who have advanced disease, with a high probability of harboring distant micrometastases.

Potential disadvantages of administering chemotherapy prior to standard local treatment are not insignificant. Although experimental models of chemotherapy plus surgery or radiotherapy do not suggest that short-term chemotherapy will preferentially select or promote the development of resistant tumor cells, complications may affect the overall treatment.[29, 40] The tumor cells may be resistant to chemotherapy, and the tumor may grow in size, making subsequent treatment more difficult. This possibility makes it mandatory that a high-response rate be achieved for any chemotherapy that is used as the initial treatment of head and neck cancer. A more difficult problem arises when chemotherapy complicates the standard treatment by causing tumor regression or normal tissue toxicity. Chemotherapy may lessen the efficacy of radiotherapy by "sensitizing" normal oral mucosa to subsequent radiation damage. Such sensitization can result in altered radiation fractionation schedules that are suboptimal for tumor control.[44] From the surgical viewpoint, tumor regression caused by chemotherapy may or may not be centripetal and tumor resection based on a smaller tumor volume may result in nests of viable tumor being left at the periphery of the unresected tissue. Such potential complications and advantages await further examination and confirmation; however, they serve as background information concerning the usefulness or limitations of chemotherapy for advanced head and neck cancer.

SINGLE AGENTS

The palliative treatment of oral carcinoma has generated extensive usage of single agent chemotherapy for this disease.[6] Squamous cell carcinoma of the oral cavity, as in other areas in the upper aerodigestive tract, is one of the most chemoresponsive of the solid tumors in humans. In Table 18–3, much of this experience is outlined. It should be noted that such response rates are obtained in patients who have had unsuccessful results with standard radiotherapy and surgery. Such patients are often debilitated following standard treatment. Certain factors that are associated with previous treatment or with the extent of disease affect response rates to chemotherapy. A list of these factors is provided in Table 18–4 and

Table 18–3. SINGLE AGENT CHEMOTHERAPY

Drug	No. of Evaluable Patients	Response Rate (%)
Methotrexate	1038	42
Hydroxyurea	18	39
Cyclophosphamide	77	36
Cis-platinum	100	34
Dibromodulcitol	81	31
Vinblastine	35	29
5-Fluorouracil	145	27
Bleomycin	435	26
Adriamycin	44	23
Cytosine arabinoside	20	20
Chlorambucil	34	15
6-Mercaptopurine	45	12
Procarbazine	31	10
Mechlorethamine	66	7

(Adapted, with permission, from Carter, S. K.: Chemotherapy of head and neck cancer. Semin. Oncol., 4:413, 1977.)

should be kept in mind when reviewing results of chemotherapy. Patients who have received prior treatment, debilitated patients with poor performance status, and patients who have had large tumor masses do not respond well to chemotherapy as palliative treatment. Most responses noted in single agent trials are of short duration, averaging 3 months. Despite the transient nature of the response, patients may benefit from such treatment by having

Table 18–4. FACTORS AFFECTING RESPONSE TO CHEMOTHERAPY

Performance Status
Ambulatory patients who are not dependent on pain medication or nutritional supplement will tolerate more chemotherapy.

Previous Treatment
Prior radiotherapy adversely affects response rate. Prior surgery may adversely affect response rate by affecting performance status.

Tumor Size
Tumors of T_3 or T_4 extent, that is, > 4 cm in diameter, respond less well to chemotherapy.

Tumor Site
Nodal metastases respond less well than do primary tumors.

Nutritional Status
Patients who have poor nutritional intake tolerate aggressive chemotherapy poorly.

Immunologic Status
Patients who have impaired cellular immunity may not respond to chemotherapy.

less pain, being better able to swallow, and, in some cases, by having prolonged survival.

Methotrexate

Methotrexate, the folic acid antagonist, is the standard single agent treatment for oral cancer. This antimetabolite has extensively been tested both in relapsed and untreated patients. Many schedules and dosages have been used. However, the standard most successful regimens employ treatment either weekly[27] or biweekly.[26] Dosages may vary widely; however, in comparative trials with calcium leucovorin, there have been no significant differences in response rate, duration of response, or survival rates at doses between 40 mg/m^2 and 3 gram/m^2 weekly.[26, 43, 47] For short treatment (up to 24 hours), it appears that the dose-response curve for methotrexate for head and neck cancer is shallow; this may reflect the large proportion of cells with prolonged cycle times or quiescent behavior.

Bleomycin

Bleomycin, an antitumor antibiotic, has been evaluated in more than 400 patients who have advanced head and neck cancer. This agent with cell cycle specific activity has been used with some benefit on both intermittent and continuous schedule. Recent experimental evidence suggests that continuous infusion bleomycin, because of its schedule-dependent cytotoxicity, may be superior to intermittent injection.[32] Cortes and associates[9] have suggested that continuous administration of bleomycin is superior to intermittent dose schedules for patients who have advanced previously treated head and neck cancer. Bleomycin is easily administered; however, one must watch for pulmonary toxicity and allergic reaction. In many cases, pulmonary toxicity may be related to the dosage given. However, it may occur at any dosage, particularly in patients who have markedly impaired pulmonary function. Bleomycin pulmonary toxicity is often not predictable in older patients and should be watched for on serial chest x-rays.[45] Serial pulmonary function tests cannot predict further bleomycin toxicity. Surgeons should be aware that patients who have been exposed to bleomycin may develop severe or fatal pulmonary toxicity if they are subsequently exposed to elevated oxygen tension. Patients who undergo surgery following bleomycin treatment should not receive inhaled oxygen concentration of more than 0.25 unless it is clinically mandated by low P_{O_2} levels.

Cis-Platinum

Cis-Platinum is a heavy metal complex that derives its antitumor activity by interacting with DNA, forming both strand breaks and intra- or interstrand cross linking.[48] The single agent activity of cis-platinum for head and neck cancer does not appear to be schedule-dependent.[17] However, a dose-response curve may be possible between 50 and 120 mg/m². Nausea, vomiting, and auditory damage may be severe following treatment, and prolonged, scheduled administration, such as continuous infusion over 24 hours or daily infusion over 5 days, may be advantageous to avoid these toxicities.[12, 38] Renal toxicity may occur and requires careful clinical monitoring of fluid and electrolytes during treatment. Pretreatment hydration is required to produce a rapid diuresis during cis-platinum administration. Both potassium and magnesium wasting occur during treatment, and these electrolytes may need to be replaced to avoid symptoms of electrolyte imbalance.

Other Agents

Several other antitumor agents are a source of significant activity in head and neck cancer. 5-Fluorouracil, vinblastine, and mitomycin C are currently in use, either singly or in combination with other drugs. These agents, like those previously discussed, have predictable side effects (see Chapter 17, Table 17–2).

COMBINATION CHEMOTHERAPY

The results of a representative sample of combination drug trials for previously treated and untreated squamous cell carcinoma are presented in Table 18–5. This list is not exhaustive, and other reviews on the topic are available.[6, 17] However, this list is useful in showing general issues regarding the efficacy of combinations of antitumor agents for head and neck cancer.

PREVIOUSLY TREATED PATIENTS

For patients who have recurrence of tumor after initial treatment with surgery or radiotherapy, in most instances, the goal of chemotherapy is palliation of symptoms. Chemotherapy alone is not a curative treatment for head and neck cancer but can, in some instances, prolong life or ameliorate symptoms such as prior or poor swallowing. Until recently, the standard chemotherapy for previously treated patients has been methotrexate. Approximately 40 percent of the patients treated with methotrexate had tumor regression for an average of three months. More recently, several combinations have been used, with encouraging results. In a randomized trial, Kaplan and colleagues[25] showed an increased duration of response in patients treated with combination chemotherapy compared with patients who received single agent methotrexate. In other nonrandomized studies, combinations of high-dose antitumor agents produced successful response rates in excess of 75 percent.[5, 12] It appears that combinations of agents may offer an advantage over single agents in selected patients (that is, those with high-performance status), but additional randomized trials are needed. At present, single agent methotrexate is the standard palliative treatment for head and neck cancer. However, for patients with favorable performance status, or those who have a chance for salvage surgery or radiotherapy, combination chemotherapy is recommended.

Table 18–5. COMBINATION CHEMOTHERAPY FOR HEAD AND NECK CANCER

Drug Regimen*	No. of Trials	No. of Evaluable Patients	% Partial Response Prior Treatment	Untreated	% Complete Response Prior Treatment	Untreated	References
CDDP, MTX-LCV-B	11	244	45	77	12	21	26–32
CDDP, B	4	93	32	76	5	23	33–36
CDDP, MTX-LCV†	1	20	—	60	—	0	31–37
CDDP, V, B	2	60	—	80	—	23	38–39
C, V, M, F, B	3	36	32	56	5	NR‡	40–42
V, M, F, B	1	30	—	87	—	NR‡	43
Vb, B, CDDP	1	45	45	74	9	22	44

*Drug abbreviations: CDDP = Cis-platinum; MTX-LCV = methotrexate–leucovorin; B = bleomycin; V = vincristine; C = cyclophosphamide; M = methotrexate; F = 5-Fluorouracil; Vb = Vinblastine.
†Dose-limiting nephrotoxicity noted.
‡Complete responses not reported.

UNTREATED PATIENTS

Chemotherapy is not a new concept for the initial treatment of advanced head and neck cancer. In earlier trials, both positive and negative results were reported for this "upfront" approach. Lustig and associates[30] noted that methotrexate used prior to radiotherapy had advantageous results, particularly for carcinoma of the oral cavity. A response to systemic high-dose methotrexate with leucovorin rescue prior to surgery or radiation has been shown to increase the disease-free survival rate at 3 years in patients who had advanced T_3 and T_4 head and neck cancers.[14] Alternatively, a randomized trial coordinated by the Radiation Therapy Oncology Group (RTOG) showed no significant advantage to preradiotherapy methotrexate in advanced T_3 and T_4 cancers of the head and neck. In this trial, however, methotrexate treatment did produce a modest but not statistically significant improvement in survival rates, particularly in patients who had tumors of the oral cavity.[16]

Despite the lack of definitive supportive evidence, many investigators have utilized drug combinations as initial treatment for advanced squamous cell carcinoma of the head and neck. The response results are listed in Table 18–5. Successful response rates for a variety of treatment combinations exceed 75 percent, and complete regression rates of 25 percent or more are common for most reports. It is not yet known whether this treatment will be of long-term benefit (that is, increased cure rates). Results of an initial report by Pennacchio and colleagues[33] suggest that initial chemotherapy utilizing cis-platinum and bleomycin prior to surgery or radiotherapy improves the disease-free survival rate at 18 months for patients who have advanced head and neck cancer. Other similar trials are now in progress; however, long-term follow-up is needed to access the efficacy of these investigations.

Certainly, initial chemotherapy as treatment of advanced head and neck cancer poses a problem with respect to potential toxicity. The toxicity of subsequent radiotherapy is mildly enhanced by prior chemotherapy.[44] The effect that chemotherapy will have on dental caries, oral mucosal healing, or osteoradionecrosis is unknown. Certainly, mucositis, an inflammation of the oral mucous membranes with or without frank ulceration, is a common effect of many drugs and is frequently seen in head and neck cancer. Such toxicities, both known and unknown, will require aggressive dental and medical management.

SUMMARY

Chemotherapy for oral cancer as well as for other squamous cell carcinomas that originate in the head and neck is a rapidly expanding field. Great progress has been made in increasing response rates, particularly in previously untreated patients. For patients who have had unsuccessful standard radiotherapy or surgery, chemotherapy in any form must be considered palliative. In this instance, the benefit of treatment must be weighed against the toxicity of the drugs given. Single agent methotrexate is the standard palliative treatment, although newer combinations that use cis-platinum, bleomycin, or mitomycin C should be considered for selected patients. For previously untreated patients who present with advanced T_3 or T_4 primary tumors or with N_2 to N_3 adenopathy, chemotherapy should be considered as the initial method of treatment. Several drug combinations that produce a greater than 75 percent chance of tumor regression are available. The results of initial reports suggest that such aggressive multidisciplinary treatment in advanced head and neck cancer will be beneficial, although controlled trials must be done to confirm the finding.

REFERENCES

1. Baker, L., and Al-Sarraf, M: A comparative trial of cis-platinum (C), oncovin (O), and bleomycin (B) vs. methotrexate (M) in patients with advanced epidermoid carcinomas of the head and neck. Proc. Am. Assoc. Cancer Res., 20:202, 1979.
2. Bianco, A., Taylor, S. G., Reich, S., et al.: Combination chemotherapy pilot studied in head and neck squamous cell cancer. Cancer Treat. Rep., 63:158, 1979.
3. Brown, A. W., Blom, J., Butler, W., et al.: Combination chemotherapy with vinblastine, bleomycin and cis-dichlorodiammineplatinum (II) in squamous cell carcinoma of the head and neck. Cancer, 45:2830, 1980.
4. Cancer Statistics, 1980. CA, 30:23, 1980.
5. Cardonna, R., Paladine, R., Ruchdechel, J. C., et al.: Methotrexate, bleomycin, and high-dose dichlorodiammineplatinum (II) in the treatment of advanced epidermoid carcinoma of the head and neck. Cancer Treat. Rep., 63:489, 1979.
6. Carter, S. K.: Chemotherapy of head and neck cancer. Semin. Oncol., 4:413, 1977.
7. Chung, T. S., and Stefani, S: Distant metastases of carcinoma of tonsillar region: a study of 475 patients. Surg. Oncol., 14:5, 1980.
8. Cortes, E. P., Amin, V. C., Artie, J., et al.: Combination of low dose bleomycin, followed by cyclophosphamide, methotrexate, and 5-fluorouracil for advanced head and neck cancer. Proc. Am. Assoc. Cancer Res., 20:257, 1979.
9. Cortes, E. P., Jagmohan, K., Annin, V. C., et al.: Chemotherapy for head and neck cancer relapsing after chemotherapy. Cancer, 47:1966, 1981.

10. Davis, S., and Kessler, W.: Randomized comparison of *cis*-diamminedichloroplatinum versus *cis*-diamminedichloroplatinum, methotrexate, and bleomycin in recurrent squamous cell carcinoma of the head and neck. Cancer Chemother. Pharmacol., *3*:57, 1979.

11. Elias, E. G., Chretien, P. B., Monnard E., et al.: Chemotherapy prior to local therapy in advanced squamous cell carcinoma of the head and neck: preliminary assessment of an intensive drug regimen. Cancer, *43*:1025, 1979.

12. Ervin, T. J., Weichselbaum, R., Miller, D., et al.: Treatment of advanced squamous cell carcinoma of the head and neck with *cis*-platinum, bleomycin, and methotrexate (PBM). Cancer Treatment. Rep., *65*:9, 1981.

13. Ervin, T. J., Miller, D., Weichselbaum, R., et al.: Chemotherapy for advanced carcinoma of the head and neck. A clinical update. Arch. Otolaryngol., *107*:237, 1981.

14. Ervin, T. J., Kirkwood, J., Weichselbaum, R., et al.: Improved survival for patients with advanced carcinoma of the head and neck treated with methotrexate-leucovorin prior to definitive radiotherapy or surgery. Laryngoscope, *91*:1181, 1981.

15. Ervin, T., Karp, D., Weichselbaum, R., et al.: The role of chemotherapy in the multidisciplinary approach to advanced head and neck cancer: potentials and problems. Arch. Otolaryngol., *90*:506, 1981.

16. Fazekas, J. T., Sommer, C., and Kramer, S.: Adjuvant intravenous methotrexate or definitive radiotherapy alone for advanced squamous cancers of the oral cavity, oral pharynx, supraglottic larynx, or hypopharynx. Int. J. Radiat. Oncol. Biol. Phys., *6*:533, 1980.

17. Glick, J. H., and Taylor, S. G.: Integration of chemotherapy into a combined modality treatment plan for head and neck cancer: a review. Int. J. Radiat. Oncol. Biol. Phys., *7*:229, 1981.

18. Goldie, J. H., and Goldman, A. J.: A mathematic model for relating the drug sensitivity of tumors to their spontaneous mutation rate. Cancer Treat. Rep., *63*:1727, 1979.

19. Goldiner, P. L., and Schweizer, D.: The hazards of anesthesia and surgery in bleomycin-treated patients. Semin. Oncol., *6*:121, 1979.

20. Helman, P., Sealy, P., and Malherde, E.: Intraarterial cytoxic therapy and x-ray for cancer of the head and neck. Lancet, *1*:128, 1965.

21. Holoye, P. Y., Byers, R. M., Gard, D. A., et al.: Combination chemotherapy of head and neck cancer. Cancer, *42*:1661, 1978.

22. Hong, W. K., Shapshay, S. M., Bhutani, R., et al.: Induction chemotherapy in advanced head and neck carcinoma with high-dose *cis*-platinum and bleomycin infusion. Cancer, *44*:19, 1979.

23. Hong, W. K.: Chemotherapy for advanced head and neck carcinoma. Clin. Cancer Briefs, *2*:3, 1982.

24. Kaplan, B. H., Vogl, S. E., Chinten, D., et al.: Chemotherapy of advanced cancer of the head and neck (HNCa) with methotrexate (M), bleomycin (B). Proc. Am. Soc. Clin. Oncol., *20*:384, 1979.

25. Kaplan, B. H., Schoenfeld, D., Vogel, S. E.: Treatment of recurrent or metastatic squamous cancer of the head and neck with methotrexate plus corynebacterium parvum or methotrexate plus bleomycin plus diamminedichloroplatinum. Proc. Am. Soc. Clin. Oncol., *22*:780, 1981.

26. Kirkwood, J. M., Canellos, G. P., Ervin, T. J., et al.: Cancer, *47*:2414, 1981.

27. Leone, L. A., Albala, M. M., and Rege, V. B.: Treatment of carcinoma of the head and neck with intravenous methotrexate. Cancer, *21*:828, 1968.

28. Leone, L. A., and Ohnuma, T.: Combined high dose MTX rescue, bleomycin, and *cis*-platinum for untreated stage III and localized stage IV advanced squamous carcinoma of the head and neck. Proc. Am. Soc. Clin. Oncol., *20*:374, 1979.

29. Looney, W. B., Ritenour, E. R., and Hopkins, H. A.: Solid tumor models for the assessment of different treatment modalities. Cancer, *47*:860, 1981.

30. Lustig, R. A., Demore, P. A., and Kramer, S.: Adjuvant methotrexate in the radiotherapeutic management of advanced tumors of the head and neck. Cancer, *37*:2703, 1976.

31. Lyman, G. H., Armistead, S., Williams, C. C., et al.: Bleomycin and prolonged infusion *cis*-diamminedichloroplatinum (CDDP) in advanced squamous cell carcinoma of the head and neck. Clin. Res., *27*:759, 1979.

32. Peng, Y., Alberts, D. S., and Wood, D. A.,: Antitumor effects and pharmacokinetics of continuous infusion (CON) vs. intermittent (INT) bleomycin (BLEO). Proc. Am. Assoc. Cancer Res., *20*:202, 1979.

33. Pennacchio, J., Hong, W., Shapsay, S., et al.: A comparison of combined modality therapy vs. radiotherapy alone in the treatment of Stage IV unresectable head and neck cancer. Proc. Am. Soc. Clin. Oncol., *21*:430, 1981.

34. Pitman, S. W., Minor, B. R., Papal, R., et al.: Sequential methotrexate-leucovorin (MTX-LCV) and *cis*-platinum (CDDP) in head and neck cancer. Proc. Am. Soc. Clin. Oncol., *20*:49, 1979.

35. Price, L. A., and Hill, B. T.: A kinetically based logical approach to the chemotherapy of head and neck cancer. Clin. Otolaryngol., *3*:339, 1977.

36. Probert, J. C., Thompson, R. W., and Bagshaw, M. A.: Patterns of spread of distant metastases from head and neck cancer. Cancer, *33*:127, 1974.

37. Randolph, V. L., Vallejo, A., Spiro, R. H., et al.: Combination therapy of advanced head and neck cancer: induction of remissions with diamminedichloroplatinum (II), bleomycin, and radiation therapy, Cancer, *41*:460, 1978.

38. Salem, P., Hall, S. W., Benjamin, R. S., et al.: Clinical phase (II) given by continuous IV infusion. Cancer Treat. Rep., *62*:1553, 1978.

39. Salmon, S. E., and Jones, S. E. (eds): Adjuvant Therapy of Cancer II. New York, Grune & Stratton, Inc., 1979, pp. 421–428.

40. Shabel, F. M.: Animal models as predictive systems. *In* Cancer Chemotherapy: Fundamental Concepts and Recent Advances. 19th Annual Clinical Conference on Cancer, 1974. University of Texas, M.D., Anderson Hospital. Chicago, Year Book Medical Publishers, Inc., 1975, pp. 323–355.

41. Spaulding, M. B., Klotch, D., and Lore, J. M.: Preoperative chemotherapy in advanced head and neck cancer. Proc. Am. Soc. Clin. Oncol., *21*:403, 1980.

42. Vogl, S. E., and Kaplan, B. H.: Chemotherapy of advanced head and neck cancer with methotrexate, bleomycin, and *cis*-diamminedichloroplatinum II in an effective out-patient schedule. Cancer, *44*:26, 1979.

43. Vogler, W. R., Jacobs, J., Moffett, S., et al.: Methotrexate therapy with or without citrovorum factor in carcinoma of the head and neck, breast, and colon. Cancer Clin. Trials, 2:227, 1979.

44. Weichselbaum, R., Posner, M. R., Ervin, T. J., et al.: Initial results and toxicity of aggressive combination therapy for advanced head and neck cancer. Int. J. Radiat. Oncol. Biol. Phys., 8:909, 1982.

45. Wheeler, R. R., Lipman, M. K., Baker, S. R., et al.: Bleomycin, vincristine and mitomycin C with or without methotrexate in the treatment of squamous cell carcinoma. Cancer Treat. Rep., 64:943, 1980.

46. Willis, R. E., Heller, K., and Randolph, V.: Cis-dichlorodiammineplatinum (II) based chemotherapy as initial treatment of advanced head and neck cancer. Cancer Treat. Rep., 63:1533, 1979.

47. Woods, R. C., and Tattersoll, S. J.: A randomized study of 3 doses of methotrexate in patients with advanced squamous cell cancer of head and neck. Proc. Am. Assoc. Cancer Res., 20:163, 1979.

48. Zwelling, L. A., and Kohn, K. W.: Mechanism of action of cis-dichlorodiammineplatinum (II). Cancer Treat. Rep., 63:1439, 1979.

19

Oral complications of chemotherapy and their management

STEPHEN T. SONIS, D.M.D., D.M.Sc.
PETER B. LOCKHART, D.D.S.

Unfortunately, more people are currently developing cancer than ever before. This fact is attributable to several factors, including increased life expectancy, pollution, and diet, as well as many variables that are unknown. It has been predicted that 850,000 Americans will develop new cancers this year. Fortunately, significant progress has been made in cancer therapy, so that there is an almost uniform increase in survival rate for the cancer patient and, in a growing number of cases, a chance for curative therapy.

At present, three major modalities are used to treat malignancies: surgery, radiotherapy, and chemotherapy. Although immunotherapy may ultimately be a significant form of treatment, it is not currently being used routinely. Of the three therapy modes available, only surgery is tumor-specific and thereby normal-tissue sparing. Contrastingly, the antitumor effects of radiotherapy and chemotherapy are based on their ability to destroy or retard cell division. Hence, rapidly proliferating tumor cells are affected by both therapeutic techniques. Because these agents are nonspecific, rapidly dividing normal tissues are also affected. The oral mucosa, as well as the remainder of the gastrointestinal tract, has a high mitotic index. Thus, the mouth is one of the major sites of nonspecific toxicity due to chemotherapy. In addition, the massive bacterial accumulation in the oral cavity "highlights" the mouth's significance as a portal of entry for infectious agents during periods of bone marrow depression. It should be understood that the mouth is potentially a major problem area in the patient who undergoes treatment for malignancy.

Before discussing the management of problems related to cancer treatment, two points must be made: first, the *frequency* of oral complications related to cancer treatment, and second, a definition of the *range* and *scope* of these problems. In a recent study of patients receiving treatment for non–head and neck malignancies, oral complications were found to affect approximately 40 per cent of the patients.[17] Similar results were obtained in a study of patients receiving chemotherapy for malignancies of the ovaries, uterus, and breast.[9] Thus, almost half the patients who receive chemotherapy can expect to develop some form of oral complication at some time during therapy. Furthermore, as the life expectancy of cancer patients increases, so too does the patient pool that receives periodic cancer therapy, which compounds the ultimate number of patients who have potential oral problems.

The noninstitutional dentist must be aware of the fact that the trend in cancer therapy is to deliver as much care as possible on an ambulatory basis. Thus, many patients who receive chemotherapy are not routinely hospitalized. Instead, they live in the community and are likely to seek advice and receive care from their family practitioner.

Young patients seem to be more susceptible to the stomatotoxic effects of chemotherapy than are adults (Table 19–1).[17] This observation is attributable to a variety of factors, including differences in the distribution of malignancies and types of chemotherapy. However, because differences in frequency are observed between young and old patients with similar malignancies and treatment regimens,

186

Table 19–1. DISTRIBUTION BY AGE OF PROSPECTIVE PATIENT SAMPLE

Age (yr)	No. of Patients	% of Total Patients	No. of Oral Complications per Total Patients	% of Oral Complications
1 to 20	10	10.7	9/10	90
21 to 40	20	21.5	12/20	60
41 to 60	36	38.7	10/36	28
61 or older	27	29.0	5/27	18
Total	93			

(From Sonis, S. T., Sonis, A. L., and Lieberman, A.: Oral complications in patients receiving treatment for malignancies other than of the head and neck. J. Am. Dent. Assoc., 97:468, 1978.)

an additional element may contribute to the differences noted. Barakat and associates,[1] utilizing animal models, have reported that physiologic regeneration of oral epithelium slows with age. It is possible that the mucosa of older patients has a lower mitotic index than that of young people and that it might be less susceptible to the effects of chemotherapy.

The oral complications of cancer therapy may be grouped into two major classes: those that are a direct result of treatment and those that are due to the myelosuppressive effects of therapy (Tables 19–2 through 19–4). The first group of complications results from the nonspecific action of therapy on rapidly dividing cells. Because the cells of the oral mucosa have a high mitotic index, they are susceptible to these effects, which result in atrophy and eventual breakdown of the integrity of the mucosa.

The major significance of the mouth in the myelosuppressed patient is as a potential portal of entry for its numerous bacterial inhabitants.

Table 19–2. ACTIONS, TOXICITIES, AND ORAL COMPLICATIONS OF SELECTED CANCER CHEMOTHERAPEUTIC AGENTS

Drug	Actions	Selected Toxicities and Oral Complications
Methotrexate	Antifolate Inhibits biosynthesis of nucleic acids	Stomatitis Oral and digestive tract ulcerations Bone marrow depression with leukopenia, thrombocytopenia, and bleeding
Bleomycin	Antibiotic Inhibits progression of cells through premitotic (G_2) and mitotic (M) phase of cell cycle Interferes with thymidine incorporation into DNA	Stomatitis and mucocutaneous ulceration
Adriamycin	Anthracyclines Leads to uncoiling of DNA helix and inhibition of DNA-directed RNA polymerase and DNA polymerase	Stomatitis Bone marrow depression
Cyclophosphamide	Alkylating agent Interferes with DNA structure—disrupts and disorganizes the cell	Depresses peripheral blood cell counts With high doses, severe bone marrow depression with leukopenia, thrombocytopenia, and bleeding
Vincristine	Plant alkaloid Mitotic inhibitor—disorganizes the mitotic spindle to arrest cell division	Mild bone marrow depression Peripheral neuritis Stomatitis
Dexamethasone	Adrenal cortical compound Alters hormonal balance and modifies growth of some cancers arising from tissues particularly susceptible to hormonal influences Important mechanism may be interference at cell membrane	Increased susceptibility to infection

Table 19–3. FREQUENCY OF ORAL
COMPLICATIONS

Complication	Number	% of Total Complications
Ulceration and mucositis	17	36
Xerostomia	10	21
Gingivitis	4	8
Cellulitis and abscesses	4	8
Generalized oral pain	3	6
Moniliasis	2	4
Lymphadenopathy	2	4
Radiation caries	2	4'
Acute necrotizing ulcerative gingivitis (ANUG)	1	2
Paresthesia	1	2
Hemorrhage	1	2
Total	47	

(From Sonis, S. T., Sonis, A. L., and Lieberman, A.: Oral complications in patients receiving treatment for malignancies other than of the head and neck. J. Am. Dent. Assoc., 97:468, 1978.)

In the cancer patient who is myelosuppressed, the oral cavity is the most frequently identifiable source of organisms that result in sepsis (Table 19–5).[8] Local infection and ulceration are common. The patient's oral health status prior to and during therapy also affects the indirect effects of therapy on the mouth.

DIRECT EFFECTS OF CHEMOTHERAPY

Cytolysis of normal tissue is one of the major side effects associated with certain chemotherapy agents. The oral mucosa is one of the target tissues that is most commonly affected by many of the agents. Clinically, the cytotoxic effects of the chemotherapy are manifested as discrete ulcerations and a generalized loss of the surface mucosa. It appears that some chemotherapeutic agents are more stomatotoxic than others. Methotrexate, Adriamycin, and the fluorinated pyrimidines are all commonly used antineoplastic drugs that have documented stomatotoxicity. The stomatotoxic effects of these agents appear to overlap and parallel the effects of these agents on the bone marrow.

The renewal time of human oral mucosal cells is approximately 10 to 14 days. Because migration and exfoliation of mucosal cells are not directly influenced by chemotherapeutic agents, the effect of stomatotoxic agents on the inhibition of DNA replication is not immediately noted in the mouth. Rather, the effects of these agents are manifested histologically as mucosal atrophy approximately 5 to 7 days following treatment. As the mucosa becomes thinned, clinical signs of mucositis become apparent and ulceration often follows. The effects of these agents are most notable on nonkeratinized mucosa such as the buccal and labial surfaces and under the tongue. The hard palate and attached gingiva are rarely involved. Similarly, it is unusual to see changes on the cutaneous areas of the lips. Clinically, one initially observes large areas of glistening erythema, which are generally sensitive. These may break down to form areas of hemorrhagic ulceration, which are extremely painful and may become secondarily infected. Generally, these areas heal without scarring in 14 to 21 days following initial chemotherapy. Diminished nutritional intake secondary to mucositis may compound the problem, because there is an overall decrease in cell migration and renewal after starvation or protein deprivation.

Table 19–4. FREQUENCY OF ORAL COMPLICATIONS IN CHILDREN

Complication	Number	% of Total Complications
Ulcers	32/45	71.1
Lip cracking	17/45	37.8
Xerostomia	5/45	11.1
Mucositis	4/45	8.9
Lymphadenopathy	3/45	6.7
Miscellaneous (pericornitis, coated tongue, erythema)	3/45	6.7
Moniliasis	2/45	4.4
Caries (radiation)	2/45	4.4
Infection	2/45	4.4
Acute necrotizing ulcerative gingivitis (ANUG)	1/45	2.2

(From Sonis, A. L., and Sonis, S. T.: J. Pedodontics, 3:122, 1979.)

Table 19–5. SITES OF MICROBIOLOGICALLY AND CLINICALLY DOCUMENTED INFECTIONS IN GRANULOCYTOPENIC PATIENTS WITH CANCER

Site	% of all Recognized Sites
Oral cavity*	19
Skin/soft tissue	14
Lung†	13
Urinary tract	11
Trachea/bronchus	8
Anus/rectum	9
Intestine/esophagus	5
Nose/sinus	3
Intravenous site/catheter	2
Other	10
Bacteremia (no primary site identified)	7
Total	100

*Mouth, pharynx, and tonsil.
†Parenchymal infection (pneumonia).
(From E.O.R.T.C. International Antimicrobial Therapy Project Group: Three antibiotic regimens in the treatment of infection in febrile granulocytopenic patients with cancer. J. Infect. Dis., *137*:14, 1978.)

Large areas of mucosa may be involved with necrosis and slough (Figs. 19–1 through 19–3). A surrounding band of erythema may be present, but its extent is variable. Tissue that is chronically irritated by teeth or dental appliances is particularly prone to ulceration. Simultaneous with their stomatotoxic effects, chemotherapeutic agents inhibit other rapidly dividing cells, especially those in the bone marrow. Thus, maximum stomatotoxicity is most frequently observed at the nadir of the white blood cell count (Fig. 19–4).

The recovery of the oral mucosa from the stomatotoxic effects of therapy often precedes that of the marrow by 2 or 3 days. An improvement in oral mucosal status is significant for predicting recovery from the nadir of myelosuppression.[13]

Elimination of mechanical irritants helps to minimize the severity of mucositis. Removable appliances should be kept from the mouth until the patient has recovered from chemotherapy. Daily mouth care should include débridement of the teeth, gingiva, and tongue with a soft toothbrush or a wet 2-in. × 2-in. sponge wrapped around a finger and frequent water rinses to keep the mucous membranes clean and moist. The aggressiveness of mouth care must be adjusted to be compatible with the status of the patient's bone marrow. Patients who are severely myelosuppressed (white blood count < 1,000, platelets < 20,000) may have to limit the extent of brushing and flossing because of the threat of bacteremia or bleeding. However, a modified oral hygiene regimen using sponges is imperative for such patients.

Relief of generalized oral pain may be accomplished by the use of frequent palliative rinses with viscous Xylocaine, Benadryl, and Kaopectate 1–1 (50 percent of each), Talacain, Dyclone, or a 2.5 to 5 percent cocaine rinse. Some patients tolerate one of these agents better than the others. The clinician should try a variety of agents until one is found that provides relief. Pain in one or more specific areas of the mouth can often be managed with topical benzocaine in orabase, applied as needed, following drying of the area with a sponge. Consideration should also be given to

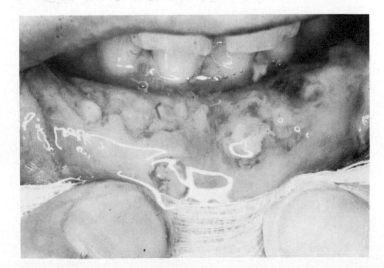

Figure 19–1. Mucositis in a 10-year-old girl who is receiving methotrexate for acute lymphocytic leukemia. Note the diffuse ulceration of the labial mucosa.

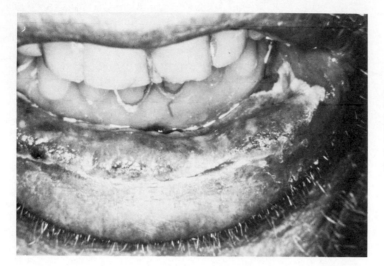

Figure 19–2. Mucositis in a 62-year-old man who has diffuse histiocytic lymphoma that is being treated with methotrexate. Note the demarcation at the mucocutaneous junction and the lack of involvement of the attached gingiva.

Figure 19–3. Mucositis in a 56-year-old man who has lymphoma that is being treated with methotrexate. Note the diffuse involvement of the labial mucosa and the demarcation at the mucocutaneous junction. The surface is covered with a necrotic slough.

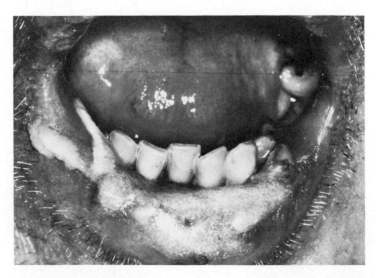

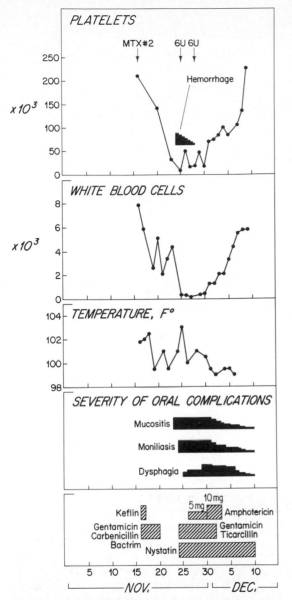

Figure 19–4. Correlation between the severity of oral complications and temperature, chemotherapy, platelet count, and white blood cell count in a 55-year-old man who has malignant lymphoma. Therapy is indicated at the bottom of the figure. Oral complications are represented diagrammatically in stepwise fashion in an attempt to quantitate their severity. (From Lockhart, P. B., and Sonis, S. T.: Relationship of oral complications to peripheral blood leukocytes and platelet counts in patients receiving cancer chemotherapy. Oral Surg., *48*:21, 1979.)

systemic analgesics and narcotics such as Tylenol elixir (not ASA), codeine, Demerol, or morphine.

Xerostomia is the second most frequent complication of nonsurgical cancer therapy and is the most common oral problem noted following radiation to the head and neck. Some forms of chemotherapy produce xerostomia. In addition to enhancing mucositis production, xerostomia promotes the accumulation of oral bacteria and, hence, the development of caries. Such caries is rapidly progressive and is usually noted in the cervical area of the teeth.

Treatment of the patient with xerostomia is aimed at stimulating salivary flow, replacing lost secretions, protecting the dentition, and reducing sucrose intake. Specifically, patients should be encouraged to stimulate salivary flow, if possible, with sucrose-free lemon drops. Some patients may prefer sugar-free chewing gum. Artificial saliva or mouth moisturizer may be helpful at mealtime. An example of such a substance is VA Oralube,[16] which approximates whole saliva in viscosity and electrolyte concentration (Table 19–6). It has been suggested that mouth rinsing with a supersaturated solution of calcium phosphate can aid in the remineralization of early carious lesions.[10] Custom trays into which 1 percent solution fluoride gel can be placed should be used daily for 4 to 6 minutes following oral hygiene in the early evening (Fig. 19–5).

Rinsing with an acidulated fluoride mouth rinse at bedtime provides an alternative means of topical fluoride application for the patient who cannot tolerate trays because of radiation or chemotherapy-induced nausea. If mucositis prevents the use of an acidulated fluoride due to burning, a nonacidulated fluoride rinse can be substituted. Patients should be recalled frequently. Diet counseling is encouraged to reduce sucrose intake.

Neurotoxicity of pulpal tissue is a rare, direct

Table 19–6. FORMULATION FOR VA ORALUBE

KCl	2.498 gm
NaCl	3.462 gm
MgCl$_2$	0.235 gm
CaCl$_2$	0.665 gm
K$_2$HPO$_4$	3.213 gm
KH$_2$PO$_4$	1.304 gm
Methyl p-hydroxybenzoate	8.0 gm
Flavoring (wintergreen-coriander spice)	16.0 gm
70% sorbitol	171.0 gm
Na carboxymethylcellulose	40.0 gm
NaF	17.68 mg
FD + C red 40 dye (2%)	1.0 ml
Water q.s. ad	

Directions: Heat water to approximately 50° C in a large blender. Add dry ingredients, attach blender lid, and mix at high setting for 2 minutes. Filter through loose glass wool prior to packaging in 4-oz soft-plastic bottles.

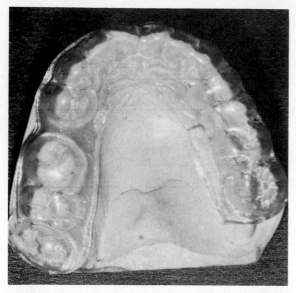

Figure 19–5. Customized fluoride tray for use in a patient who is receiving head and neck irradiation for intraoral carcinoma. The tray was made using an omnivac with niteguard material. Note the extension of the tray beyond the gingival margin.

complication of some forms of chemotherapy (vincristine). Patients present with an acute, constant, pulpitis-like pain, most frequently in the mandible. Clinical examination is usually unremarkable. Radiographic examination may reveal enlarged periodontal ligament spaces around the apices of caries-free teeth. Relief of symptoms with narcotic analgesics is the treatment of choice, because the condition seems to be drug-related and ceases when the drug is discontinued.

INDIRECT EFFECTS OF CHEMOTHERAPY

The indirect effects of chemotherapy are due to myelosuppression, which results in neutropenia and thrombocytopenia. The major oral manifestations of myelosuppression are local infection, necrosis, and hemorrhage.

Oral infection in the patient receiving myelosuppressive therapy is life threatening and must be dealt with aggressively, yet with cognizance of the patient's fragility because of bone marrow depression. The mouth is obviously an important potential portal of entry for many organisms. As in the normal individual, oral infections in the patient receiving chemotherapy are due to bacterial, fungal, or viral agents.

Bacterial Infections

Odontogenic

The diagnosis of odontogenic infection in patients who are myelosuppressed is often complicated by the lack of objective findings due to the individual's decreased ability to produce an inflammatory response. Pain and fever, however, are usually present and may be the only clinical evidence of infection.[2] The evaluation of signs and symptoms of infection thought to be of odontogenic origin should include a mirror examination for caries, percussion, palpation, pulp testing, hot and cold sensitivity, and detailed periapical and bitewing films.

Prevention and Treatment. Many chronic subacute odontogenic lesions become acute and of systemic significance following myelosuppression. Hence, the removal of teeth that have a questionable prognosis *prior* to chemotherapy is recommended. If odontogenic infection is suspected at a time of myelosuppression, it is the degree of suppression that largely determines therapy. At the patient's nadir, medical rather than surgical management is indicated and should include appropriate antibiotic and pain medication. If the use of antibiotics does not result in the resolution of the infection and an extraction is necessary, the patient should be covered with high-dose broad spectrum parenteral antibiotics and, depending upon the platelet count, platelet transfusions. Attempts to manage oral infection in neutropenic patients who are immunosuppressed, particularly when they are febrile, with antibiotics taken by mouth often fail and necessitate parenteral antibiotic therapy for a worsening situation. Surgery should be as atraumatic as possible, with an attempt at primary closure with sutures over the socket. Packing material placed in the socket for hemostasis should not be used routinely in the patient who is myelosuppressed, because it may act as a bacterial breeding ground. Clinical judgment is necessary in evaluating patients for extraction versus root canal treatment. Patients who have falling peripheral counts and who present with pulpitis should be evaluated in terms of the hopelessness of the tooth, the ability of the patient to maintain his or her mouth, and the potential for overt infection during the patient's nadir. In our experience, initiating root canal treatment just prior to or during a falling white blood cell count is risky and may force an extraction at a time when the patient is unable to tolerate the inevitable

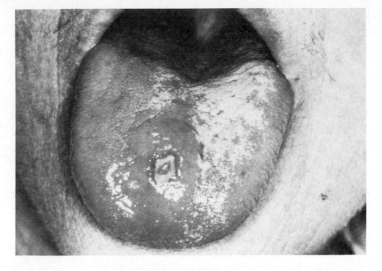

Figure 19–6. Ulceration with secondary infection of the tongue of a 57-year-old woman who has acute leukemia and who was myelosuppressed from chemotherapeutic agents. Note the raised margins around the ulceration, the depth of the ulceration, and the loss of lingual anatomy. The patient was febrile to 102°F secondary to the ulceration.

hemorrhage and bacteremia. Patients who have low counts and a pulpal abscess, however, may be best managed with a pulpectomy, because drainage and pain relief may be accomplished without the bacteremia associated with an extraction. In addition, this procedure may "buy time" until the patient's counts permit more definitive treatment.

Soft-Tissue Infection

Cancer chemotherapy may predispose patients to bacterial infection by several mechanisms. Myelosuppression results in decreased production of white blood cells, most importantly polymorphonuclear leukocytes (PMNL), and thus interferes with the most effective means of host resistance. The degree and duration of granulocytopenia often determines the incidence and severity of infection.

These infections often originate from the normal oral flora but may also be acquired from the hospital environment. In the immunocompetent host, the predominant oral flora are gram-positive cocci (Staphylococcus and Streptococcus). Data from several studies suggest that during myelosuppression the oral flora is altered to a predominantly gram-negative opportunistic coccus, such as Pseudomonas, Klebsiella, Serratia, Enterobacteriaceae, *Escherichia coli,* and *Bacillus proteus.*[10, 6] Oral infections can be caused by pure isolates of one organism or a mixture of the previously mentioned organisms with other species. They are usually similar in appearance, being grayish white, slightly exudative, and mildly erosive lesions on an erythematous base (Figs. 19–6 and 19–8). Ulcerations of the oral mucosa may be very small (2 to 3 mm) and difficult to visualize, even with good lighting. In spite of

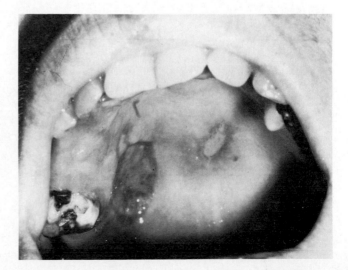

Figure 19–7. Palatal ulceration in a 53-year-old woman who has leukemia who was neutropenic secondary to chemotherapy. Note the broad, deep ulcer with a granulating base on the right side of the palate and the newer ulceration with a necrotic base on the left side of the palate. Both ulcers reveal minimal surrounding inflammatory infiltrate or erythema secondary to the myelosuppression.

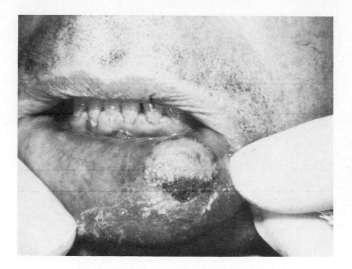

Figure 19–8. Secondarily infected labial ulcer in a 66-year-old man who has diffuse histiocytic lymphoma and was myelosuppressed secondary to chemotherapy. Note the large, necrotic area that is swollen. The lesion was extremely sensitive and had areas of hemorrhage.

their seemingly innocuous size, they may be acutely painful and serve as a portal of entry for pathogenic organisms (Fig. 19–9). Isolation of oral organisms from the blood of patients with sepsis is an important corroboratory procedure in those who are suspected of having oral infection.

Prevention and Treatment. It is often difficult to determine which mucosal lesions require antibiotic coverage. Factors to consider are the location and appearance of the lesion, the degree and duration of neutropenia, and the patient's temperature. If infection is suspected, the patient should be started on broad spectrum antibiotics to cover gram negatives and anaerobes. Such treatment should be continued until the lesions have resolved, the patient is afebrile, and the PMNL count shows

a significant rise (1000 cells per mm^3). Results of efforts to eliminate microorganisms from the mouth with broad spectrum nonabsorbable antibiotics have been disappointing, even when patients are maintained in laminar flow rooms. These opportunistic infections, therefore, are not always preventable, but their early recognition will decrease the incidence of morbidity and mortality.

Necrotizing Ulcerative Gingivitis

Necrotizing ulcerative gingivitis is a frequent oral complication of chemotherapy-induced neutropenia (Fig. 19–10). As with typical ANUG (Vincent's disease), the patient presents with painful necrosis of the marginal and papillary gingiva. There is loss of normal gin-

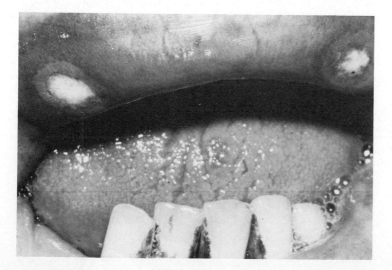

Figure 19–9. Bilateral, traumatic labial ulcerations in a myelosuppressed patient who has leukemia.

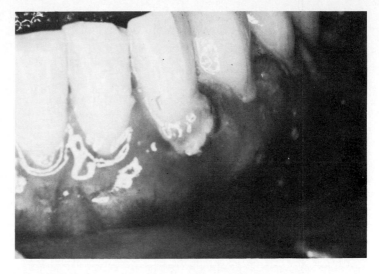

Figure 19–10. Necrotizing gingivitis in a 54-year-old woman who has acute myelogenous leukemia. At the time of the marginal ulceration and necrosis, the patient was significantly neutropenic. Note the clinical signs of pre-existing gingival inflammatory disease, which underlies the development of necrotizing gingivitis in these patients.

gival architecture. A necrotic pseudomembrane is usually present. The lesions frequently expand to include extensive areas of attached gingiva and palatal tissue. Bleeding may be noted. The causative organism involved in this lesion has not been determined. However, the shift to a predominantly gram-negative flora in patients who are myelosuppressed is well documented. Therefore, a variety of organisms, including *B. proteus,* Klebsiella, Serratia, Pseudomonas, Enterobacteriaceae, Bacteroides, and *E. Coli,* as well as spirochetes and fusiform organisms, must be considered as potential etiologic agents of ANUG. Patients who have pre-existing gingival inflammatory conditions appear to be at a higher risk of development of neutropenia-induced ANUG.

Treatment of chemotherapy-related ANUG is aimed at minimizing the systemic risk of infection, controlling local tissue destruction and palliation. Patients who are neutropenic (white blood count [WBC] < 1000) and febrile should be aggressively managed with broad spectrum parenteral antibiotics. Locally, tissue should be gently debrided with cotton swabs soaked in hydrogen peroxide and water. The mouth should be rinsed frequently. Recent evidence suggests that fluoride rinses may be helpful in reducing bacterial accumulation. Palliative rinses or systemic analgesics should be prescribed as needed. A soft diet may be recommended.

Salivary Gland Infection

Bacterial infections of the salivary glands most often affect the parotids. These infections are serious, especially in the cancer patient who is immunosuppressed or debilitated. Acute bacterial sialadenitis is usually found in a patient who is dehydrated, with decreased salivary flow and poor oral hygiene. Patients with severe vomiting, stomatitis, or other debilitating conditions that prevent adequate oral intake are also predisposed to this type of infection. The development of antibiotic-resistant bacteria and the use of drugs that decrease salivary flow have been suggested as a cause. *Streptococcus viridans* has been implicated in some cases, but penicillin-resistant *Staphylococcus aureus* is believed to be the most prevalent organism. Eighty to 90 percent of the reported cases of acute bacterial parotitis are unilateral. Patients usually complain of pain of sudden onset. Clinically, patients may have leukocytosis (if not myelosuppressed) in addition to fever and other signs of infection. The gland may be enlarged, red, and tender and may feel warm. If purulent material can be milked from Stensen's duct, the diagnosis is confirmed.

Prevention and Treatment. To prevent salivary gland infection, one must practice good oral hygiene and maintain adequate hydration. Cancer patients who have suspected or confirmed parotid bacterial infection should be treated aggressively. Specimens of the purulent discharge should be sent to the laboratory for culture and determination of antibiotic sensitivity. The patient should be started on parenteral antibiotics that are active against penicillin-resistant Staphylococcus before receiving sensitivity results. Oral hygiene should be instituted. Salivary flow can be stimulated with glycerin-lemon swabs or artificially sweetened lemon candy. Surgical drainage may be necessary if antibiotics do not result in rapid improvement.

Fungal Infections

There are several organisms that can cause fungal infections in the patient who is myelosuppressed, the most common being *Candida albicans* (Fig. 19–11). *Candida albicans* is a normal member of the oral microbiota in 20 to 50 percent of the population.[19] In the normal individual, the presence of this organism is of little clinical consequence, because its growth is kept in check by competitive inhibition by other organisms and by normal host defense mechanisms. However, in the patient who is compromised by disease or aggressive myelosuppressive or immunosuppressive therapy or whose oral microflora has been altered by antibiotics, Candida may overgrow and invade local tissue, may spread to the esophagus and/or lungs, or may involve hematologic spread. It has been proposed that any patient whose WBC falls to 200 cells per mm³ or below will develop oral candidiasis.[7]

Clinically, Candida infection may take on a variety of appearances. Classically, the lesion is described as being a white, raised, curdy cottage cheese–like growth that scrapes off, leaving a red, raw hemorrhagic base. Patients who have Candida are uncomfortable. Candida may also appear as an erythematous or white plaque that may also be discolored by exogenous forms of pigmentation. Patients rarely develop fever from Candida, which is localized in the mouth. Frequently, Candida infection may be noted on the palate under a denture. Other common sites include the dorsal surface of the tongue and the buccal mucosa.

Candida infections may also involve or spread to the esophagus or respiratory tract. Such involvement may occur secondary to oral candidiasis or may manifest *without* oral infection. The patient who is myelosuppressed and complains of dysphagia and is febrile should be considered for an esophagram.

Diagnosis of candidiasis is usually based on clinical appearance. Smears of infected areas will reveal mycelia when stained with gram stain or periodic acid-Schiff stain.

Prevention and Treatment. Although the value of prophylactic nystatin in the treatment of patients who do not have Candida is controversial,[4, 11, 14] its use does not pose a threat to the patient and may offer protection by postponing the onset of oral candidiasis as the patient proceeds to his or her nadir. The degree and duration of neutropenia seems to influence the incidence and extent of candidiasis. Therefore, the longer the time that candidiasis can be prevented or controlled, the less time the disease will have to manifest extension to the esophagus or lungs before the return of neutrophils to the peripheral blood. Patients in whom myelosuppression is anticipated should be placed on 300,000 units of nystatin (in suspension), to be swished and swallowed t.i.d. both at the initiation of and throughout chemotherapy treatment until the white blood cell counts return to near normal. Once Candida is clinically apparent intraorally,

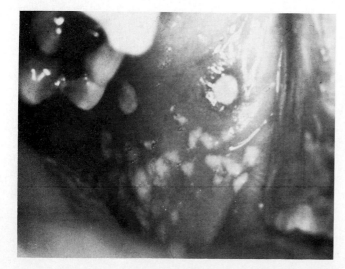

Figure 19–11. Candida infection in a 54-year-old woman who has acute leukemia. Note the raised, white areas along the buccal mucosa. The lesions could be scraped off, leaving a raw, bleeding base.

the nystatin dose can be raised and the patient may be started on Mycostatin lozenges (vaginal suppositories for use as lozenges), if tolerated, to prolong the contact of the antifungal agent with the oral mucosa. Popsicles of diluted nystatin are useful in the treatment of children. Oral candidiasis may also respond to topical gentian violet. The major disadvantage of gentian violet is that the purple stain that it imparts to the oral mucosa makes it very difficult for the clinician to visualize and follow oral lesions. A newly introduced antifungal troche, clotrimazole, 10 mg (Mycelex) may be used as an alternative to rinses. A troche is dissolved in the patient's mouth five times daily for 2 weeks. Throughout chemotherapy patients should be watched carefully for the onset of dysphagia. Esophageal or disseminated candidiasis must be treated early and aggressively with a systemic antifungal agent such as amphotericin B.

Viral Infections

The two most common viral infections seen in and about the oral cavity in the compromised patient result from the herpes simplex and varicella-zoster viruses.

Herpes Simplex

Herpes virus infections usually manifest in the adult as a result of reactivation of the virus from a latent state in regional nerve ganglia (Fig. 19–12). Infection appears as a singular or crop of vesicular lesions that are extraoral at or beyond the mucocutaneous junction. Although rare in the healthy patient, intraoral herpes lesions seem to occur with greater frequency and grow to a much larger size in the patient who is immunosuppressed. A cytologic smear of the base of the vesicle may reveal large epithelial cells that have an increase in the nuclear-cytoplasmic ratio and lobulation of the large nuclei. Viral inclusion bodies can be shown with special stains. Patients who have herpes simplex may have lymphadenopathy and may be febrile. Secondary bacterial infection of the virally involved site with local hemorrhage is not uncommon in patients who are myelosuppressed.

Herpacin-L ointment may be helpful in preventing the occurrence of new herpetic vesicles. Steroids are to be avoided. The lesions should be kept lubricated with ointment, such as Neosporin or Vaseline, to prevent drying and cracking of the mucosa. Patients who have herpes simplex should be followed closely for secondary infection, especially if they are neutropenic. The lesions normally regress within 7 to 10 days, depending upon host resistance, but have the potential to progress to multiple lesions in and around the mouth, pharynx, and esophagus.

Herpes Zoster

Herpes zoster infections are infections of varicella that remain latent in posterior root ganglia. Clinically, patients complain of sensitivity and present with unilateral vesicular lesions that follow the distribution of a branch of the trigeminal (V) nerve. Depending upon

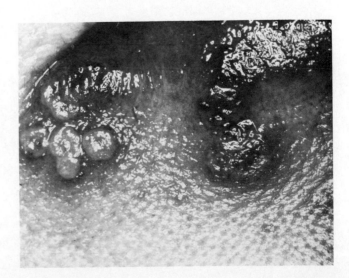

Figure 19–12. Herpes labialis in a 56-year-old woman who has acute leukemia. Note the raised, croppy vesicular areas at the corner of the mouth. There are also indications of secondary hemorrhage in and around other vesicles, probably as a result of the patient's thrombocytopenia.

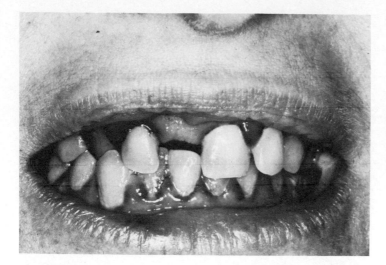

Figure 19–13. Gingival bleeding in a patient made thrombocytopenic secondary to myelosuppression from chemotherapy. Note the blood oozing from the gingival sulcus. There is evidence of pre-existing gingival disease and poor oral hygiene.

when they are seen, many lesions have ulcerative areas. Treatment is usually palliative.

Gingival and Submucosal Hemorrhage

Bleeding may occur anywhere in the mouth and may be spontaneous or may result from trauma to compromised tissue. Thrombocytopenia from chemotherapy-induced bone marrow suppression and pre-existing gingival pathology predispose patients to gingival bleeding (Fig. 19–13). Even minor trauma to the mucosa may result in submucosal bleeding and hematomas (Figs. 19–14 through 19–16). Bleeding may also occur from disseminated intravascular coagulation, an acquired disorder in which clotting factors and platelets are consumed in widespread coagulation within the blood vessels. The platelet count is not the sole indicator of the potential for hemorrhage; qualitative changes in the platelets also occur.[12] However, spontaneous gingival bleeding is usually indicative of a platelet count of about 15,000 cells per mm^3 or less.[18]

Prevention and Treatment. As mentioned previously, all potential sites of trauma, such as sharp teeth and appliances, should be eliminated prior to chemotherapy. An attempt should be made to create as healthy a gingival situation as possible in order to reduce the potential for hemorrhage. Gingival bleeding can usually be controlled with the use of

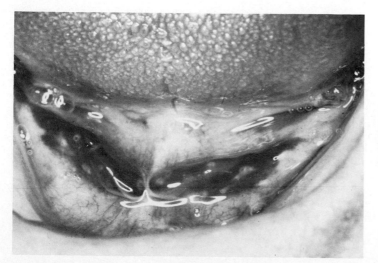

Figure 19–14. Submucosal hemorrhage in a patient made thrombocytopenic secondary to chemotherapy. Note the bilateral hemorrhagic appearance under the tongue.

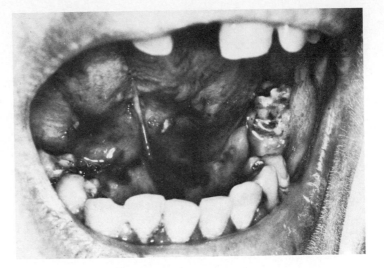

Figure 19–15. Sublingual area of the patient shown in Figure 19–14. Note the hematoma, especially on the left side of the tongue.

sponges soaked in topical thrombin and applied to the area. The clots formed should not be disturbed by chewing food or by rinsing or other mouth care, because these areas will continue to bleed if not managed carefully. Toothbrushing should cease when patients first note oozing or when the platelet count drops below 10,000 to 20,000 cells per mm³. Gingival enlargement secondary to leukemic infiltration may be seen in patients who have acute myelogenous leukemia. These patients are more prone to gingival trauma and bleeding, and radiotherapy is sometimes indicated to shrink the tissue.

Hematomas should be watched carefully for evidence of secondary infection because these collections of blood in a septic environment

such as the mouth can serve as a medium for growth of organisms. Hematomas in the floor of the mouth, oropharynx, or posterior tongue should be followed carefully for the development of a compromised airway. Healing hematomas may exhibit surface necrosis, followed several days later by the extrusion of granulationlike tissue from the area. These plugs of tissue should not be disturbed and will eventually exfoliate from a healing base. These problems of hemorrhage resolve with the return of platelets to the peripheral blood.

The use of platelet transfusions in thrombocytopenic patients is based on the threat of continued blood loss and potential for bleeding into the brain, gastrointestinal tract, or other vital organs. Overuse of platelet transfusions

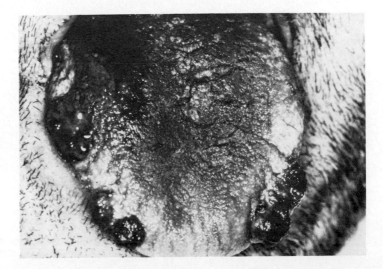

Figure 19–16. Hematoma formation on the lateral borders of the tongue in a thrombocytopenic 42-year-old man who has acute leukemia. Note that the hematoma formation appears to be localized to areas on the lateral border of the tongue, which are subject to trauma.

may result in antiplatelet antibodies and a decreased response to platelet therapy.

GENERAL PRINCIPLES OF PREVENTION

The primary goal in the management of oral cancer patients should be prevention. Ideally, these patients should be seen for complete dental evaluation soon after diagnosis and, if possible, prior to instituting chemotherapy or (head and neck) radiotherapy. If the patient's blood counts and overall condition permit, teeth that cannot be saved should be extracted and those remaining should be restored to prevent an acute situation at a time when dental manipulation may be contraindicated.

Endodontic therapy should be considered as an alternative to extraction for those patients who will maintain their dentition and hygiene at a high level of care. However, endodontic therapy involves risk in those patients who are expected to reach their nadir with consequent granulocytopenia and thrombocytopenia before the endodontic treatment can be completed. Temporary restorations may have to be placed in teeth to "buy time" until the patient's counts return to acceptable levels and until time is available for the placement of more permanent restorations. Patients who are too ill or whose counts are too low and who have unresolved carious lesions of the teeth should be started on a fluoride rinse in an effort to arrest the carious lesions. Sharp teeth and appliances should be adjusted. In addition, if time and blood counts permit, the patient should have a thorough oral prophylaxis to remove all local irritants from the teeth. At this time, the relationship between the patient's mouth and his or her overall health during the proposed chemotherapy should be discussed and proper emphasis should be placed on scrupulous oral hygiene. Patients often become highly motivated in mouth care when they understand that the incidence and severity of oral problems are often proportional to oral hygiene and health.

The systemic and local effects of chemotherapy also predispose these patients to nutritional disorders. Careful consideration of the patient's diet, including sucrose and refined carbohydrate intake, should be made on a continuing basis. Oral complications and cancer therapies may cause the patient to either lose interest in food or actually prevent eating or drinking. Stomatitis, secondary to chemotherapy-induced folic acid deficiency, contributes to mouth pain and decreased oral intake.

Nausea and vomiting also inhibit nutritional intake and increase the loss of proteins and water-soluble vitamins necessary for epithelial cell structure.[6] These considerations are also important in the patient who receives radiation that involves the salivary glands.[11, 15] Dreizen found that there was a measurable decline in food consumption and serum albumin during radiotherapy due to mucosal pain, anorexia, nausea, taste loss, and swallowing difficulties.[5] Foods to be avoided are those that are rough (for example, toast) and may abrade the mucosa, those too thick for the minimal saliva present, those too spicy or hot, and those that sting or burn the oral mucosa (for example, citric juices and alcoholic beverages). Generally, patients are best able to tolerate frequent feedings of high-protein and carbohydrate foods.[3] Cold foods and fluids are well tolerated and often soothing. Topical anesthetic rinses, topical benzocaine in orabase, and systemic analgesics should be used as needed to prevent mouth pain from limiting the patient's oral intake.

Although the decreased mortality rates among cancer patients are very encouraging, the frequency of morbidity associated with the treatment of cancer remains discouraging. As previously mentioned, oral complications from various treatment protocols are very significant, because they may account for compromised nutritional intake and patient discomfort, and, in the case of oral infection, they may indicate a threat to survival. The dentist can significantly help the cancer patient, not only in prolonging his or her life but also, and most importantly, in improving the quality of life. The patient who cannot speak, eat, or control secretions because of complications of therapy clearly cannot enjoy life to the extent of the patient who, in addition to having his or her malignancy controlled, is free of the side effects of therapy.

REFERENCES

1. Barakat, N., Toto, P., and Choukas, N.: Aging and cell renewal of oral epithelium. J. Periodontol., 40:599, 1977.
2. Bodey, G. P., Rodriguez, V., Chang, H. Y., et al.: Fever and infection in leukemic patients: a study of 494 consecutive patients. Cancer, 41:1610, 1978.
3. Bruya, M. A., and Madeira, N. P.: Stomatitis after chemotherapy. Am. J. Nurs., 75:1349, 1975.
4. Carpentieri, U., Haggard, M. E., Lockhart, L. H., et al.: Clinical experience in prevention of candidiasis by nystatin in children with acute lymphocytic leukemia. J. Pediatr., 92:593, 1978.

5. Dreizen, S.: Dental oncology at the University of Texas Dental Branch. Cancer Bull., *29*:61, 1980.
6. Dreizen, S., Bodey, G. P., and Rodriguez, V.: Oral complications of cancer chemotherapy. Postgrad. Med., *58*:75, 1975.
7. Edwards, J. E.: Severe candidal infections—clinical perspective, immune defense mechanisms, and current concepts of therapy. Ann. Intern. Med., *89*:91, 1978.
8. E.O.R.T.C. International Antimicrobial Therapy Project Group: Three antibiotic regimens in the treatment of infection in febrile granulocytopenic patients with cancer. J. Infect. Dis., *137*:14, 1978.
9. Hannigan, A., Sonis, S. T., and Lockhart, P. B.: Unpublished data.
10. Johanson, W. G., Pierce, A. K., Sanford, J. P.: Changing pharyngeal bacterial flora of hospitalized patients—emergence of gram-negative bacilli. N. Engl. J. Med., *281*:1137, 1969.
11. Keys, H. M., and McCasland, J. P.: Techniques and results of a comprehensive dental care program in head and neck cancer patients. Int. J. Radiat. Oncol. Biol. Phys., *1*:859, 1976.
12. Lisiewicz, J.: Mechanisms of hemorrhage in leukemias. Sem. Thromb. Hemost., *4*:241, 1978.
13. Lockhart, P. B., and Sonis, S. T.: Relationship of oral complications to peripheral blood leukocytes and platelet counts in patients receiving cancer chemotherapy. Oral Surg., *48*:21, 1979.
14. Pizzuto, J., Conte, G., Ambruz, R., et al.: Nystatin prophylaxis in leukemia and lymphoma. N. Engl. J. Med., *298*:279, 1978.
15. Rotman, M., Rogow, L., DeLeon, G., et al.: Supportive therapy in radiation oncology. Cancer, *39*:744, 1977.
16. Shannon, I. L., Trodahl, J. N., and Starcke, E. N.: Remineralization of enamel by a saliva substitute designed for use by irradiated patients. Cancer, *41*:1746, 1978.
17. Sonis, S. T., Sonis, A. L., and Lieberman, A.: Oral complications in patients receiving treatment for malignancies other than the head and neck. J. Am. Dent. Assoc., *97*:468, 1978.
18. Stafford, R. F., Lockhart, P. B., Sonis, A. L., et al.: Hematologic parameters as predictors of oral involvement in the presentation of acute leukemia. J. Oral Med., *37*:38, 1982.
19. Taschdjian, C. L., Kozinn, P. J., and Tuni, E. F.: Opportunistic yeast infections with special reference to candidiasis. Ann. N.Y. Acad. Sci., *174*:606, 1974.

20

Immunology and immunotherapy of cancer

JOEL L. SCHWARTZ, D.M.D., D.M.Sc.

The health of the oral tissues, like other tissues in the body, is dependent upon their ability to resist infection. One of the ways that the body defends itself is through its immune system.

In the head and neck region and throughout the body, the immune defense system is composed of certain organ systems that produce the immune effector cells.

The thymus is composed of a series of lobules of epithelial cells. In each lobule, there are packed aggregates of lymphocytes. The outer cortical area is formed of actively mitotic lymphoid cells and surrounds an inner medullary region of reticular epithelioid cells, fewer lymphocytes, and isolated Hassall's corpuscles. The lymphocytes derived from the thymus are referred to as T cells (thymus-derived cells). The loss of a thymus results in the decreased circulation of lymphocytes (T cells), reduced ability to reject grafted tissue, impairment in the humoral immune response or formation of antibodies to some foreign materials (antigens), and reduced ability to destroy some cancer cells.

In chickens, there is another lymphoid organ called the bursa of Fabricius. It is from this organ that cells capable of producing antibody are derived, and therefore are called B cells (bursa-derived cells). The equivalent of the bursa in man and other mammals has not clearly been defined; however, results of studies using the bone marrow or fetal liver indicate that there is hematopoietic induction of precursors of B cells.

Morphologically, the B and T lymphocytes are similar in appearance and size. Morphologic criteria can only be utilized when the B lymphocyte matures into a plasma cell. The

plasma cell exhibits a striking histologic picture, with an eccentric nucleus that contains a cartwheel arrangement of nucleolar material and a clear area that surrounds a prominent Golgi complex situated close to the nucleus.

T and B lymphocytes can be isolated and identified with fluorescein-labeled anti-immunoglobulin. Results of these immunofluorescent staining techniques have shown that T lymphocytes do not possess immunoglobulin (Ig) on their cell surface, but they do have Thy 1 (theta) antigen. Additionally, in studies using antisera that are directed against the T-lymphocyte cell surface, the Ly 1, 2, and 3 antigen system, a complex of three antigenic determinants on the cell surface of T lymphocytes, has been defined. The identification of this system has disclosed that there are subsets to the T-lymphocyte population. The T helper cell, which helps the B cell to produce antibody (Ly 1^+, 2^-, 3^-); the T suppressor cell, which reduces the formation of antibody (Ly 1^-, 2^+, 3^+); the cytotoxic T cell, which can lyse tumor cells (Ly 1^-, 2^+, 3^+); and the progenitor T cell, which matures into any of the other types of T cells, especially the T suppressor cell, after antigen stimulation (Ly 1^+, 2^+, 3^+) and thereby modifies the antibody response.[6]

The B-lymphocyte population lacks the Ly cell surface antigens; instead, they have various antibody classes on their cell surface. The most prominent antibody class found on the surface is IgM. After stimulation following antigen presentation, IgG, IgA, or IgE will be formed. Another class of antibody, IgD, is formed early in development, particularly in the notochord. Its function is not well understood, and its relationship to IgM production is unclear.[74]

202

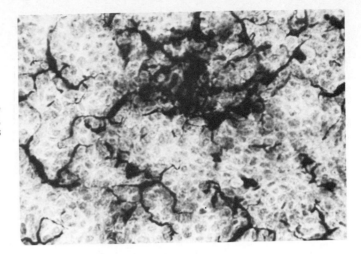

Figure 20–1. Epithelial whole mount of the buccal pouch of a normal Syrian hamster, showing the distribution of Langerhans cells (ATPase-Pb stain × 600).

Another important effector cell in the immune response is the macrophage. The macrophage is a widely distributed phagocytic cell that processes antigen and then presents this molecule to the T cell. The macrophage can also release various chemical products to either stimulate colony production of immune effectors (CSF, colony stimulating factor) or produce prostaglandin products, complement proteins, or collagenase, elastase, and lysosomal proteases, as a small example of the large secretory capacity of these cells.[6]

The Langerhans cell, a particular type of macrophage, is regarded as the functional equivalent in the skin and mucosa.[65] This macrophage-like cell is critical in antigen processing as well as in the presentation of antigen to the T cell.[53] These cells have the same functional characteristics as macrophages; they bear the Fc receptor (the biologic active crystalline portion of immunoglobulin) and the C_3 receptor (C3b), which is a blood protein that is important in the lytic activity of antibody. Additionally, they have Ia antigen on their cell surface and respond to alloantigen in a manner similar to macrophages.[43]

Schwartz and colleagues[58] have recently shown that these cells are found in a nonrandom pattern in the oral mucosa of the Syrian hamster. That is, there are both focal aggregates of these cells and a diffusely arranged interfocal dendritic network of the Langerhans cells.[58] It has also been found that the distribution and morphology of these cells are affected by various exogenous agents.[58, 70] Results of recent investigations have shown that the carcinogen 7,12-dimethylbenz(a)anthracene (DMBA) and 13-cis-retinoic acid affect the density and alter the morphology of the Langerhans cells (Figs. 20–1 through 20–4).

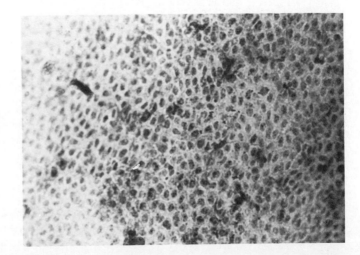

Figure 20–2. DMBA-treated buccal pouch of a Syrian hamster, showing absence of Langerhans cells (ATPase-Pb stain × 600).

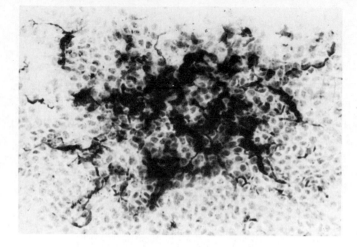

Figure 20–3. Focal distribution of Langerhans cells in the buccal pouch of a normal hamster (ATPase-Pb stain × 600).

These agents may then alter the antigen processing by the Langerhans cells and therefore affect the immune response to antigen.

In addition to the primary lymphoid organs previously described, there are other sites of immune activity. The lymph nodes, with their structure of germinal centers, cortical regions (B-lymphocyte region), and paracortical regions (T-lymphocyte region), represent a major site of immune activity. In the spleen, another important site, there is activity in the region of the white pulp, particularly in the cortical arterial sheath region (T lymphocytes) and in the peripheral arterial sheath region (B lymphocytes). Additionally, in the spleen, one finds germinal centers like those of the lymph nodes. Another site is the diffuse lymphoid system of the gastrointestinal tract, which takes the form of Peyer's patches, consisting of isolated germinal centers and lymphoid follicles, composed of B and T lymphocytes and macrophages.[67]

In the oral cavity, there are extraoral lymph nodes derived from lymph capillaries. These lymph nodes drain the tongue, floor of the mouth, palate, cheeks, lips, gingiva, and pulp of the teeth. In addition to these areas, there are lymphoid masses between the glossopalatine and pharyngopalatine arches (palatine tonsils), lingual tonsils on the posterior lateral border of the tongue, and pharyngeal tonsils (adenoids) under the mucosa of the nasopharynx. In the head and neck region, there is also major lymph node drainage through the jugular and digastric system.[28]

Immunity is not a single host response but may involve several different patterns, including:

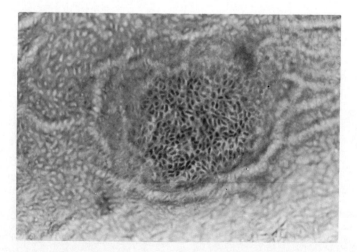

Figure 20–4. Epidermal elevation in the buccal pouch, showing absence of Langerhans cells following treatment with DMBA (ATPase-Pb stain × 600).

1. The humoral response in which antibody is produced through the activation of the B lymphocytes.

2. Cell-mediated immunity in which T or B cells are activated to produce various chemical products (lymphokines) that modulate and elaborate the immune response.

3. Macrophage response, which elaborates its phagocytic ability to become cytotoxic to cancer cells, and processes antigen to initiate the cell-mediated response and antibody formation. The macrophage as well as other effectors (null lymphocytes, K cells, and killer cells) are also involved in a cytotoxic response, which does not require a cell to cell interaction but only antibody. This antibody (IgG or IgM) acts as a bridge, via an Fc receptor from the effector cell to the target cell,[13, 46] and is called *antibody dependent cellular cytotoxicity (ADCC)*.

Results of recent studies have indicated that in animal tumor models and in some human cancers there are tumor specific antigens located on the tumor surface.[20] It has been hypothesized that the immune response that actively protects the host from tumor development (immune surveillance theory) also recognizes these tumor specific antigens.[16] Evidence for this theory has come from observations of tumor formation following the use of immunosuppressive agents in patients and in animals.[66] However, it is clear that tumors do escape this defense by a variety of mechanisms. To fully comprehend how this occurs and how immunotherapy might help to alleviate the tumor load of the host, one must understand the immune response and regulatory mechanisms.

Early in the formulation of the immune surveillance theory, it was determined that the basis for resistance to both allografts and syngeneic tumor grafts was cellular in nature. In a classic experiment, it has been shown that immune (sensitized) lymphoid cells can protect a syngeneic recipient from the appropriate tumor. Additionally, using a leukemia system in vivo, antisera from tumor-bearing animals have protected non-immune animals from the identical tumor.[6]

MECHANISMS OF HOST IMMUNE RESPONSE

Humoral Immunity—B-Lymphocyte Response

B lymphocytes, as previously stated, are concerned with antibody production. Specifi-

cally, this antibody could be directed toward a tumor antigen on the cell's surface. Additionally, this antibody can also combine with the Fc receptors of effector cells and mount an ADCC reaction. Therefore, with the production of antibody, there is not only a proliferation of a specific B-cell line but also an elaboration of the immune response, so that other effectors are excited and have a heightened immune responsiveness. Additionally, through a blood protein system called *complement* (C1 to C9), there is an increase in phagocytosis (opsonization) through the activity of C3b and an increase in chemotactic migration with C3a and C5a of macrophages and polymorphonuclear leukocytes. Additionally, this protein system causes the lytic activity of IgG immunoglobulin to target cells.[1] It has also been shown that this system elaborates the immune response by releasing an anaphylotoxin, which is a small fragment of C3a or C5a that is capable of degranulating mast cells and liberating vasoactive amines.[1]

In head and neck cancer patients, changes in humoral immunity have not been found to be dramatic. The regional lymph nodes of these patients seem to have a decreased number of B lymphocytes.[64] To date, there is no increase in ADCC activity,[63] and there appears to be only a poorly understood variable response to pokeweed mitogen, a B-lymphocyte stimulator of antibody production to various antigens.[73]

It is interesting to note that, in general, head and neck cancer patients have increased titers of serum IgA and IgE, whereas there are normal levels of IgG, IgM, and IgD.[15, 59] In addition, it has been found that salivary IgA and IgG is increased, although the levels are variable.[15] It has been hypothesized that the selective increase of the IgA class of immunoglobulin could be associated with IgA's capacity to alter the adherence of foreign antigen (*Streptococcus mutans*). In relation to its role as the immunoglobulin of greatest concentration in saliva derived from the submaxillary and sublingual glands, the increase in IgA may be associated with the observation of a localized accumulation of plasma cells (mature B lymphocytes) in draining submaxillary and sublingual lymph nodes of head and neck tumors.[38] It would be interesting to know if oral sensitization by tumor might stimulate B cells in the gut associated lymphoid tissue (GALT), mucosal associated lymphoid tissue (MALT), or bronchial associated lymphoid tissue (BALT) systems.

Antibody has been observed on the cell

surface of squamous cell carcinomas derived from the oral mucosa.[69] Whether the antibody was deposited directly on the tumor surface or in the form of an antigen-antibody complex is unknown.[50] Immune complexes of antigen-antibody have been found to be circulating in the blood stream of more than 50 percent of the head and neck cancer patients in one study.[45] Antibody has been found to be directed against viral specific antigens of the Epstein-Barr virus and herpes type I virus in head and neck cancer patients.[40, 61] It is interesting to note that the Epstein-Barr virus is currently thought to be the etiologic agent in Burkitt's lymphoma and nasopharyngeal carcinoma.[30, 33]

In addition to the complement system, other blood proteins, including immune reactive proteins (IRP); glycoproteins, such as haptoglobin and acid glycoprotein; and an antitrypsin have been found to alter the humoral immune response.[1, 4] However, their specific effects on antibody production is, as yet, undefined.

Cell-Mediated Immunity—Cell to Cell Interaction

Cell-mediated immunity involves the activation of an effector cell without the activity of antibody. One effector of great importance in this form of immune response is the T lymphocyte, which is used routinely for in vitro tumor assays. The development of a cytotoxic lymphocyte (CTL) is derived from the presence of the Ly surface phenotype, which is Ly 1^-, 2^+, 3^+, and was previously described. Using such assays as the Winn assay or chromium release assay (CRA) that involve the adoptive transfer of recognizable tumor cells of the host, the effector CTL T cells cause the lysis of the target tumor cells as a result of their capacity to respond to a foreign major histocompatibility antigen (Ia response gene products on the cell surface).[6]

Another effector that has recently become important in cellular tumor immunity has been the heterogenous null lymphocyte population. One prominent cell involved is the killer cell. Using spleen cells from young (2- to 4-week-old) normal rats and mice and after separating out the killer population, these cells have been shown to be cytotoxic to Moloney leukemia virus-transformed cells and Yac-lymphoma target cells.[50] Additionally, it has been shown that a mouse-derived null cell population will preferentially migrate to the site of a Moloney sarcoma virus–induced tumor[57] and that this population as well as other killer- and K-cell

populations can lyse specific tumor target cells by ADCC.[34, 37]

The macrophage is the most important non-lymphocyte effector cell in tumor immunity. Recent evidence indicates that after activation of the macrophage by various antigens or by lymphokines, produced by T and B lymphocytes, such as macrophage activating factor and macrophage inhibitory factor, the macrophage becomes cytotoxic. The cytotoxic macrophage can discriminate between malignant cells that lack contact inhibition and normal cells that show inhibition.[22]

Other lymphokines produced by activated T or B lymphocytes elaborate the immune response by increasing the production of other immune effectors and by producing chemotactic factors that direct the migration of these immune effectors.[52]

In head and neck cancer patients, there seems to be a defect in the cell-mediated immunity. This defect in cell immunity has been determined through the use of skin sensitivity to dinitrochlorobenzene (DNCB). In 56 to 70 percent of head and neck cancer patients, a decrease was shown in delayed skin hypersensitivity to DNCB compared with only a 5 percent loss of this reaction in patients in a control group.[17] It has been said that this anergic reaction to DNCB correlates with the regression of the tumor following radiotherapy and with the ability to remain tumor free.[11, 12]

Another antigen, purified protein derivative of tuberculin (PPD), produces a secondary delayed hypersensitivity in normal patients, and studies indicate that it is a better predictor of short-term survival than is reactivity to DNCB.[44] This antigen and others such as mumps antigen, candidal antigen, or streptokinase-streptodornase (SK-SD) antigen have been used to show anergic responses in 45 percent of head and neck cancer patients compared with 8 percent of non–tumor-bearing patients.[3] It is of interest that this lack of response to antigen is found in head and neck cancer patients at an earlier stage than in sarcoma or melanoma patients.[51]

Experimentally, in vitro assays of T lymphocytes indicate that there is a decrease in T-cell rosette formation and in mitogen and blast response to concanavalin A (Con A) and phytohemagglutinin (PHA).[36, 54] Additionally, the mixed lymphocyte reaction (MLR), which produces a cytotoxic T lymphocyte, shows a 47 to 67 percent reduction in activity in ability to lyse a cancer target cell.[23] A depression of the peripheral T lymphocytes is also indicated.[18]

Other factors that may be involved in the immune response are the presence of primary or secondary immune deficiencies and the age of the patient.[29, 71] In particular, there is indirect evidence that the incidence of head and neck cancer increases with age and that there is a depression of delayed hypersensitivity to DNCB and PPD. In addition, it has been noted that there is a reduction of blast formation and proliferation by PHA and Con A.[26] In patients who are immunosuppressed, specifically in those receiving grafts, it has been noted that there is an increase in the development of squamous cell carcinoma of the lip.[48] Immune reactivity can also be affected by the quantity of alcohol consumed daily,[8] liver damage,[9] malnutrition,[39] smoking,[19] chemotherapy,[10] and radiotherapy.[63]

Although the immune response appears to be well developed for defending the host from tumor development, a variety of mechanisms are used by tumors to circumvent these defenses.

Tumor Evasive Mechanisms

The first means through which the tumor escapes destruction is by a lack of a recognizable foreign tumor cell surface. This end result is achieved through the development of a state of tolerance[42] or a lack of immune response gene activity (Ia) by immune effectors (T, B, or macrophage cells).[16] Although an immunologic reaction is produced, it is also possible that it is too weak to destroy the tumor burden.[2] A correlate to the previously mentioned escape path is that the tumor growth rate surpasses the immune capacity.[2]

Other mechanisms that are used by tumors to evade immune surveillance include various blocking factors, which are secreted by tumor cells.[31] These factors enhance tumor growth by either directly blocking effector cell receptors (Fc or C3b) with antigen-antibody complexes or by tumor antigen, which is released by the tumor.[35, 62] Recently it has been found that tumors can alter the immune response by altering blood vessel formation (angiogenesis factor, leukotriene release) and developing a fibrous, fibrin network that surrounds a developing tumor and by protecting the tumor from antibody or interaction with immune effectors.[25] Antigen-antibody complexes have been isolated from head and neck cancer patients, as well as eluted from the cell surface of lymphoma cells.[41] An unblocking antibody has

been found that counteracts the effects of free antigen blocking the immune response.[62]

The activation and elaboration of the immune response may also result in the proliferation of T suppressor cells, reducing antibody formation. This population has been found to be active in animals that have growing tumors.[47]

It has been hypothesized that the depletion of blood complement levels decreases the lytic ability of antibody and the elaboration of the immune response.[16]

IMMUNOTHERAPY

Many attempts have been made to augment the immune response. Immunotherapy is divided into the following categories:

1. Prophylactic immunization with normal or treated tumor cells. These tumor cells may be identical or may share antigens with the tumor possessed by the host.

2. Treatment with a variety of non–tumor-related adjuvants that increase the immune response nonspecifically, such as *Corynebacterium parvum* (*C. parvum*).

3. Inoculation directly into the accessible tumor with agents that augment the tumor immunity of the host, such as bacillus Calmette-Guérin (BCG) or attenuated *Mycobacterium tuberculosis*.

4. Passive immunotherapy involving inoculation of antibody or modified antibody specific for the tumor's antigenic surface.

5. Adoptive immunotherapy using activated T lymphocytes or immune reactive products. These substances include transfer factor, immune RNA, thymus extracts and interferon.

Experimentally, tumor cells have been inoculated into animals in small doses to produce growth, then regression of the tumor. This response has provided the host with a relatively strong resistance to secondary challenge to the original tumor. In addition, if the tumor is first irradiated to eliminate mitotic division and if it is given in small doses, a prophylatic immunization by the host can be seen towards the tumor.[7] It has also been shown that if tumor cells are chemically treated, slightly altering their cell surface with chemicals such as dinitrophenol, iodoacetate, or vibrio cholera neuraminidase, a rejection of untreated identical tumor cells is noted.[21, 68]

Currently, adjuvant immunotherapy is being investigated in several studies. Substances such as BCG and *C. parvum*, which nonspecifically activate macrophages to become cytotoxic,[55, 56] have been injected intralesionally into squamous cell carcinoma of the oral cavity. The results indicate that there is a reduction in the number and concentration of infiltrating tumor cells in these patients.[5] Another study noted a reduction in tumor mass in 65 percent of 52 patients who had malignant melanoma of the mucosa, following x-irradiated neuraminidase and BCG treatment of melanoma cells.[60] In animal tumor model systems, particularly in the hamster buccal cheek pouch, BCG has been shown to inhibit the growth of squamous cell carcinoma induced by DMBA.[27] Using an antihelmintic drug, levamisole, and the hamster pouch tumor model, there was a reduction in the tumor size and number induced by DMBA compared with those in the control group.[24] In a recent study in human patients, levamisole was given to patients who had squamous cell carcinoma, with the thought of stimulating the cell-mediated immune system. The results indicated that the only significant effect of this drug was a reduction in the tumors of patients who had stage II oral cancer.[72]

Using a multimodal therapy approach, thymosin was injected into lesions of the head and neck after the patients had received a course of radiotherapy. The unfortunate observation was made that there was no difference between the thymosin treated group and a similar untreated group in terms of their immune function and death rate.[75]

Recently, human leukocyte interferon has been used to treat tumors of the head and neck. Interferon application appears to prevent dispersal of tumor cells during surgery and decreases metastatic spread after treatment.[14]

As we become more knowledgeable about the immune process and tumor rejection, it is hoped that immunotherapy will play a more useful role in the treatment and eradication of tumors.

REFERENCES

1. Austen, K. F.: The classical and alternative complement sequence. In Benacerraf, B., and Unanue, E. R. (eds.): Textbood of Immunology, Chapter 12. Baltimore, The Williams and Wilkins Co., 1979, pp. 218–239.
2. Baldwin, R. W.: Immunological aspects of chemical carcinogenesis. Adv. Cancer Res., 18:1, 1973.
3. Banner, R. L., Vaughn, W. K., Hagey, K. A., et al.: Cyclic adenosine monophosphate - phosphodiesterase (CAMP-PDE) in lymphocytes from patients with stage III and IV squamous cell carcinoma of the head and neck. J. Surg. Oncol., 9:61, 1977.
4. Baskies, A. M., Chretien, P. B., Wolf, G. T., et al.: Correlation of serum immune-reactive proteins with clinical tumor stage in patients with squamous carcinoma of the head and neck and nasopharyngeal carcinoma. Surg. Forum, 30:516, 1979.
5. Bast, R. C., Jr., Zbar, B., Borsos, T., et al.: BCG and cancer. N. Engl. J. Med., 290:1458, 1974.
6. Benacerraf, B., and Unanue, E. R.: The cellular basis of immunity. In Textbook of Immunology, Chapter 5. Baltimore, The Williams and Wilkins Co., 1979, pp. 76–108.
7. Benacerraf, B., and Unanue, E. R.: Tumor immunology. In Textbook of Immunology, Chapter 11. Baltimore, The Williams and Wilkins Co., 1979, pp. 196–217.
8. Berenyi, M. R., Straus, B., and Crux, D.: In vivo and in vitro studies of cellular immunity in alcoholic cirrhosis. Am. J. Digest. Dis., 19:199, 1974.
9. Bernstein, I. M., Williams, R. C., Webster, K. H., et al.: Reduction in circulating T-lymphocytes in alcoholic liver disease. Lancet, 2:488, 1974.
10. Bitter, K.: Immunity suppression by bleomycin-methotrexate combined treatment in patients with epidermoid carcinoma of the oral cavity. J. Maxillofac. Surg., 2:35, 1974.
11. Bosworth, J. L., Ghossein, N. A., and Brooks, T. L.: Delayed hypersensitivity in patients treated by curative radiotherapy. Cancer, 36:353, 1975.
12. Bosworth, J. L., Thaler, S., Ghossein, N. A.: Delayed hypersensitivity and local control of patients treated by radiotherapy for head and neck cancer. Am. J. Surg., 132:46, 1976.
13. van Boxel, U. A., van Stobo, J. D., Paul, W. E., et al.: Antibody-dependent lymphoid cell mediated cytotoxicity for requirement for thymus derived lymphocytes. Science, 175:194, 1971.
14. Brodarec, I. D., Padovan, I., Knexevic, M., et al.: Applications of human leukocyte interferon in patients with tumors of the head and neck. Lancet, 1:1025, 1981.
15. Brown, A. M., Lally, E. T., and Frankel, A.: IgA and IgG content of the saliva and serum of oral cancer patients. Arch. Oral Biol., 20:359, 1975.
16. Byers, V. S., and Levin, A. S.: Tumor Immunology. In Fudenberg, H. H., Stites, D. P., Caldwell, J. L., et al. (eds.): Basic and Clinical Immunology, Chapter 21. Los Altos, California, Lange Medical Publications, 1976, pp. 242–259.
17. Catalona, W. J., Sample, W. F., and Chretien, P. B.: Lymphocyte reactivity in cancer patients correlation with tumor histology and clinical stage. Cancer, 31:65, 1973.
18. Check, I. J., Hunter, R. L., Lounsberg, B., et al.: Prediction of survival in head and neck cancer based on leukocyte sedimentation in Ficoll-Hypaque gradients. Laryngoscope, 90:1281, 1980.
19. Chretien, P. M.: The effects of smoking on immunocompetence. Laryngoscope, 88:11, 1978.
20. Coggin, J. H., Jr., and Anderson, N. G.: Cancer, differentiation and embryonic antigens: some central problems. Adv. Cancer Res., 19:105, 1974.
21. Cunningham, T. J., Amtemann, R., Paonessa, D., et al.: Adjuvant immuno- and/or chemotherapy with neuraminidase-treated autogenous tumor vaccine and bacillus Calmette-Guérin for head and neck cancers. Ann. N. Y. Acad. Sci., 277:339, 1976.
22. David, J. R., and David, R. R.: Cellular hypersensitivity and immunity: Inhibition of macrophage migration and the lymphocyte mediators. Prog. Allergy., 16:300, 1972.

23. Deegan, M., Coulthard, W., Qualman, S. J., et al.: A correlative analysis of in vitro parameters of cellular immunity in patients with squamous cell carcinoma of the head and neck. Cancer, *37*:4475, 1977.

24. Eisenberg, E. and Shklar, G.: Levamisole and hamster pouch carcinogenesis. Oral Surg., *4*:562, 1977.

25. Folkman, J., and Cotran, R.: Relation of vascular proliferation to tumor growth. Int. Rev. Exp. Pathol., *16*:207, 1976.

26. Giannini, D., and Sloan, R. S.: A tuberculin survey of 1285 adults with special reference to the elderly. Lancet, *1*:525, 1957.

27. Giunta, J. L., Reif, A. E., and Shklar, G.: Bacillus Calmette-Guérin and antilymphocyte serum in carcinogenesis. Arch Pathol., *98*:237, 1974.

28. Gray, H.: *In* Goss, M. C. (ed.): Anatomy of the Human Body, Chapter 10. Philadelphia, Lea and Febiger, 1973, pp. 741–747.

29. Gross, L.: Immunologic defect in an aged population and its relationship to cancer. Cancer, *18*:201, 1965.

30. Heimer, R., and Klein, G.: Circulating immune complexes in sera of patients with Burkitt's lymphoma and nasopharyngeal carcinoma. Int. J. Cancer, *18*:310, 1976.

31. Hellström, K. E., and Hellström, I.: Lymphocyte mediated cytotoxicity and blocking serum activity to tumor antigen. Adv. Immunol., *18*:209, 1974.

32. Henle, W., and Henle, G.: Comparison of immune responses and viral markers in herpes virus-associated carcinomas: a review. IARC Sci. Publ., *24*: 801, 1978.

33. Herberman, R. B., and Holden, H. T.: Natural cell mediated immunity. *In* Klein, G., Weinhouse, S., (eds.): Advances in Cancer Research. New York, Academic Press, Inc., 1978.

34. Herberman, R. B., Munn, M. E., and Lavrin, D. H.: Natural cytotoxic reactivity of mouse lymphoid cells against syngeneic and allogenic tumors. I. Distribution of reactivity and specificity. Int. J. Cancer, *16*:230, 1976.

35. Jeejeebhoy, H. F.: Stimulation of tumor growth by the immune response. Int. J. Cancer, *13*:665, 1974.

36. Jenkins, V. K., Ray, P., Ellis, H. H., et al.: Lymphocyte response in patients with head and neck cancer. Arch. Otolaryngol., *102*:596, 1976.

37. Kiessling, R., Petranyi, G., Kane, K., et al.: Killer cells, a functional comparison between natural immune T cell and antibody dependent in vitro systems. J. Exp. Med., *143*:772, 1976.

38. Kvneval, T., Applebaum, E., Popovic, D., et al.: Demonstration of immunoglobulin in tumors and marginal tissues of squamous cell carcinoma of the head and neck. J. Natl. Cancer Inst., *59*:1089, 1977.

39. Law, D., Dudrick, S., and Abdow, M. I.: Immunocompetence of patients with protein-caloric malnutrition. Ann. Intern. Med., *79*:545, 1974.

40. Levine, P. H., Ho, J. H., Nkrumah, F., et al.: Evaluation of delayed hypersensitivity reactions to lymphoid cell lines and antibodies to Epstein-Barr virus. IARC Sci. Publ., *24*:893, 1978.

41. Lichtenstein, A., Sighelboim, J., Dorey, F., et al.: Comparison of immune derangements in patients with different malignancies. Cancer, *45*:2090, 1980.

42. Linscott, W. D.: Specific immunologic unresponsiveness. *In*: Fudenberg, H. H., Stites, D. P., Caldwell, J. L., et al. (eds.): Basic and Clinical Immunology, Chapter 13. Los Altos, California, Lange Medical Publications, 1976.

43. Lynch, D. H., Genish, M. F., Daynes, R. A.: Relationship between epidermal Langerhans cells density,

44. Mandel, M. A., and Kiehn, C. L.: The prognostic significance of delayed cutaneous reactivity in head and neck cancer patients. Plast. Reconstr. Surg., *53*:72, 1974.

45. Maxim, P. E., Veltric, R. W., Sprinkle, P. M., et al.: Soluble immune complexes in sera from head and neck cancer patients. A preliminary report. Otolaryngology, *86*:428, 1978.

46. Moller, G., and Svehag, S. E.: Specificity of lymphocyte-mediated cytotoxicity induced by in vitro antibody-coated target cells. Cell. Immun., *4*:1, 1972.

47. Nakayama, E., Shiku, H., Stockert, E., et al.: Cytotoxic T cells: Ly$^+$ phenotype and blocking of killing activity by Ly$^+$ antisera. Proc. Natl. Acad. Sci., *74*:76, 1977.

48. Penn, I.: Immunosuppression and cancer importance in head and neck surgery. Arch. Otolaryngol., *101*:667, 1975.

49. Pisciotta, A. V., Westring, D. V., DePrey, C., et al.: Mitogenic effects of phytohemagglutinin at different ages. Nature, *215*:193, 1967.

50. Popovic, D., Gill, L., Sisson, G., et al.: Detection and localization of tumor-associated immune complements of head and neck squamous cell carcinomas. Trans. Am. Acad. Opthamol., *82*:119, 1976.

51. Potvin, C., Tapley, J. L., and Chretien, P. B.: Thymus derived lymphocytes in patients with solid malignancies. Clin. Immunol. Immunopathol., *3*:476, 1975.

52. Rocklin, R. E.: Mediators in cellular immunity. *In* Fudenberg, H. H., Stites, D. P., Caldwell, J. L., et al. (eds.): Basic and Clinical Immunology, Chapter 10. Los Altos, California, Lange Medical Publications, 1976, pp. 102–113.

53. Rowden, G., Phillips, T. M., and Delovitch, T. L.: Expression of Ia antigen by murine keratinizing epithelial Langerhans cells. Immunogenetics, *7*:465, 1978.

54. Sample, W. F., Gertner, H. R., and Chretien, P. B.: Inhibition of phytohemagglutinin-induced in vitro lymphocyte transformation by serum from patients with carcinoma. J. Natl. Cancer Inst., *46*:1291, 1971.

55. Schlesinger, S., Pickartz, H., and Bier, J.: Quantitative changes in the intratumoral and peritumoral cell population after BCG cell wall therapy for squamous cell carcinoma of the oral cavity. Dtsch. Zahna. Z., *35*:118, 1980.

56. Schuller, G., Squire, C., Moy, C., et al.: Presurgical intratumor immunotherapy of carcinoma of the head and neck. Proc. Am. Assoc. Cancer Res., *19*:223, 1978.

57. Schwartz, J. L., Reinisch, C. L.: Migration of null lymphocytes to murine sarcoma virus induced tumors. Clin. Immunol. Immunopathol., *20*:74, 1981.

58. Schwartz, J. L., Solt, D. B., Pappo, J., et al.: Distribution of Langerhans cells in oral mucosa undergoing carcinogenesis. J. Dermatol. Surg. Oncol., *7*:1005, 1981.

59. Scully, C.: The immunology of cancer of the head and neck with particular reference to oral cancer. Oral Surg., *53*:157, 1982.

60. Seigler, H. F., Cox, E., Mutzner, F., et al.: Specific active immunotherapy for melanoma. Ann. Surg., *190*:366, 1979.

61. Shillitoe, E. J., and Silverman, S.: Oral cancer and herpes simplex virus: a review. Oral Surg., *48*:216, 1979.

62. Sjögren, H. O., Hellström, I., Bansal, S. C., et al.:

Suggestive evidence that the "blocking antibodies" of tumor bearing individuals may be antigen-antibody complexes. Proc. Natl. Acad. Sci., 68:1372, 1971.

63. Stefani, S. S., and Kerman, R. H.: Lymphocyte response to phytohemagglutinin before and after radiation therapy in patients with carcinoma of the head and neck. J. Laryngol. Otol., 91:605, 1977.

64. Stefani, S. S., Kerman, R. H., and Abbate, J.: Serial studies of immunocompetence in head and neck cancer patients undergoing radiation therapy. Am. J. Roentgenol., 126: 4:880, 1976.

65. Stingl, G., Katz, S. I., Shevach, E. M., et al.: Analogous functions of macrophages and Langerhans cells in the initiation of the immune response. J. Invest. Dermatol., 71:59, 1978.

66. Stutman, O.: Immunodepression and malignancy. Adv. Cancer Res., 22:261, 1975.

67. Taylor, K. B.: Gastrointestinal and liver disease. In Fudenberg, H. H., Stites, D. P., Caldwell, J. L., et al. (eds.): Basic and Clinical Immunology, Chapter 30. Los Altos, California, Lange Medical Publications, 1976, pp. 449–466.

68. Taylor, S. G., Sisson, G. A., Bytell, D. E.: Adjuvant chemoimmunotherapy of head and neck cancer. Recent Results Cancer Res., 68:297, 1978.

69. Teshita, A., Wanebo, H. J., and Pinsky, C.: Circulating immune complexes detected by 125 I-CIq de-

viation test in serum of cancer patients. J. Clin. Invest., 59:1134, 1977.

70. Toews, G. B., Bergstresser, P. R., and Streilein, J. W.: Epidermal Langerhans cell density determines whether contact hypersensitivity or unresponsiveness follows skin painting with DMFB. J. Immunol., 124:445, 1980.

71. Waldorf, D. S., Wilkens, R. F., and Decker, J. L.: Impaired delayed hypersensitivity in an aging population. J. A. M. A., 203:111, 1968.

72. Wanebo, H. J., Hilal, E. Y., Strong, E. W., et al.: Adjuvant trial of levamisole in patients with squamous cancer of the head and neck: a preliminary report. Cancer Res., 68:324, 1979.

73. Wanebo, H. J., Young, M. J., Strong, E. W., et al.: T cell deficiency in patients with squamous cell cancer of the head and neck. Am. J. Surg., 130:445, 1975.

74. Wang, A. C.: The structure of immunoglobulins. In Fudenberg, H. H., Stites, D. P., Caldwell, J. L., et al. (eds.): Basic and Clinical Immunology, Chapter 2. Los Altos, California, Lange Medical Publications, 1976, pp. 15–31.

75. Wara, W. M., Wara, D. W., Anmann, A. J., et al.: Immunosuppression and reconstruction with thymosin after radiation therapy. Int. J. Radiat. Oncol. Biol. Phys., 5:997, 1979.

21

Maxillofacial prosthetics in the rehabilitation of the oral cancer patient

JOSEPH B. BARRON, D.M.D.

Maxillofacial prosthetics, by definition, is the art and science in dentistry of the replacement by artificial material of those intraoral or paraoral structures that are missing, mutilated, or distorted as a result of surgery, trauma, or birth defects. It also involves "devices" that can be used during surgery as an integral part of the surgical procedures. These prostheses (implants, implant scaffolding, splints, and stents) are basically constructed prior to surgery and can be modified during surgery.

With the increasing number of treatments by radiation and chemotherapy, prostheses are often used as adjuncts to these therapeutic modalities.

Maxillofacial prosthetics seeks to restore the intraoral topography as it was prior to surgery, prior to the discovery of the lesion, and prior to the existence of the lesion.

It is extremely difficult to give a simple explanation or demonstration of the exceedingly complex interplay of all the disciplines, that is, anatomy, neurophysiology, and psychology involved in the healthy patient. It is almost impossible to do so in the patient who has had oncologic disease.

The oral cavity is a space that is contained within the lips, cheeks, maxilla (hard and soft palate), mandible, tongue, and the other muscular and glandular structures that are located within the lower jaw, cheeks, and pharynx. In addition, both jaws normally contain teeth. The unique articulation of the temporomandibular joints, the complexity of muscular actions, the proprioceptive involvements, and the various types of "normal" salivary secretions, all make treatment by prosthetics challenging.

Normal physiology, speech, swallowing of saliva, mastication of foods, and esthetics demand the integrity of all the structures and the cooperative interplay of the nerves, muscles, and glands of these structures.

The complexity of the neuromuscular physiology of these structures, the form and shape of the hard and soft structures, and the dynamic actions of the movement of these structures, both voluntary and involuntary, are what make the oral cavity unique.

Of considerable importance is the proprioceptive response that each individual has acquired to his or her own awareness and use of the oral cavity. Humans are very adaptable creatures. If this were not true, most prostheses would not be acceptable.

To be able to speak normally, there must be integrity of all structures involved, not only the neuromuscular action of the tongue, soft palate, and pharyngeal muscles, but also the shape and form of the hard structures with which these muscles are involved. Any perforation of the hard or soft palate allows the escape of air, which consequently alters certain sounds and, if the perforation is too large, speech becomes unintelligible. Any limitation or restriction in tongue position or movements because of postsurgical adhesions, scarring, or absence of tongue structure or adjacent tissues prevents normal speech. If the condition is severe in extent or is not retrainable, speech may become unintelligible. Any limitation of mandibular movement because of postsurgical trismus owing to the elimination of the disease around the temporomandibular joint, loss of muscle structures that affect joint movements, or the effects of radiation to the joint or tissues adjacent to the joint or those involved with movements of articulation, or if the trismus is induced by the patient's desire to reduce the pain initiated by mandibular movement, severely alters the physiology of speech and deglutition.

The acts of mastication, chewing and swallowing a bolus of food, liquids, and saliva, require anatomic as well as neuromuscular integrity. The quantity and quality of saliva are affected by the disease as well as by the various methods of treatment used to eliminate the disease. Retraining may be possible. Artificial saliva can be added. Prostheses may be helpful. But, just as water cannot be carried in a sieve or a container with a hole, neither can the functions of the oral cavity be carried out adequately if the oral cavity has a "leak" in it or if the proprioceptor reflexes are thoroughly confused.

An intraoral prosthesis that can seal the leak and restore the presurgical normal anatomy and that can be physiologically and psychologically tolerated is successful in a static condition. However, problems arise concerning the functional aspect of the prosthesis. If one could predetermine and control the functional and dynamic forces to which each prosthesis could be subjected, it is possible that all properly constructed prostheses would work well. This is the ultimate goal of intraoral maxillofacial prosthetics.

Normally, in order to chew efficiently and to speak clearly, there must be the proper relationship between the upper and lower teeth, and all other oral structures must be intact and functioning normally. If some or all the teeth of either or both jaws are defective or missing, good dental treatment can usually restore the patient to a more normal condition. Esthetics may be of secondary importance and can generally be restored at the time that the maxillofacial prosthesis is constructed.

However, if parts of the lip, cheeks, or hard or soft palate are missing because of oncologic surgery, the patient cannot or will not speak intelligibly, swallow fluids, or chew efficiently. Foods, fluids, and air escape via the nose and onto the face, exit through the lips, or may be aspirated. The patient may become a maxillofacial cripple. Surgical closures or corrective prosthetics may be required.

When, as a result of surgery, part of the mandible and often part of the tongue is removed, the situation becomes much worse. The remaining segment of the lower jaw may swing markedly to the side of surgery, muscle control is greatly reduced, and the normal positional relationship of the upper to lower jaw may be completely lost. No matter how much the patient tries, he or she usually cannot voluntarily force the mandible to move into any position required to masticate properly. Nutritional problems may develop. The distortion of the "normal" position of the chin results in loss of esthetics and often causes severe psychological problems.

In addition, because the remaining part of the tongue may be limited in motion and size, swallowing of foods that have been processed in a blender and even liquids such as saliva requires extreme conscious effort. The patient's remaining muscles are not put to function because of the pain following surgery, and consequently, the futility of trying to compensate without success can become psychologically destructive. Trismus and inability to adequately control the movements of the remaining jaw segment ensue.

Because so many structures have been removed or mutilated, the remaining part of the tongue has no place to be positioned and must be retrained to facilitate swallowing and to aid in speech. Often, the only answer is tongue-positioning prostheses (Fig. 21–1).

The problems of the prosthetic care associated with oral cancer have been well documented. Maxillofacial prosthetics can be related to oncology as presurgical, surgical, and postsurgical prostheses, preradiation, radiation, and postradiation prostheses, and prostheses used during and following chemotherapy.

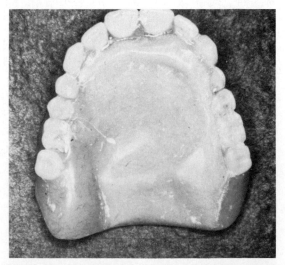

Figure 21–1. Palatal drop tongue positioner, a prosthetic aid in speech and deglutition following partial resection of the tongue.

Maxillofacial prosthetics is an integral part of the treatment in many cases of oral cancer. The prosthodontist should be consulted in all cases in which deformity may occur following surgical treatment. This consultation should occur before treatment in order to construct proper prosthesis and presurgical topographic records. Prostheses can be used in each treatment modality and can be modified as required by each phase of treatment.

Surgery may or may not create severe defects that require prostheses.

1. Removal of small intraoral lesions of the soft or hard tissues may not require prostheses except to replace missing bone, tissue, or teeth.

2. Removal of larger lesions followed by properly placed grafts may require only temporary stents to assist in graft retention and to facilitate healing of the tissues.

3. Removal of parts of the palate, hard, or soft or both, usually results in oronasal or oroantral deformities that require prostheses if surgery does not result in complete closure (Fig. 21–2).

4. Removal of sections of the mandible followed by bone grafts or alloplastic implants or both may initially require only the surgical prosthesis, followed by conservative prosthetics, postsurgically.

5. Removal of parts of the mandible that are not repaired by implants or grafts results in moderate to severe deformities and impairment of function. Prostheses are usually required.

6. Removal of sections of the tongue, depending upon the location and extent of the glossectomy, may cause problems in speech and deglutition. Respiratory distress and dysphagia may occur.

Re-establishing occlusion in function is a primary goal. However, in most instances, intraoral oncologic surgery may create other defects that require intraoral maxillofacial prostheses more urgently than occlusal reconstruction. The type of malignant lesion that is removed is secondary to the extent of the tissues and structures that are removed. The type of prosthesis used is determined by the state of health of the tissues upon which the prosthesis will rest and by the dynamic forces applied to the prosthesis.

In all cases that require intraoral prostheses, stabilization of the prosthesis is directly proportional to the number, location, and health of the teeth and the supporting tissues available for primary and secondary anchorage of

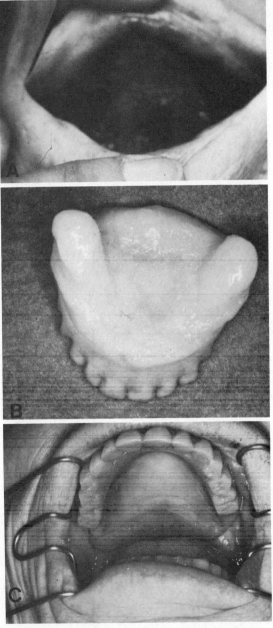

Figure 21–2. Bilateral maxillary resection. A, Intraoral surgical defects. B, Prosthesis with bilateral obturators. C, Prosthesis in place.

the prosthesis. If possible, endodontics, periodontics, and restorative procedures should be initiated and completed prior to surgery, radiation, or chemotherapy. If there is not sufficient time to do all the planned work, every effort should be made to salvage key teeth, with the sacrifice of those teeth with questionable prognoses, prior to initiation of radiation therapy. Because prosthetic treatment is usually carried out in three phases, immediate, transitional and definitive, temporizing treatments are acceptable in the overall treatment planning.

Unfortunately, the design of the definitive prosthesis is often dictated by the limitation of finances rather than by the requirements of the case.

Multiple clasping, broken stress attachments, and fixed partial prostheses with precision attachments can increase stabilization and esthetics. The jaw that is opposite the jaw with the defect must be incorporated into any consideration of stabilization, especially during occlusal function. This is termed *antagonistic stabilizing occlusion* and justifies the need for the construction of such an occlusion with fixed or removable prostheses whenever necessary.

The type of prosthesis that is required in an edentulous jaw demands a well-constructed opposing occlusion. The location and the extent of the surgery, and the amount of usable tissue and bone undercuts determine stabilization without function. Function and directions of applied forces are the final determinants of the area of coverage and the amount of stabilization to be achieved. When a prosthesis is placed over irradiated areas or areas in which surgery has been done these areas must be scrupulously and constantly monitored for soft tissue or bone breakdown. Paresthesia often results from oncologic treatment. Patients who feel no pain because of this may be unaware of traumatic lesions caused by a prosthesis.

Because almost all intraoral postsurgical prostheses are removable, proper design is imperative. Unfortunately, the principles and laws of "normal" prosthodontics are often violated, but not out of choice. They are forced upon the operator because of the demands of the case. The ideal of tripodal tooth stabilization of a removable partial prosthesis is lost if the teeth remaining are only on one side or are relatively unstable. The ideal of auxiliary tissue stabilization by maximum coverage over edentulous areas of palatal ridges and palate is lost when there are no palate or bony ridges left.

In addition, because of the extent and location of the defect to be obliterated, almost all intraoral prostheses must be cantilevered, making stability even less attainable. Multiple clasping may increase retention, but not necessarily stability. Relieving the occlusal forces on the side of the defect may aid in minimizing unwanted stressful movements, but this is true only when teeth are present. When the jaw to be treated is edentulous, the problems of stabilization are even more difficult to overcome. Tissue tolerance and patient acceptance and adaptability are prerequisites to any properly designed and functioning prosthesis.

The clinician must be able to modify the "inflexible" rules of occlusion and to bend to the desires and comfort of the patient within the parameters of the prosthetic and physiologic requirements of the treatment of the defect (Fig. 21-3).

In more complicated situations, transitional and definitive prostheses may be required. Transitional or interim prostheses are constructed faster and often indicate modification or design alterations required in the more sophisticated definitive prostheses. The transitional prosthesis may be acrylic with wrought wire clasps and used on teeth that have been treated, provisionally. The definitive prosthesis may have a cast metal base with semiprecision clasping and broken stress attachments on crowned or splinted teeth.

The following are some illustrative cases of intraoral prostheses.

MAXILLA

Partial resections of ridges without loss of basal bone structure or oroantral perforations are treated by adding denture base material to an already existing prosthesis or by constructing a fixed or removable prosthesis, incorporating those areas that have been removed into the pontic areas or denture base material.

Resection of Soft Palate: Partial or Total (Figs. 21-4 through 21-6)

Problems.
1. Pharyngeal muscle action.
2. Gagging.
3. Speech difficulty.
4. Difficulty in swallowing of fluid and food.

Recommended Solutions. Because of the location of the defect, all prostheses that supply retropharyngeal extensions are subject to cantilever forces. Muscle function can help to seat the prosthesis if the case is properly designed. Sequentially and segmentally placed extensions may reduce gagging reflexes by allowing the patient gradually to become accustomed to the "unnatural" prosthetic projection into the posterior wall of the pharynx.

The defect is obturated with a bulb that extends posteriorly from a removable partial

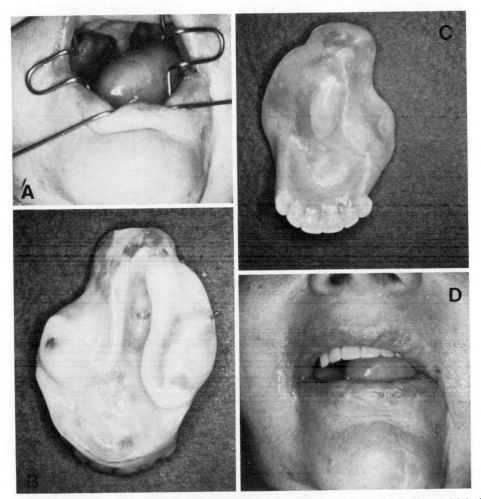

Figure 21–3. Total palatal resection. *A*, Defect, vomer exposed. *B*, Hollow bulb prosthesis (tissue side). *C*, Hollow bulb prosthesis (intraoral view). *D*, Prosthesis in place (speech and swallowing improved).

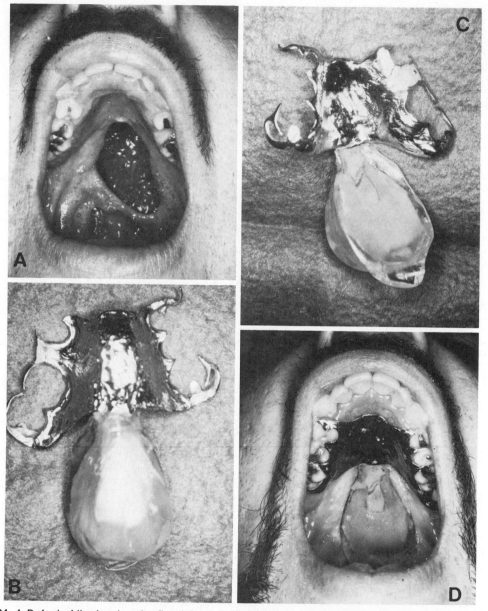

Figure 21–4. Defect of the hard and soft palate. *A,* Surgical defect. *B,* Cast metal base with soft and hard hollow acrylic bulb (superior side). *C,* Prosthesis (inferior surface) with multiple clasps to overcome displacement by cantilever action. *D,* Prosthesis in place; peripheral seal accomplished by functional impressions.

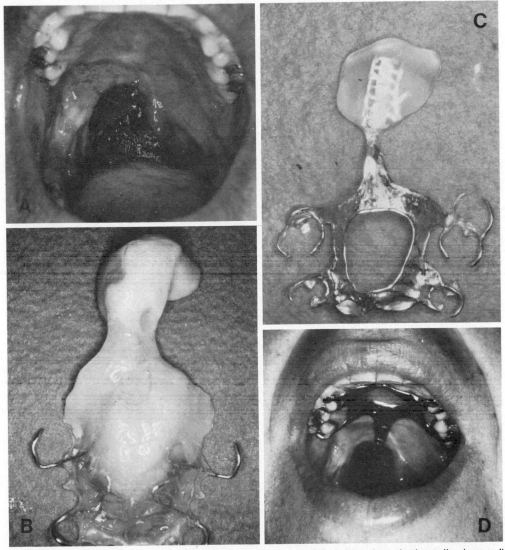

Figure 21–5. Soft palate resection (dentulous). *A,* Surgical defect. *B,* Transitional surgical prosthesis, acrylic and tissue conditioning functional reline. *C,* Definitive multiclasped obturating prosthesis. *D,* Prosthesis in place.

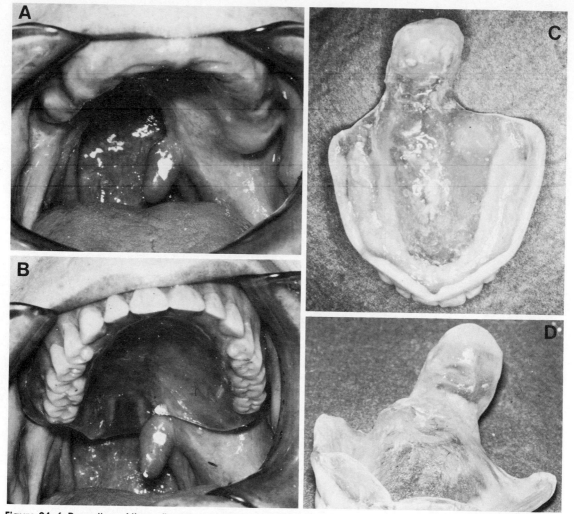

Figure 21–6. Resection of the soft palate—edentulous. *A,* Surgical defect. *B,* Prosthesis in place. *C,* Obturating bulb (tissue surface). *D,* Position of the bulb, determined by speech and function.

or complete denture. The proper location, size, and shape of this bulb are achieved by functional impression techniques using the muscle actions and speech requirements as determinants. This correct registration can overcome the leaking of air and fluids, making speech and deglutition more normal. If the weight of the bulb is excessive, it should be made hollow.

If part of the soft palate exists, the remaining muscle action may assist in sealing as well as aiding in the relearning of proprioceptive tongue-palate positions in speech and swallowing.

Resection of Maxilla: Dentulous
(Figs. 21–7 through 21–9)

Problems.
1. Trismus.
2. Size and location of defect.
3. Location, health, and stability of remaining teeth.
4. Weight of prosthesis.
5. Peripheral seal of prosthesis.
6. Relining and rebasing of obturating prosthesis.

Recommended Solutions. In attempting to achieve a properly extended impression of the

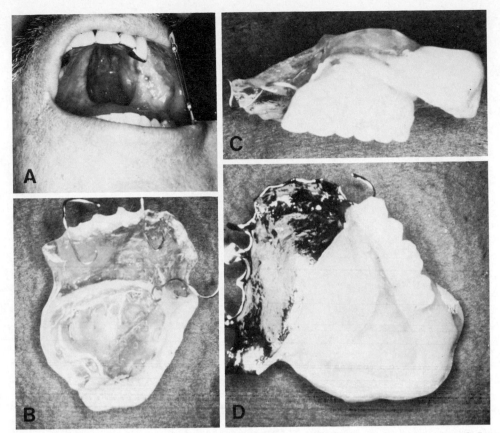

Figure 21–7. Hemimaxillectomy—dentulous. *A,* Palatal defect. *B,* Immediate surgical obturator. *C,* Transitional prosthesis (teeth added for function and esthetics). Distolateral extensions were obtained by functional impressioning. *D,* Definitive prosthesis, cast metal multiclasped base with hollow bulb obturator and teeth.

defect areas as well as of the teeth and adjacent healthy tissues, impression trays of the proper size are required. If trismus is severe, conventional stock trays may not be able to be inserted without being modified. Sectional impressions may be required. These are best constructed on presurgical casts. When these are not available, they must be constructed at the time that the impression is taken. Treatment for reducing trismus should be instituted before attempting to take an impression. Often, some reduction in the height of the mandibular anterior teeth may be required in order to insert even the smallest of trays.

If the size of the defect is not too large and is confined within the hard palate or part of the soft palate but is surrounded by healthy tissue, the obturation of the defect (Fig. 21–10) can be accomplished without too much

discomfort to the patient or peripheral leakage. Relining can overcome most deficiencies, and the pressure of the patient's tongue against the prosthesis often aids in sealing the margins during swallowing.

If the remaining teeth are not in severe malocclusion and are healthy or can be restored to health and periodontal stability, multiple clasping or coronal splinting or both can markedly increase retention and stabilization. Enthusiastic overloading of the existing teeth and the excessive forces of cantilever action unfortunately may loosen these teeth. Therefore, no fixation should be attempted that is beyond the requirements of each case.

The weight of the prosthesis should be proportional to the size of the defect and the volume of bulb to be used. Hollow bulb prostheses or prostheses with only limited

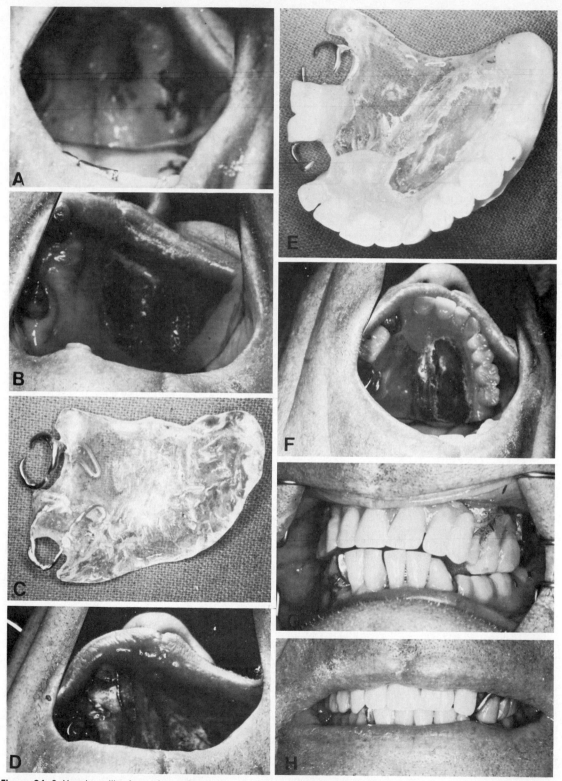

Figure 21–8. Hemimaxillectomy for melanoma—dentulous. *A,* Presurgical intraoral view showing pigmented tumor. *B,* Postsurgical view showing large defect. *C,* Immediate surgical obturator. *D,* Obturator in place. *E,* Transitional hollow bulb prosthesis. *F,* Prosthesis in place, intraoral view. *G,* Prosthesis in place, occlusion defective. *H,* Prosthesis in place, facial view.

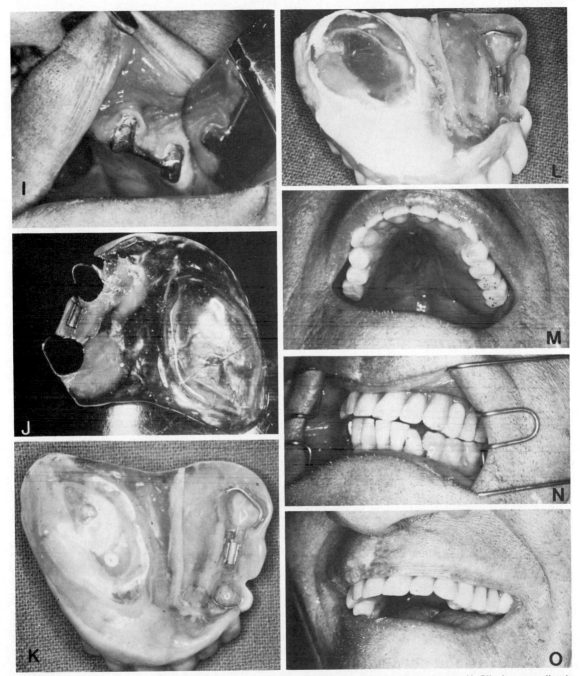

Figure 21–8 *Continued. I,* Clip-bar retention. *J,* Clip-bar prosthesis with auxiliary clasps. *K,* Clip-bar prosthesis, including hollow bulb, converted to overlay prosthesis. *L,* Relining of hollow bulb for peripheral fit. *M,* Prosthesis in place. *N,* Prosthesis in place, occlusion satisfactory (mandibular overlays used). *O,* Prosthesis in place, facial view.

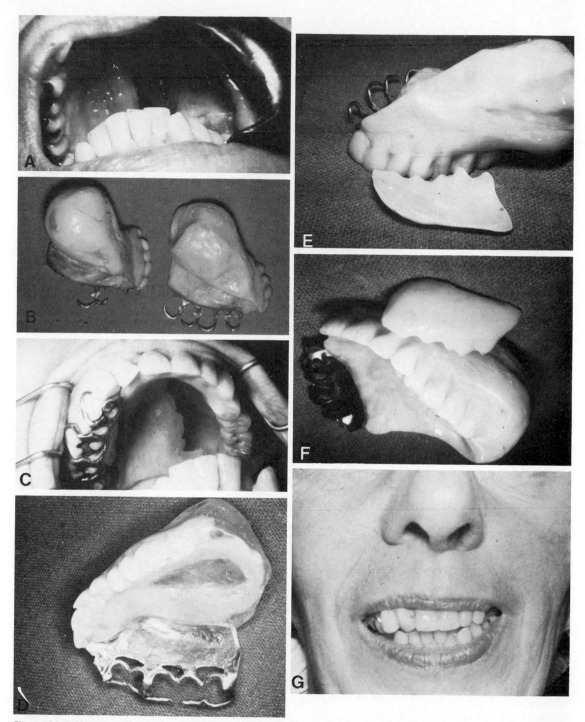

Figure 21–9. Hemimaxillectomy—dentulous. *A*, Surgical defect. *B, Left,* prosthesis (inadequate clasping and hollow bulb adaptation). *C,* Prosthesis in position in mouth. *D,* Multiclasped cast metal hollow bulb prosthesis with clear acrylic monitoring section. *E,* Labial plumping section for prosthesis. *F,* Labial plumping section for prosthesis with sequentially enlarged sections to restore facial contour. *G,* Completed prosthesis, facial view.

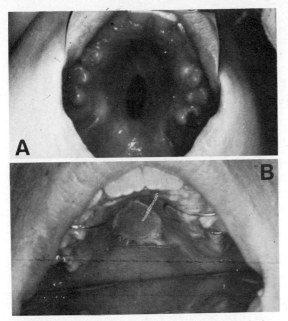

Figure 21-10. Surgical defect after treatment of pleomorphic adenoma of palate. A, Residual surgical defect. B, Immediate postsurgical prosthesis in position. Palatal prosthesis is transparent acrylic except for the defect area.

flange extensions into the defect area dramatically lighten the weight, thus increasing comfort and stability.

The medial seal of the defect utilizes the undercuts of the bone of the palate created by the surgery, but in only limited amounts, which are determined by the direction of the insertion of the prosthesis and the tolerance of the tissues that cover the bone in this area to the functional forces applied. The lateral and anterior seal is determined by the location of the intraoral scarband following surgery, the elasticity of this tissue, and the displacing forces caused by the movements of these structures during function. The posterior seal is determined by the amount of the remaining soft palate, the relation of the distopalatal extension to the movements of the coronoid process of the mandible during function, and the ability of the patient to tolerate the additional volume of material required to close the defect.

Minor defects of leakage of air and fluids and overenthusiastic adjustment for "sore" spots can be corrected by additions of functional soft lining material. These can be transferred to hard denture base material when necessary. If deficiencies exist only in the obturating section, only this area should be modified. Total rebasing of the prosthesis is not usually necessary in the removable partial

prosthesis if the original prosthesis was seated correctly. Arbitrarily, to rebase completely may result in loss of proper seating of the retention clasps or precision attachments.

Resection of Maxilla: Edentulous (Figs. 21-11 and 21-12)

Problems.
1. Trismus.
2. Size and location of defect.
3. Weight of prosthesis.
4. Peripheral seal of prosthesis.
5. Relining and rebasing of obturating prosthesis.

Recommended Solutions. Although presenting a problem, trismus is not as frequent a problem in the edentulous impression as it is when some maxillary teeth are present. The latter situation requires impression trays of larger dimension to register the anatomy of the existing teeth. In the edentulous case, trays of wafer-thin thickness can be used and provide adequate casts for the construction of custom sectional trays in the laboratory. Presurgical casts greatly reduce the problems of tray fabrication.

Problems that pertain to the size and location of the defect and to the weight and peripheral seal of the prosthesis are resolved similarly to those in dentulous maxillectomy cases. Relining and rebasing must be done very often, not only in the bulb area but also over the entire tissue base area so that the initially achieved occlusal relationship to the mandibular teeth is not disturbed.

MANDIBLE

Prosthetic treatment following the horizontal removal of part of the mandible without any partial resection of the tongue and in which the body of the mandible remains intact is comparable to that of the maxillary resection with similar surgically created bone and tissue defects. Fixed or removable partial or complete prostheses may be used to restore the missing hard and soft structures with additional denture base material or increased length of the pontics. When a partial resection of the tongue has also been done, a tongue resection prosthesis is the prosthetic therapy of choice.

If a condyle or part of the ramus has been removed, the prosthetic treatment is accomplished by the replacement of the condyle with an alloplastic implant. If this is not done, occlusal guide planes can be used in the re-

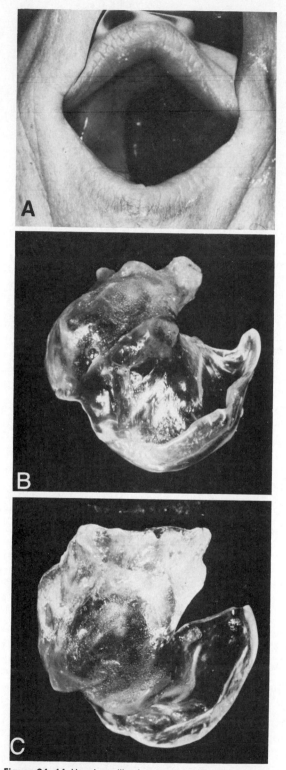

Figure 21–11. Hemimaxillectomy and soft palate resection—edentulous. *A*, Surgical defect. *B*, Extensive palatal obturator (immediate). *C*, Palatal view of the extent of the obturator.

maining teeth to guide the mandible into a more normal centric relationship with the maxillary dentition.

If a condyle, ramus, and a section of the body of the mandible have been removed, properly constructed autogenous or alloplastic implants can surgically be placed to restore the mandibular integrity. Restoration of the presurgical occlusion is a prerequisite to this procedure.

If the residual muscle forces cause excessive torquing on the implant, the implant may fail.

Most prosthetic intervention in this type of hemimandibular resection is in the form of guide plane prostheses (Fig. 21–13). Constructed presurgically, these prostheses can be inserted immediately following surgery. The patient then has little deviation of the residual mandible in the closed and rest positions.

The guide planes prevent lateral mastication and guide the mandible into relatively successful vertical masticatory positions. After surgical healing, patients may continue to wear the guide plane; however, they can usually retrain themselves to chew vertically and laterally with efficiency and comfort. A motivated patient can place the remaining mandible in voluntary occlusal positions and may use the guide plane as an occlusal splint during sleeping or resting hours.

Following healing and depending upon the number of teeth lost during surgery, prosthetic reconstruction of occlusion or esthetics can be performed. If a sufficient number of teeth exist in the remaining healthy mandible and if there is a continuous occlusion through the molar area, no prosthesis, other than the guide plane, may be necessary.

If there are an insufficient number of mandibular teeth for efficient mastication, a removable partial prosthesis that incorporates guide planes can be used. If many teeth must be added over non–bone-supported areas, cantilever forces may be excessive. This requires multiple anchorage on the existing teeth, with clasps, semiprecision attachments in fixed partial prostheses, and if feasible, broken stress attachments. Occlusion must be adjusted to reduce excessive forces on the cantilevered section of the prosthesis.

When mandibular resection results in the removal of part of the body of the mandible, leaving bilateral sections of the body, rami, and condyles intact, prostheses are essential.

Surgical implants of the proper size and that

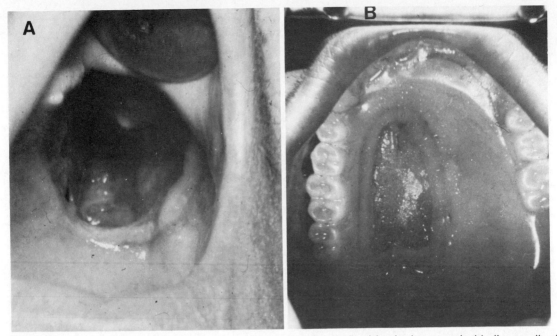

Figure 21–12. Hemimaxillectomy—edentulous. *A,* Defect. *B,* Hollow bulb obturator incorporated in the prosthesis and a clear window, used to monitor the integrity of the bulb.

are properly stabilized can be placed, repositioning the remaining sections of the mandible into normal presurgical positions, resulting in proper maxillomandibular relations and occlusion. After healing, fixed or removable partial prostheses or combinations of each can be used for auxiliary stabilization of the bone segments and for occlusal function and esthetics. Sometimes, when partial glossectomies have been performed, the prostheses can provide new areas for residual tongue positioning. They aid in swallowing and in the return of intelligible speech as well as in reducing the amount of saliva that may pool in the floor of the mouth. Proprioception returns after varying amounts of time, and the patient acquires compensatory movement of the tongue which, in turn, can lead to more normal oral physiology.

Resection of Mandible: Dentulous

Problems.

1. Trismus.
2. Deviation of remaining mandible at rest position and function.
3. Amount and location of mandibular bone removed.

4. Occlusal deviation.
5. Impression problems.
6. Stability during function, unilateral and bilateral.

Recommended Solutions. The presurgical registration of maxillomandibular relation is imperative for proper surgical and postsurgical prosthetic treatment. In the dentulous case, presurgical occlusal relationships are mandatory if the postsurgical occlusion is to be restored to "normal." Gross malocclusion can usually be minimized with the properly constructed presurgical or surgical prosthesis.

Following mandibular surgery, the trauma caused by the surgery, edema, and the limitation of motion because of pain experienced during deglutition and speech often results in severe trismus. The acentric and eccentric movements of the residual mandibular section or sections may cause the nonstabilized fragments to impinge upon the teeth or ridges of the maxilla. This can result in painful traumatic lesions, which in turn may restrict movements of the jaw. The patient may limit movements of the jaw to reduce the pain, and this may compound the trismus. Controlled jaw exercises and prostheses used to treat trismus may be required.

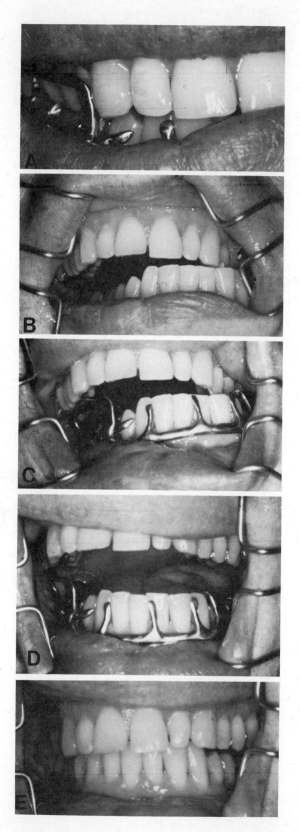

Figure 21–13. Hemimandibulectomy—dentulous. *A,* Mandibular occlusal guide plane (presurgically). *B,* Mandibular deviation (postsurgically). *C,* Guide plane in the malpositioned mandible. *D,* Sliding of the mandible to the right to correct occlusion. *E,* "Retrained" mandible in centric position without the use of a prosthesis (occlusion on the left is slightly open).

The mandible is essentially a horseshoe shaped bone (body) with projections of bone (rami) extending at almost right angles from the body of the bone and hinged at both ends to the skull via a complicated joint system. Like most joints, the extent of motion of this hinged bone is limited by the anatomy of the joint and its surrounding structures. The mandible is attached beneath the maxilla by ligaments and a complex system of muscles. These muscles can elevate, depress, and rotate the mandible into several positions that act in concert with each other or independently. In addition to the proprioceptor actions of the occlusion and the tongue, these muscles cause the voluntary movements that are essential in mastication and speech. These movements, resultant muscular forces, and the dynamics of occlusion make the mandible the most versatile single bone in the body. Impairment of the function of any of the muscles or directly attached to the mandible results in limitation or alteration of motion, to some degree, for example, in cases of trismus, dyskinesia, and myasthenia gravis.

If the mandible is intact, whether the impairment of muscle function is unilateral or bilateral, the symptoms are usually interpreted as temporomandibular joint problems. And, conversely, temporomandibular joint problems per se can limit or alter movements of the jaw. Simple prostheses such as occlusal splints or guide planes may alleviate the oral problems related to the condition.

However, if the integrity of the mandible is destroyed by the complete removal of a section of bone, that part of the musculature that is related to the mandibular movement can no longer function. The fine antagonistic balance associated with "normal" position or motion no longer exists. The remaining bone tends to move somewhat erratically toward the area of surgery.

This deviation of the position of the mandible from its normal tooth to tooth and bone to bone relationship to the maxilla in "rest" and "functional" positions is, in large part, proportionately related to the location and amount of bone removed and the amount of muscle attachments lost during surgery. The remaining attached muscles function with no oppositional muscles and with no limitations of motion found when the mandible is intact. The remaining bone segment or segments become "overpositioned," limited by the extent of muscle force and the restrictions of the soft tissue that surrounds the bone segment or segments.

If the section of bone removed has had little or no muscle attachment removed, as in the removal of a temporomandibular joint, the deviation may not be severe.

If a mandibular resection involves the unilateral removal of a ramus and a contiguous part of the body of the mandible, the remaining mandibular positions are controlled by the actions of the remaining muscles that are attached to the mandible and the anatomic limitations of the remaining joint.

At first, the deviation is uncontrolled and erratic. Medial rotation muscles over-rotate medially. The elevator muscles overclose in this medial position. The depressor muscles, also unbalanced in kinetic positions, add to the confusion. The brain stimulates nerves that have no muscles to activate.

The pterygoid complex, masseter, temporal, digastric, platysma, and hyoid complex of muscles function without a sound mandible and with two limiting joints; thus, the remaining mandible positions itself according to the directional pull of the functioning muscles.

If the mandible is lost from the midline

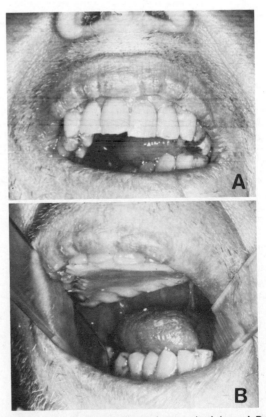

Figure 21–14. Hemimandibulectomy—dentulous. *A*, Deviation of the mandible to the left, severe malocclusion. *B*, Maxillary acrylic splint with palatal guide plane for occlusion and mandibular guidance to the right.

unilaterally, including the ramus and temporomandibular joint, the midline deviation at the "rest" position is not too severe. The same number of elevator and depressor muscles remain as have been removed, and although unilateral in position, the remaining mandible seems to have some balance. However, the rotational movements, being unilateral and without an opposing joint to limit lateral motion, cause occlusal malrelation in any position

of mastication other than in a vertical direction. In essence, the patient who does not have a reconstructed mandible and joint must retrain occlusion positioning, and the prosthodontist must be prepared to alter the occlusal tables as they are generated in positions of function.

When a section of the body of the mandible has been removed (Figs. 21–14 and 21–15) and both temporomandibular joints, rami, and

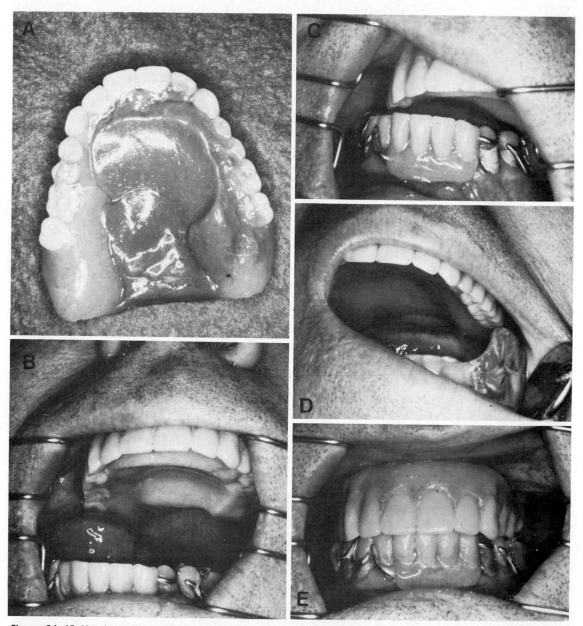

Figure 21–15. Hemimandibulectomy—dentulous—and partial glossectomy—edentulous maxilla. *A,* Tongue stop position is incorporated into the palatal prosthesis by using functional impressions (thermolabile wax). *B,* Maxillary palatal drop tongue positioner in place. Deviation of the mandible toward the side of surgery (open position). *C,* Deviation of the mandible (closed position). *D,* Acrylic guide plane incorporated into the left side of the removable prosthesis. Minimizes deviation on closure. *E,* "Normal" closed centric position with the aid of guide planes.

contiguous sections of the body of the mandible are intact, the malposition of the remaining mandibular sections creates even more complications. Both remaining mandibular sections move medially and superiorly and rotate inferiorly in such a position that the resulting occlusal plane tilts lingually to "normal." Mastication becomes a very uncontrolled and painful procedure. Swallowing saliva and speaking become difficult. This physical pain coupled with facial distortion and consequent mental depression creates problems that must be solved.

If presurgical diagnostic casts have been made, they can be used for the construction of surgical splints, guide planes, and provisional prostheses. Custom impression trays can be made that can be sectioned and reassembled in and out of the mouth postsurgically.

Postsurgical impressions are often difficult to achieve because of the severe displacement of the remaining mandible, trismus, and lack of tongue mobility. Often, the side of the tongue that is adjacent to the surgical site is sutured to the cheek, thus eliminating the vestibular and submaxillary spaces. Sectional trays are almost mandatory, because when the patient opens his or her mouth to receive the tray, the fragments move medially, and when the patient closes his or her mouth during the setting of the impression material, the fragments move laterally. In hemisections, the movement is not particularly significant. In resections with normal posterior bilateral mandibular bone, the independent movements of each section negate a one-piece impression, because the residual mandibular sections are not registered in any true relationship.

Stability of prostheses during function is extremely difficult to achieve. If each remaining section is independently impressed and reassembled out of the mouth using the opposing occlusion as a guide, repositioning of the sections in their correct relations may be possible. However, completely stabilizing the sections with fixed or removable partial prostheses usually requires occlusal adjustments and some compromise to achieve "ideal" occlusal harmony.

If the forces of torsion exceed the retentive and stabilizing action of the clasps, attachments, or fixed prostheses because of muscular action during occlusion, the prosthesis may act destructively as an orthodontic prosthesis. The anchor teeth may loosen or the cement seal may break loose from the crowns, resulting in the failure of the fixed prosthesis. Broken stress attachments may be used to allow each mandibular fragment to move independently and thus minimize the torquing action of each independently moving mandibular section.

If one bone section contains teeth and the other is edentulous, stabilization of the edentulous section is exceedingly difficult. Often, the best that can be hoped for is merely to base the edentulous segment sufficiently with soft reline material. This will prevent this section of the jaw from moving superiorly and medially to such an extent that it impinges on the occlusal surfaces of the opposing maxillary molar and premolar teeth, which could result in traumatic ulcers. In some cases, protective occlusal splints may be used on the maxillary posterior teeth. In extreme cases, the posterior maxillary teeth that cause the traumatic ulcers may need to be extracted.

Resection of Mandible: Edentulous

Problems.
1. Trismus.
2. Deviation of remaining mandible at rest position and function.
3. Amount and location of mandibular bone removed.
4. Occlusal deviation.
5. Impression problems.
6. Stability during function, unilateral and bilateral.

Recommended Solutions. Trismus is usually not as severe in edentulous cases as in dentulous cases. This is probably only a relative observation, because the absence of teeth provides a larger maxillomandibular space and allows easier insertion of sectional impression trays. However, unlike dentulous cases, antitrismus prostheses or exercises are difficult, because the remaining malpositioned edentulous mandible is usually too elusive for prosthetic aids. More successful exercises employ the fingers to grasp and move the fragments into various positions.

The deviation of the remaining mandible follows that of dentulous cases but may be greater, because the lack of teeth results in the loss of occlusal stops. The rotational distortion is often so severe that the external oblique ridge is the most occlusally placed mandibular bone in contact with the maxilla.

If a hemisection of the mandible has been performed and no mandible, ramus, or condyle exists unilaterally, a hemidenture is the initial attempted prosthesis. This denture base is carried as far as possible into the area of surgery. Limitations of this extension are from tongue-cheek impingement on the denture base extension, lack of any submaxillary and vestibular space, and cantilevered occlusal forces, which tend to displace an already unstable denture base.

Guide planes for this type of prosthesis are usually ineffective, and the patient must form his or her own occlusal patterns in centric and function. Often, this means increasing the occlusal table of the maxillary teeth. If a maxillary denture is present, an acrylic occlusal table may be placed in the palatal vault of the denture. If the maxilla is dentulous, an acrylic palate similar to a removable partial prosthesis is constructed, and an acrylic occlusion is incorporated. Occlusal wax registrations against the occlusal surfaces of the eccentrically moving mandibular hemidenture are recorded. These are transferred into clear acrylic, and the patient soon learns how to utilize this occlusion that has been generated via the hemidenture and controlled by the actions of the remaining mandibular muscles. Eventually, ramping of the maxillary and mandibular occlusion can be instituted. Gradually, the patient may retrain his or her mandible to reorient its location into a more normal position. The ramping must be done sequentially and never at the expense of overloading the mandibular occlusion, with consequent displacement of the denture base.

If the resection of the mandible results in leaving bilateral condyles, rami, and sections of the body of the mandible, sectional impressions of the prosthetically usuable mandible are taken. These are assembled in the laboratory. A denture base with a provisional occlusal plane is constructed. Tissue conditioning and functional impressions are sequentially made over the mandibular stumps. The mandibular anatomic landmarks usually found in complete removable prosthodontics become only of academic concern. Underextensions of the flanges may be required because of occlusal interference from the maxilla, and overextensions of the soft denture base material, if tolerated, must be used. Reduction of occlusal forces, retraining for mastication against an unusually placed maxillary occlusion, and a positive psychological approach can make a person who has dental handicaps feel less hopeless and become more cooperative.

Occlusal deviations may never be overcome unless implant surgery is attempted. If this is not possible or if it has been done without success, the maxillofacial prosthodontist must construct prostheses for the condition that the patient presents. The ingenuity of the prosthodontist, the cooperation of the patient, and the ability of both to compromise often yield success and an improved quality of life for the patient.

Impression problems are complicated by loss of anatomic landmarks. The fabrication of uniquely designed custom trays and impressing around a tongue that has severe restriction of movement must be done. Clear denture bases are recommended, because the clinician has more visual knowledge of denture base stability, overextensions and underextensions, and overcompressed and undercompressed or displaced tissues.

In addition to the problems of the positions of the remaining bone and the muscle action transmitted to this bone, often the resection of mandibular bone involves removing part of the floor of the mouth and some of the tongue tissue and contiguous musculature. Suturing of these structures often results in the loss of vestibular and submaxillary space. In some cases, the surgical side of the tongue is sutured to the cheek. This means that any removable prosthesis not only has no solid base but also rests on freely movable tissue or is limited in extent by the displacing actions of the tongue-cheek-scar movements. In those cases in which a graft has been used in the floor of the mouth, excessive space may be created in non–denture-supporting tissue. Pooling of saliva and foods in the artifically created pouch may further complicate prosthetic reconstruction.

In all cases of intraoral maxillofacial prostheses, maxillary or mandibular or both, proper occlusion is probably the best stabilizing force utilized. Therefore, it is imperative that a proper occlusion be constructed, not only for the jaw in which surgery was performed but also for the opposite jaw. This prosthesis is an integral part of the rehabilitation and is termed an *antagonistic stabilizing prosthesis*.

Resection of Tongue

Problems.
1. Speech.
2. Salivation.
3. Mastication.

Recommended Solutions. With partial resections of the tongue, the amount of the remaining tongue determines the degree of loss of function. The tongue may be restricted in motion because of suturing and scarring. Corrective surgery may provide a more freely moving residual tongue and make prostheses more acceptable and successful.

Impaired tongue function limits certain speech sounds. The tongue requires solid tongue-positioning stops to make certain sounds. When the tongue has no stop, improperly made sounds are the result. By creating maxillary and mandibular stops in properly constructed removable prostheses, the proprioceptor responses are soon relearned, and proper speech therapy allows retraining by compensatory positioning of the residual tongue.

Salivation problems result from the inability of the residual tongue to move into areas in which saliva pools. Normally, the tongue rests on the floor of the mouth and completely fills in the area bounded by the lingual surface of the lower teeth and mandible. The space that exists between the inferior surface of the tongue and the floor of the mouth is a "potential" space. A space is created when the tongue is in function and moved from its rest position. The space disappears when the tongue returns to the rest position. Any fluid that pools in this space is forced out and appears on the superior and lateral surfaces of the tongue, areas from which it can easily be swallowed. When a partial glossectomy is performed, there is suddenly much less tongue volume and the "potential" space no longer exists and becomes a "dead" space.

What has occurred is the formation of an actual space into which fluids and foods can pool. Because of the diminished size of the residual tongue as well as the restrictions of motion as a result of surgical scarring and loss of musculature, the patient can no longer express the pooled fluids onto the dorsum of the tongue for reflex swallowing.

Because artificial material cannot be attached to the tongue, the dead space volume must be reduced by adding hard or soft material to the removable prostheses. The size, shape, and location of the material can be generated in thermolabile wax by the movements of the residual tongue. The dead space is thus eliminated, and the residual tongue has positive stop areas from which relearned swallowing actions can function.

Mastication is primarily the function of the teeth in which the food is ground into masses that can be swallowed. Saliva liquifies the bolus. By proprioceptor actions, the cheek and tongue muscles push the food back onto the grinding areas of the teeth. Normally, neither the cheek nor tongue get caught between the occluding teeth.

A tongue that is limited in motion or suddenly decreased in size as a result of surgery cannot function properly in masticatory activities. Food collects in the "dead" space of the floor of the mouth and cannot be thrust to the back of the mouth by the residual tongue. As is the case in reducing the pooling of saliva, a removable prosthesis with tongue-positioning stops can help restore tongue function. Thermolabile wax is placed on the lingual surface of the denture base in the area in which there once was tongue structure. The residual tongue establishes its own impression on the lingual denture base surface and creates a tolerable floor of the mouth extension to the denture. This wax addition is transferred into hard or soft acrylic. This is also done on the palatal prosthesis for the creation of palatal tongue stops. These tongue stops created by the dynamic action of the residual tongue enable better deglutition and minimize the pooling of food and fluids. The use of fingers or silverware as "oral shovels" becomes less essential. As the patient redevelops more tongue movement and proprioceptive responses, mastication and deglutition become more tolerable. As a result of this increased manipulative skill, nutrition markedly improves.

The total resection of a tongue is similar to a total maxillectomy. The prognosis for prosthetic reconstruction is essentially negative. Some progress has been made, but not enough successful cases have been reported to warrant discussion of a positive treatment modality.

Resection of Cheeks and Lips

Problems.
1. With partial loss or mutilation of an external surface of the oral cavity, escape of air, fluids, or food results.
2. Mutilation of external features.

Recommended Solutions. Loss of cheek and lip structures must be repaired, preferably by surgery. If surgery cannot be performed, one must attempt to use extraoral prostheses. The use of large surgical dressings is not well tolerated by many patients. No extraoral prosthesis can be so closely adapted to and adhere at its peripheral margins so well as to provide a leak-proof prosthesis. The movements of the cheeks and lips during changes of facial expressions and the jaw movements of eating and speaking make the size of the peripheral seal excessive, with the resultant loss of esthetics. Because of the large size required, most prostheses look like immobile, expressionless masks. For a prosthesis to be effective, the patient must condition himself or herself to restrictive motions during speaking, mastication, and deglutition.

Atresia-Microstomia

Problems.
1. Impression.
2. Insertion of prostheses.

If severe problems of scarring of the lips are a result of surgery, correction by surgery is desired, but it may require intraoral stents for scaffolding or guides. Therefore, intraoral impressions may be required.

Recommended Solutions. Depending upon the extent of surgery, the intraoral topography may be completely normal or normal in the jaw in which surgery has not been performed. The problems of impressing large intraoral areas through the very small opening of the existing scarred lip structures can be overcome by the use of sectional impressions with reassembly outside the mouth.

Problems related to insertion of the final prosthesis can be overcome if the prosthesis is made in sections, inserted in sections, and reassembled intraorally with definitive locking sections.

If further lip surgery is not being considered, prostheses may be used for sequential plumping of scarred or deficient labial tissues. Over a period of time and with the use of progressively larger plumping wafers placed over the labial flanges of the denture or over intact anterior dentition and labial sulcus, it may be possible to loosen the scars and create more pliable labial structures. Problems of trismus usually associated with microstomia are reduced. This is evident by the fact that after a period of time, the sectional prosthesis can be converted into a one-piece prosthesis and inserted and removed from the mouth without excessive stretching of the labial tissues.

Submandibular or Sublingual Sinuses

Due to disease or failure of surgical closure, sinuses may occur that lead from the floor of the mouth and exit extraorally under the chin or under the lateral and posterior body of the mandible. This escape of liquids, food, and saliva out to the neck is best relieved by proper surgery. When surgery is not performed, excessive leaking into gauze packs is unsightly, inconvenient, and foul smelling.

This problem can be relieved by the construction of a series of silicone plugs or stoppers that are made sequentially smaller as healing progresses. A large sinus may often shrink to the size of a small fistula. At this point, surgical repair can be more easily managed.

Adjunctive Maxillofacial Prosthetics

Adjunctive maxillofacial prosthetics are often used in the nonsurgical aspects of intraoral cancer treatments.

Radiation Therapy

Radiation therapy, used alone or in conjunction with surgery, often requires prostheses as an adjunct to therapy.

Radiation Shields. These can be constructed with lead or lead-impregnated acrylic or silicone, allowing only selected intraoral structures to receive x-ray therapy while protecting the healthy surrounding tissue from scatter or unwanted radiation.

Radon Seed Carriers. These carriers can be constructed with receptacles for the correct placement of enclosed radon seeds and worn by the patient for determined periods of time.

Docking Devices. These devices are constructed to assist the radiotherapist in precise, repeatable localization of radiation cones.

Flexible Trays. For carrying fluoride and other medication, flexible trays can be easily constructed and modified for the application of prescribed medication over teeth. The only equipment and materials required are accurate study casts, a vacuum forming press, and flexible mouth-guard material. This treatment, in addition to good dentistry and proper home care, reduces the effects of tooth breakdown and possible osteoradionecrosis.

Protective Devices. During and following radiation therapy, intraoral soft tissues may swell and impinge upon sharp cusps on teeth, spaces created by missing teeth, or diastemas. Traumatic ulcers of the tongue, cheek, or labial mucosa may be prevented by the construction of flexible or acrylic stents placed over these potentially irritating areas.

Chemotherapy Appliances

Similar in constructiom to flexible fluoride tray carriers, chemotherapy appliances can be made and used by the patient to alleviate and treat the problems of the mucosa that are often seen in those who receive chemotherapy.

CONCLUSIONS

Obviously, the medical management for the eradication of the intraoral lesion is of prime importance. The quality of treatment and the quality of life are often enhanced by the use of prostheses. With the increasing number of physicians who use the services of qualified maxillofacial prosthodontists, patients are able to receive a more complete treament with less psychological and physiological trauma than in the past. Thus, the return to "society" can be an attainable reality for the patient.

REFERENCES

1. Beumer, J., Curtis, T. A., and Firtell, D. N.: Maxillofacial Rehabilitation: Prosthodontic and Surgical Considerations. St. Louis, The C. V. Mosby Co., 1979.
2. Chalian, V. A., Drane, J. B., and Standish, S. M.: Maxillofacial Prosthetics: Multidisciplinary Practice. Baltimore, The Williams and Wilkins Co., 1972.
3. Dreizen, S., Brodey, G. P., and Rodriguez, V.: Oral complications of cancer chemotherapy. Postgrad. Med., 58:75, 1975.
4. Rahn, A. O., and Boucher, L. J.: Maxillofacial Prosthetics: Principles and Concepts. Philadelphia, W. B. Saunders Company, 1970.

22

Role of the speech pathologist in the rehabilitation of oral cancer patients

DEBORAH GEORGIAN KOCH, M.A., CCC-SP

The speech pathologist has long been an integral member of the team of health professionals who care for patients who have head and neck cancer. Traditionally, this involvement has centered on the laryngectomee who suffers a total loss of phonation as a result of surgery. However, even cancer patients who undergo less radical resection sustain significant impairment to speech and swallowing. In these cases, consultation with the speech pathologist may be less automatic, yet it can be of great benefit.

As the length of survival of oral cancer patients increases, disabilities resulting from the loss of portions of the structures for mastication, deglutition, salivary control, phonation, and articulation become more significant. These functional handicaps, in addition to cosmetic disfigurement, cannot be hidden and frequently add to social and psychological disability.[8]

Deprivation of speech is devastating for the patient who has undergone ablative surgery for oral cancer. In society, a premium is placed upon effective communication. Verbal skill is particularly rewarded in our highly competitive culture. It is paramount to social and vocational success and conformity. Van Riper describes speech as the essence of man, as he writes, "because we can speak, we can think symbolically; and it is this which has enabled man to conquer the world and space and every other creature."[13] The experience of normal eating is also marred for oral cancer patients. The tastes, smells, and textures of food once enjoyed are suddenly lost. At the same time,

the social pleasures that surround mealtimes are reduced because of the blatant changes in eating habits resulting from surgery. Thus, two major goals of the rehabilitative process must be the attainment of communication skills and deglutition, both of which allow for social adaptation and an improved quality of life.[10] The speech pathologist who has had extensive training in these disciplines is well equipped to facilitate the rehabilitation of both functions in oral cancer patients.

Successful rehabilitation requires the efforts of a multidisciplinary health team, which includes surgeons, radiotherapists, prosthodontists, speech pathologists, social workers, psychologists, vocational counselors, dieticians, physical therapists, and nurses. Intervention by the health team must include preoperative counseling, early evaluation and treatment, ongoing support, and long-term planning and follow-up.

SWALLOWING

It is important to help the patient achieve consistent swallowing prior to specific speech intervention. Adequate nutrition is necessary for proper healing and restoration of strength. Also, for many patients, the removal of the nasogastric tube is an important psychological milestone. Furthermore, stimulation of improved oral function for swallowing actually begins the speech rehabilitation process, because these two processes have many of the same anatomic and physiologic features.

Physiology of Normal Swallowing

To understand the postoperative dysphagia that frequently occurs in oral cancer patients, it is first necessary to review normal swallowing. This may be divided into three stages: oral, pharyngeal, and esophageal. In the oral phase, the lips, cheeks, tongue, floor of the mouth, teeth, and palate participate in the preparation of a food bolus. The preparatory functions include oral continence, lateralization of material for mastication, and bolus formation. Lingual peristaltic action then propels the prepared bolus posteriorly to the faucial arches. The tongue maintains its retracted position to prevent the bolus from returning to the anterior oral cavity.

At the faucial arches, the swallowing reflex, a multifaceted muscular activity, is initiated. In this involuntary pharyngeal phase, the soft palate simultaneously elevates and retracts to prevent nasopharyngeal regurgitation. The lateral and posterior pharyngeal walls constrict to begin the pharyngeal peristalsis, which is necessary for propelling the food downward. The larynx moves upward and forward to close against the posterior tongue, which moves backward and downward. Three levels of sphincter activity function to protect the airway against aspiration. The epiglottis moves back to cover the top of the trachea, the false vocal cords approximate, and the true cords close completely. Pharyngeal peristalsis ends in relaxation of the cricopharyngeal sphincter.

In the esophageal phase, the bolus is carried by peristalsis through the esophagus. This complex mechanism of swallowing is a well-coordinated activity that is accomplished rapidly. Oral and pharyngeal transit times are each approximately 1 second in duration, and esophageal transit time is 8 to 10 seconds.[1]

With so many structures involved in this complex process, resection of oral cancer at a variety of sites may result in postoperative difficulties. Patients who have undergone significant resection of the tongue, palate, lips, faucial arches, mandible, maxilla, or floor of the mouth benefit from early intervention by a speech pathologist.

Evaluation

The patient's medical record is reviewed to determine the extent of ablative and reconstructive procedures and the amount of preoperative radiotherapy. A detailed interview with the patient is invaluable, not only to delineate functional defects but also to assess the patient's alertness and orientation. This is important because the patient's ability to follow a sequence of 3 or 4 instructions and his or her emotional restraint and behavior control are fundamental to the success of treatment. By the time of the interview, many patients have attempted to swallow but have experienced some difficulty. Often, they can give a surprisingly accurate description of the problems encountered. It is also important to note the patient's ability to control secretions.

The speech pathologist then completes an oral motor examination that assesses the range, speed, accuracy, and strength of speech and nonspeech movements. The palatal reflex is tested using a cold laryngeal mirror at the juncture of the hard and soft palates. A gag is elicited by stimulating the base of the tongue or the posterior pharyngeal wall. Sensation within the oral cavity to light touch, temperature, taste, and texture is determined. This is important because deficits in sensation and function often coincide.

Before swallowing is attempted in the evaluation, the patient's ability to protect the airway must be noted. Airway protection depends upon the patient's strength to produce an adequate cough and to maintain vocal cord adduction. The latter is assessed by analysis of vocal quality, pitch, and intensity and the duration of phonation. Pulmonary function studies are important, because decreased pulmonary reserves restrict the amount of aspiration that is tolerable.

If the above examinations reveal limited or severely impaired function, particularly in laryngeal control, the clinical bedside swallowing evaluation should be deferred. If it has been determined that the patient may have some aspiration during the evaluation, the surgeon's clearance should be obtained prior to continuation.

The evaluation continues with observation of the patient's swallowing. Patients are usually apprehensive, so it is important to proceed slowly, providing continual reassurance. The choice of liquid or soft food for the initial swallow is based upon the ability to protect the airway and to propel a bolus. This decision requires the expertise of the speech pathologist. A small amount of material, no more than 1 or 2 ml, is given, and the patient is instructed to swallow when he or she is ready. Notation is made of the timing and motility throughout the stages of swallowing. The speech pathologist does this by placing a hand with fingers spread from the patient's mandible to the thyroid cartilage. In this position, movements of the hyoid bone, base of the tongue and larynx, as well as the triggering of the swallowing reflex, may be ascertained. After the swallow is completed, the oral cavity is examined for residual material. Aspiration is indicated by excessive coughing, copious secretions, and a gurgly vocal quality. Examples of specific difficulties that may occur are listed in Table 22–1.

Videofluoroscopic evaluation may provide further information. Lateral and anteroposterior film views of the oral cavity and pharynx during swallowing of contrast material reveal movement patterns and timing. This is especially helpful in assessing pharyngeal function which cannot be determined in the clinical examination and in defining the presence, amount, and etiology of aspiration.

Treatment

A variety of treatment techniques are attempted, and those that are most successful are incorporated into ongoing therapy. Most oral cancer patients experience the greatest difficulty in the preparation to swallow and oral transit phase. Pharyngeal or esophageal abnormalities are seen in only a few patients. Positioning of the food in the oral cavity and

Table 22–1. CLINICAL EXAMINATION OF SWALLOWING

Preparation to Swallow
  Mastication
    Unable to lateralize material
    Unable to mash material
  Bolus formation
    Unable to form bolus
    Unable to hold bolus
    Unable to hold food in mouth
    Abnormal hold position

Oral Transit Time
  Stasis in anterior sulcus
  Stasis in lateral sulcus
  Stasis in midtongue depression
  Adherence to hard palate
  Disturbed lingual peristalsis
  Uncontrolled bolus or premature swallow
  Piecemeal deglutition
  Late velar elevation

Pharyngeal Transit Time
  Diffuse falling over base of tongue
  Vallecular stasis
  Late swallowing reflex
  Reduced laryngeal elevation
  Reduced laryngeal closure
  Aspiration

posturing of the head can improve oral transit time. For example, in cases of oral incontinence and reduced tongue mobility, food is placed posteriorly in the oral cavity. If the patient has adequate airway protection, he is then instructed to tilt the head back slightly and swallow. In addition, the head should be tilted away from the side of ablation, thus favoring the most efficient pharyngeal passage. If airway protection is marginal, a simple "supraglottic swallow" regimen can be taught to the patient. Before swallowing, the patient should take a breath and hold it tightly. He then must swallow while holding his breath and cough afterward to clear any residual material from the vocal cords.

Food should be positioned away from the intraoral site of ablation or sensory deficit. A straw, used pipette fashion, allows for discrete placement of the liquid and control of timing.

A tongue blade is effective for putting food onto the tongue posteriorly. A syringe will function similarly and will also allow for administration of larger amounts of material when the patient's function has improved. Cold materials and carbonated beverages provide the patient with enhanced sensation so that he can learn to place food properly by himself. Alternating solids and liquids helps to reduce oral stasis by washing down any remaining material.

For some patients, a maxillary prosthesis may aid swallowing rehabilitation. It may serve to prevent reflux into the nasal cavity in cases of palatal resection. After partial glossectomy, the prosthesis enables the tongue stump to reach the hard palate to remove material and to help provide a contact for bolus formation and peristalsis.

Patients who were deferred from swallowing attempts during initial assessment should still receive intensive treatment. Range of motion exercises are provided to increase the mobility of the remaining oral structures. Airway protection can be improved by strengthening vocal cord adduction through manipulation of vocal pitch and exercises for repeated glottal attacks and increased tension in the neck muscles. The palatal and swallowing reflexes can be stimulated using an iced nasopharyngeal mirror. Repeated contact with the cold mirror should be made at the base of the anterior faucial arches. After 10 to 15 times, 1 to 2 ml of water is placed by straw (pipette fashion) at the site that has been stimulated. Upon release of the water by the therapist, the patient is instructed to swallow.

A structured program should be provided for patients who drool. The patient is given the responsibility for daily recording of the amount of time the lips are closed. An initial goal of closure for 30 seconds at a time is appropriate with subsequent increases of 1 minute per day. The patient is instructed to swallow when he feels the saliva collecting in his mouth. Cues to maintain a slightly retracted head posture may aid those patients for whom mouth closure is extremely difficult.

Attempted feeding in the presence of a tracheostomy is not necessarily contraindicated. Adequate precautions must be taken, and approval must be obtained by the surgeon. A tracheostomy permits more direct observation of aspiration and facilitates suctioning. Also, the patient can easily eliminate aspirated material. The speech pathologist must work closely with the nursing staff in suctioning both before and after the swallowing attempts.

If oral and pharyngeal transit times are increased threefold, oral feeding is probably not a realistic consideration, because the process is too slow to allow for adequate nutrition. If more than 10 per cent of swallowed material is consistently aspirated or if the patient is losing weight, tube feeding may be required to augment or to replace oral feeding. Nonoral feeding methods include use of a nasogastric tube, gastrostomy, or esophagostomy. These methods help to maintain nutrition while swallowing therapy continues. The patient can better relax and concentrate on the instructions given knowing that he is not yet dependent upon successful oral feeding for necessary caloric intake.

It is critical to do everything possible to help encourage and motivate the patient in his eating attempts. Here the ongoing involvement, training, and support of the nursing staff and family members are invaluable. The labored nature of eating, the deprivation of favorite foods, and the lack of appeal of a soft diet can quickly lead to depression and even loss of the will to live. The oral cancer patient can make significant gains in swallowing given sufficient time, careful instruction, and maximal support.

COMMUNICATION

Ablative surgery may damage or destroy function of the articulatory structures, resulting in impaired speech intelligibility. Speech is produced by a stream of air that passes through a vibratory source, the vocal cords. Resulting sound waves then resonate in a series of cavities. The breath stream is shaped by a variety of articulatory valves that serve to modify sound into phonemes. There are both mobile and fixed articulators that form the labial, dental, alveolar, palatal, velar, lingual, and glottal valves. Patients who present with significant lesions involving any of these sites in the vocal tract may be expected to have communication problems postoperatively. In these cases, preoperative assessment by a speech pathologist is appropriate.

Evaluation

The preoperative evaluation begins with a detailed history that focuses on the patient's dependency on verbal communication at home, with friends, at work, on the telephone, and in other social situations. (At the same time, questions are asked regarding eating habits and food preferences.) This information helps in planning treatment goals based on the patient's expectations, motivation, and communicative needs. A tape recording of conversational speech, oral reading, and a standardized sentence articulation test are obtained. This is to provide a baseline of the patient's speech, documenting any dialectal variations and pre-existing speech, language, or oral motor deficits.

Postoperative evaluation begins when the surgeon determines that intraoral healing is sufficient to tolerate exploration of compensatory movements of the remaining oral musculature. Information about the extent of resection and the mode of reconstruction is reviewed from the operative report. This provides an estimate of the impact of surgery on the structures of the vocal tract and on the strength and control of the muscles necessary for articulation and phonation. The patient is then assessed clinically to determine the functional deficits resulting from surgery. Once again, a tape recording is made of conversational speech, oral reading, and articulation in structured sentences. This test battery is used to obtain an overall intelligibility rating, which can help to gauge progress made in therapy. Careful analysis of articulatory patterns is made to determine the sites of dysfunction. Next, some trial treatment techniques are introduced in order to judge the patient's comprehension, cooperation, and capacity for improved function.

Treatment

The major goal of treatment is to restore communication. Most often, such restoration is achieved by teaching substituted articulatory movements that compensate for the loss of tissue and mobility of the articulators. Dental prostheses may also significantly aid in the improvement of speech intelligibility by filling in cavities or providing points of contact and closure with the remaining articulators (see Chapter 21). In some patients, near-normal articulation can be re-established through systematic training of a reduced speaking rate and improved monitoring of phoneme production. Effective communication may be furthered by the development of gestural and visual cues to accompany speech. Training of both the patient and family members in the use of contextual cues and key words also helps to facilitate communication and reduce frustration.

Lips

The lips, the most distal of the articulatory valves, must have adequate ability to round, spread, constrict, close, and open rapidly. When the lips are surgically removed, shortened, or immobilized, perhaps in conjunction with a partial mandibulectomy or maxillectomy, the bilabial and labiodental phonemes are affected (Table 22–2). If the lower lip has undergone resection, the tongue tip may be used to contact the upper lip or anterior maxillary teeth, thus forming a substitution for the normal valving mechanism. The resultant compensatory sounds are generally identifiable and moderately intelligible when embedded in a linguistic context.[6]

Maxilla

Removal of any part of the maxilla will in some way affect production of the labiodental, linguodental, linguoalveolar, or linguopalatal phonemes. These articulatory placements account for 16 of the 25 consonants used in American speech (see Table 22–2). In addition, removal of any portion of the soft palate may result in hypernasality, which is usually coupled with nasal emission. A modified dental prosthesis can often be used both to restore a surface for dental and alveolar contacts and to separate the oronasal and nasopharyngeal cavities (see Chapter 21). The speech pathologist may aid the prosthodontist in assessing the effectiveness of the prosthesis in providing for adequate resonance and articulatory contacts.

Objective gains in intelligibility may be documented and measured using audio taping of single words and conversational speech. This is done prior to the placement of the prosthesis, when the wax contour is completed and again when the final prosthesis has been worn for 4 to 6 weeks. In some medical centers, the speech pathologist, in cooperation with the radiologist and prosthodontist, may utilize videofluoroscopy. Lateral views are obtained during single syllable word production. The selected words contain both initial and final consonants that require close approximation or contact of the tongue tip to the maxillary teeth, tongue blade to alveolar ridge, tongue blade to prepalatal area, and back tongue to the posterior palate and velum.[14] If there is insufficient prosthetic material to complete a necessary contact, this can be detected and modified.

Tongue

Partial or total glossectomy results in changes in the size of the resonating oral cavity as well as in the mass and mobility of the tongue. Tongue flaps or other reconstructive techniques that may limit the flexibility of the residual tongue stump may be as important as the extent of resection in determining the prognosis for restored speech.

After sufficient healing has occurred, range of motion exercises are provided to improve the excursion and control of the tongue stump. It is recommended that the exercises be done 10 times each day, 4 to 5 times in each direction. In addition, tongue manipulation of licorice and hard lollipops helps to strengthen the musculature, thus increasing the range and rate of movement.

Specific compensatory articulation patterns are explored and taught for each lingual phoneme. Such compensatory adjustments may include movements of the lips, cheeks, and pharyngeal wall. For example, pharyngeal constrictions may be taught in order to obtain a resonable /k/ and /g/. The consonants /t/ and /d/ may be formed by approximation of the upper teeth and lower lip. Consistency in phoneme substitution is established through intensive drills. Through these measures, even patients who have had total glossectomies have been reported to achieve intelligible speech.[5, 11]

A maxillary prosthesis may be made to reshape the palatal vault in order to complement the remaining range of tongue function. Again, evaluation by videofluoroscopy will aid in the shaping of the palatal structure. Here, anter-

Table 22–2. CONSONANT PHONEMES CHART

Place of Articulation	Manner of Formation					
	Plosive	Fricative	Affricate	Glide	Lateral	Nasal
Bilabial	p b	hw		w		m
Labiodental		f v				
Lingual dental		th(voiced) th(unvoiced)				
Lingual alveolar	t d	s z			l	n
Lingual palatal		sh zh	ch j	y r		
Lingual velar	k g					ng
Glottal		h				

oposterior film views, in addition to the lateral views, are important to account for any asymmetry in the tongue-alveolus seal.[14] Replacement of tongue bulk by myocutaneous flap or artificial tongue may also improve resonance and facilitate articulatory adjustments.

Treatment techniques for the oral cancer patient must be individually tailored. The extent of resection is only one factor to be considered in the formulation of treatment plans and goals. Consideration must also be given to the patient's overall health, neurological and mental status, and motivation. Prognosis for maximal rehabilitation is limited by depression and lack of cooperation. The length of treatment varies with the individual patient. Rehabilitation usually extends from 2 to 6 months, with an average of 3 months. When the patient is undergoing prosthetic management, a longer period of follow-up may be necessary.

Recent advances in augmentative, nonvocal communication systems have provided a variety of options for patients who are depressed, unmotivated, or so severely impaired that sufficient rehabilitation of speech is not possible. Written language, use of idea-signaling systems such as American Indian Sign, or hand held word processors with written printout may be used.

CONCLUSION

The most important aspect in the management of the oral cancer patient is the attempt at curative therapy, whether through surgery, radiotherapy, or a combined approach. However, many patients are equally concerned with recovery of function and return to as normal a lifestyle as possible. The speech pathologist plays an important role in the rehabilitation of speech and swallowing, two of the most significant postoperative concerns. Most patients should be able to develop some form of functional verbal or nonverbal communication. Optimally, most patients should leave the hospital with the capability of swallowing liquids and soft foods without aspiration. The ability to tolerate solid, textured foods depends upon the presence of a significant remnant of the structures necessary for mastication. Although some return of function may occur spontaneously, most patients require the assistance of a trained professional to reach their full potential. Thus, the speech pathologist plays an integral role in the rehabilitation process.

A well-organized team approach is in the best interests of the oral cancer patient. The surgeon should coordinate the provision of services by timely referral to the appropriate professionals. Clear, ongoing communication among the team members is vital for consistent reinforcement of treatment goals. This will serve to shorten the length of hospitalization and to optimize the return of the patient's functional abilities.

REFERENCES

1. Aguilar, N. V., Olson, M. L., and Shedd, D. P.: Rehabilitation of deglutition problems in patients with head and neck cancer. Am. J. Surg., *138*:501, 1979.
2. Amerman, J. D., and Laminack, C.: Evaluation and rehabilitation of glossectomy speech behavior. J. Commun. Disord., 7:365, 1974.
3. Batsakis, J. G.: Tumors of the Head and Neck. Baltimore, The Williams & Wilkins Co., 1979.
4. Conley, J. J.: Swallowing dysfunctions associated with radical surgery of the head and neck. A.M.A. Arch. Surg., *80*:602, 1960.
5. Duguay, M. J.: Speech after glossectomy. N.Y. State J. Med., *64*:1836, 1964.

6. Hufnagle, J., Pullon, P., and Hufnagle, K.: Speech considerations in oral surgery parts I and II. Oral Surg., 46:349, 1978.
7. Lauciello, F. R., Vergo, T., Schaaf, N. G., et al.: Prosthodontic and speech rehabilitation after partial and complete glossectomy. J. Prosthet. Dent., 43:204, 1980.
8. Light, J.: Psychological aspects of disability and rehabilitation of cancer patients. N.Y. J. Dent., 46:293, 1976.
9. Logemann, J. A., and Bytell, D. E.: Swallowing disorders in three types of head and neck surgical patients. Cancer, 44:1095, 1979.
10. Meyerson, N. D., Johnson, B. H., and Weitzman, R. S.: Rehabilitation of a patient with complete mandibulectomy and partial glossectomy. Am. J. Otolaryngol., 1:256, 1980.
11. Skelly, M.: Glossectomee Speech Rehabilitation. Springfield, Illinois, Charles C Thomas Publisher, 1973.
12. Trible, W. M.: The rehabilitation of deglutition following head and neck surgery. Laryngoscope, 77:518, 1967.
13. Van Riper, C.: Speech Correction. Englewood Cliffs, Prentice-Hall, Inc., 1972.
14. Wheeler, R. L., Logemann, J. A., and Rosen, M. S.: Maxillary reshaping prostheses: effectiveness in improving speech and swallowing of postsurgical oral cancer patients. J. Prosthet. Dent., 43:313, 1980.

23

Tumors and tumor-like lesions of the jaws

ELLEN EISENBERG, D.M.D.

Accurate diagnosis is the product of a sequential process that demands logic and discipline. In addition, it requires the acquisition, correlation, and synthesis of a thorough knowledge of the patient; the history of the problem; the clinical and, where appropriate, radiographic features of the lesion; and finally, the results of pertinent laboratory studies, particularly the biopsy. In the clinical approach to problem-solving, microscopic studies may provide the critical information upon which a diagnosis is established. More frequently however, microscopic findings alone are of only limited diagnostic value, because without clinical and clerical supportive data, the pathologic perspective is narrowed such that even the most elegant details of cytology are reduced to meaningless descriptives. Thus, it may be hazardous to base diagnosis on the isolated interpretation of microscopic slides.

With regard to problems in bone pathogenesis, probably more so than any other tissue, it is essential that the clinician recognize that, like the impressions generated from analysis of the radiographic findings, those derived from the biopsy alone can neither determine the diagnosis nor be the primary basis upon which treatment is predicated. Additionally, the biopsy can neither supersede nor substitute for good radiographs and complete familiarity with the clinical picture for purposes of orientation and for demonstrating the topographic and behavioral characteristics of the lesion. Therefore, it is incumbent upon the pathologist to reserve diagnostic judgment of any bone tissue specimen until it has been carefully reviewed by all three methods.

It is not the intent of this chapter to give a detailed treatise on the histopathology of all neoplastic and tumor-like conditions of the jaw bones. Rather, it is to provide descriptions of the microscopic features of a few frequently encountered lesions and some important but less common conditions to offer comments on factors that may be useful in distinguishing these entities from others with which they may be confused; and to urge the reader to keep in mind that among the data required for the diagnosis and, ultimately, the treatment of a bone lesion, histopathology alone is insufficient and may be dangerous.

GIANT CELL LESIONS

Varying numbers of multinucleated giant cells may be found in virtually any specimen that contains osseous tissue; thus, just the fact of their presence is of little diagnostic significance. They represent osteoclasts, the cells normally responsible for the dynamic process of bone resorption. Characteristically, osteoclasts are of a variety of shapes and sizes, have basophilic cytoplasm, and have impressive numbers of nuclei which, regardless of the number per cell, usually appear distinct, with well-demarcated nuclear membranes and single, clearly discernible nucleoli.

Several diverse benign pathologic entities featuring increased numbers of osteoclast-like multinucleated giant cells as their microscopic hallmark, manifest in the jaw bones. These include the central giant cell ("reparative") granuloma; the osteolytic lesions of hyperparathyroidism; cherubism; and the true giant cell tumor, which occurs more commonly in the long bones. Based on microscopic appearance alone, it may be difficult, if not impossible, to categorically distinguish any one of these conditions from the others. However, with adequate clinical, radiographic, and laboratory data accompanying the histologic description, it is possible to separate the lesions diagnostically (Fig. 23–1).

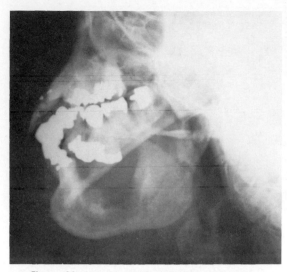

Figure 23–1. Giant cell lesion of the mandible.

Giant Cell "Reparative" Granuloma

Giant cell "reparative" granuloma is a common oral lesion. It manifests in the jaws as either a "peripheral" lesion that affects oral mucosa (gingiva, in particular) or a "central" lesion, which is an intraosseous process from inception but may extend into and involve the overlying mucosa. Stratified squamous epithelium covers the surface of the peripheral type; otherwise, the forms are histologically identical.

Central giant cell granuloma classically appears in people who are younger than 25 years of age, with a predilection for the primary tooth-bearing regions of both dental arches. Trauma, such as a blow to the jaw, or a recent tooth extraction is frequently documented preceding the development of the lesions (thus the descriptive "reparative"), but this is not a consistent historical factor in all patients. Like neoplasms or infectious processes, the lesions may grow rapidly, show dramatic radiographic evidence of osteolytic destruction, give rise to considerable jaw deformity, and demonstrate a propensity to persist and recur. However, there is little to support the impression that central giant cell granuloma represents an infectious (granulomatous) or neoplastic process. Rather, the evidence suggests that the lesion is more likely an exuberant, reactive process. The amenability of the lesion to conservative treatment modalities confirms this impression.

Microscopically, central giant cell granuloma is a nonencapsulated process. It is characterized by a richly vascular fibroangiomatous stroma that contains abundant, plump fibroblastic cells. Throughout, multinucleated giant cells are distributed in varying concentrations, often closely associated with delicate vascular channels. Fresh hemorrhage, hemosiderin deposition, and phagocytic activity are common features. Scant infiltrates of lymphocytes may be present, and in keeping with the alleged "reparative" nature of the lesion, there is often evidence of osteoid deposition in the stroma as well as reactive bone formation at the periphery (Figs. 23–2 and 23–3).

Giant Cell Lesions of Hyperparathyroidism

A similar histologic picture is seen in the focal bone lesions of hyperparathyroidism. In this condition, lytic osseous changes that re-

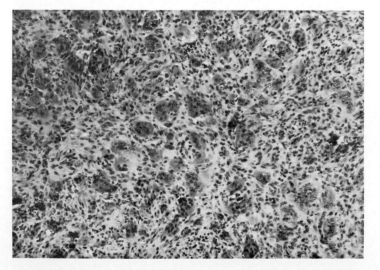

Figure 23–2. Giant cell granuloma. Multinucleated giant cells within a characteristic fibroangiomatous stroma (hematoxylin and eosin, × 250).

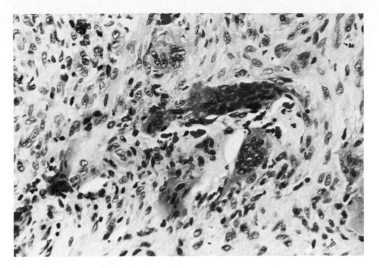

Figure 23–3. Higher-power view of multinucleated giant cells with uniform nuclei (Hematoxylin and eosin, × 450).

sult from parathormone-mediated osteoclastic bone resorption may be generalized for areas throughout the skeletal system (osteitis fibrosa cystica generalisata or von Recklinghausen's disease of bone), accompanied by corresponding hypercalcemia. Systemic sequelae of hyperparathyroidism include renal failure, hypertension, and lethargy.

Bone lesions of hyperparathyroidism have been grossly described as "brown tumors" because of their brown coloration due to extensive stromal hemorrhage. These radiographically cystic lesions appear microscopically identical to central giant cell granulomas; thus, when the nature of a giant cell lesion is in question, demonstration of elevated serum calcium is a useful differential diagnostic indicator of hyperparathyroidism.

In contrast to the "cystic" lesions that are abundant in multinucleated giant cells, other osseous lesions of hyperparathyroidism may contain few, if any, giant cells and may appear more radiographically diffuse. Histologically, these lesions show replacement of bone by cellular, delicate fibrovascular tissue. Within this stroma, new bone trabeculae show plump, single layers of osteoblastic cells and only scant numbers of osteoclasts on their surfaces.

The primarily nonsurgical management of giant cell osseous lesions in hyperparathyroidism is predicated on documentation of the underlying endocrine disturbance. After the source of excessive parathormone secretion has been eliminated either medically or by surgical excision of hyperplastic or adenomatous parathyroid tissue, the secondary bone lesions resolve.

Giant Cell Tumor of Bone

Controversy exists as to whether there is a jaw bone counterpart of the "true" giant cell tumor of long bones. When subjected to critical diagnostic review, most jaw lesions as well as long bone lesions so designated fail to satisfy the criteria that would qualify them as neoplasms; instead, they appear more consistent with reactive, inflammatory processes (that is, giant cell granulomas). However, some researchers are convinced that in selected cases there is justification for favoring a diagnosis of giant cell tumor rather than giant cell granuloma, based on the degree to which the lesion shows local aggressiveness, ominous radiographic findings, and documented evidence of metastasis.

Based on histopathology only, it is not always possible to make a confident distinction between giant cell tumor and giant cell granuloma. Allegedly, the lesions differ primarily with regard to the morphology and distribution of their multinucleated giant cells. In the "tumor," the giant cells are larger and rounder and tend to be more densely prevalent within the stroma. Additional contrasts to what is seen in giant cell granuloma include the conspicuous lack of inflammatory infiltrates and vascular changes compatible with inflammation and the absence of both internal new bone deposition and peripheral reparative bone formation.

Cherubism

Cherubism is a hereditary disturbance of bone development that is characterized by childhood onset of multiquadrant jaw deformity with corresponding distortion of surrounding facial structures and aberrant eruption patterns of the dentition. Frequently, other family members have similar symptoms.

The microscopic features of cherubism are variable and are not pathognomonic. Although the condition is classified among the jaw lesions that are composed of multinucleated giant cells, in some specimens these cells may be rare or present in relatively high concentrations only in areas in which intralesional hemorrhage has taken place. The stroma consists of very loose, delicate vascular fibrous connective tissue with little evidence of osteoblastic activity and corresponding new bone formation.

Diagnosis is based primarily on the correlation of clinical and radiographic features rather than on microscopy. The latter may be helpful to confirm the diagnosis in a suspected case, but, alone, it is of little value.

FIBRO-OSSEOUS LESIONS

Bone lesions in the fibro-osseous category are among the most commonly encountered benign pathologic conditions of the jaws. Clinically, manifestations of these lesions range from trivial incidental radiographic findings to impressive deforming lesions that are frequently accompanied by evidence of multisystem involvement. Despite their clinical diversity, which includes the entire spectrum of pathologic processes from developmental to neoplastic, fibro-osseous lesions are so designated because of their similar histologic features, the common denominator being the replacement of bone by fibrous connective tissue that contains varying quantities of mineralized tissue and osteoid.

Although the lesions have been subclassified exhaustively according to microscopic character, morphology, and extent of their individual calcified components, in most cases taxonomic efforts in this regard appear to be of greater academic than diagnostic or prognostic value. For the most part, the histologic details of a single fibro-osseous lesion provide significantly less information about the lesion's disposition than that which may be derived from the correlation of its clinical and radiographic features. In most cases, impressions formulated from studying the latter are sufficiently diagnostic as to obviate completely the need for biopsy.

The fibro-osseous processes can be subclassified into the following categories:

1. Lesions of uncertain etiology such as the cementoma, which is known by many other names, including periapical fibrous dysplasia, periapical cemental dysplasia, gigantiform cementoma, and benign fibro-osseous lesion of periodontal ligament origin (BFOPDL).

3. True neoplasms (ossifying fibroma, cementifying fibroma, and cemento-ossifying fibroma).

3. Fibrous dysplasia.

The latter deserves attention as a separate fibro-osseous process, because it is, unlike the others, clearly developmental in origin.

Cementoma (BFOPDL)

In the jaws, the so-called "cementoma," or periapical cemental dysplasia, in all its dimensions, represents the most familiar presentation of fibro-osseous disease. The lesions are classically asymptomatic curiosities that are detected on routine radiographic survey, where they appear as focal conglomerates of mixed radiolucency and radiopacity. These changes in radiodensity are usually well demarcated from surrounding normal bone trabeculae and located in the vicinity of the periodontal ligament. Although the term *cementoma* implies a neoplastic derivation, these lesions do not behave as such. It has been suggested that they are either developmental in origin and represent an attenuated form of fibrous dysplasia (a specific fibro-osseous process with definite hamartomatous features) or represent reactive, sclerosing osteomyelitis, the result of low-grade chronic inflammation in the periodontal ligament. Because of this uncertainty, perhaps the most appropriate diagnostic term for these lesions and their apparently hereditary variant (familial gigantiform cementoma) is *benign fibro-osseous lesion of periodontal ligament origin* or *BFOPDL,* because it most closely describes the involved abnormal tissue without implicating a specific inciting factor. From here on, they will be referred to as BFOPDL.

Histologically, BFOPDL lacks a capsule and merges with the surrounding normal bone. The connective tissue stroma may be densely collagenous or more loose and areolar. Within this stroma, fibroblasts are generally plump or fusiform and there are no mitotic figures. In keeping with the proposed low-grade inflammatory etiology, it is not unusual to find focal aggregates of lymphocytes and fibrohistiocytic

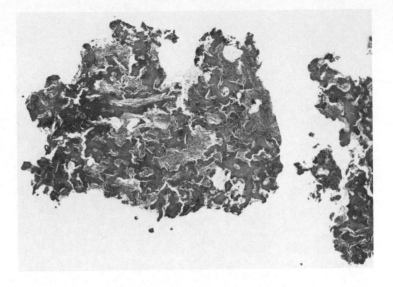

Figure 23–4. Benign fibro-osseous lesion ("cementoma," BFOPDL). Delicate osseous trabeculae in fibrous stroma (Hematoxylin and eosin, × 100).

cells; however, just as often, the stroma may show no evidence of chronic inflammatory activity.

The morphology and distribution of the calcified tissue components in BFOPDL may be remarkably varied, consisting of combinations of more or less cellular osteoid, bone, and cementum. They may appear in a heterogeneous mixture of trabeculae, islands, and droplets (cementicles) or may be more uniform, in which case one or another form prevails. The degree of osteoblastic activity may vary throughout the lesion. Regardless of the extent to which osteoblastic activity is evident or differences with regard to size and shape, the mineralized elements are characteristically well defined and appear to stand out against the stromal background. Further, they may be sparse and widely separated or closely arranged and anastomose with one another to form a syncytium or broad sheet of lamellar bone or cementum (Figs. 23–4 and 23–5).

Ossifying Fibroma, Cementifying Fibroma, and Cemento-ossifying Fibroma

These terms are reserved for the much less commonly seen fibro-osseous lesions that are true benign neoplasms. In most respects, these tumors are characterized by microscopic features that are virtually identical to those of BFOPDL. Unlike BFOPDL, however, the neoplasms are demarcated from surrounding normal bone by a dense fibrous capsule. Stromal cells in these lesions may be more

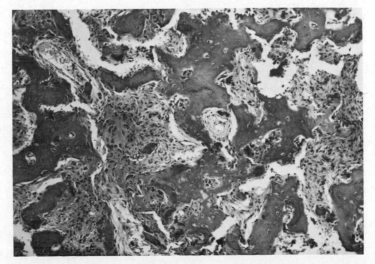

Figure 23–5. Benign fibro-osseous lesion. Note the tendency for the trabeculae to interconnect. Osteoblasts and osteoclasts are present on the trabecular surfaces (Hematoxylin and eosin, × 250).

uniformly spaced apart from one another and may reveal more spindly or stellate forms than are seen in BFOPDL; mitotic activity is not generally seen. In the lesions in which cementum predominates, the cement lines of the mineralized tissue may be quite prominent.

Fibrous Dysplasia

The term *fibrous dysplasia* refers to a specific fibro-osseous hamartoma. Such lesions typically manifest in very young children and progress through the years of active skeletal growth. Frequently, they arise in older children or in late adolescence and tend to cease in growth with adulthood. Clinical manifestations of fibrous dysplasia may be confined to a single bone (monostotic) or may be multifocal (polyostotic), affecting several bones throughout the skeletal system. The polyostotic form may be accompanied by extraskeletal disturbances such as skin pigmentation and endocrine abnormalities.

Jaw lesions are more prevalent in the maxilla and manifest as a unilateral swelling, sometimes with extension into the maxillary antrum. Occasionally, the mandible is also affected. There may be multiple quadrant involvement, resulting in minor facial asymmetry or considerable deformity. In contrast to the benign fibro-osseous neoplasms, which are encapsulated, or the lesions of BFOPDL, which tend to be well demarcated even when they involve more than one location in a single jaw bone, fibrous dysplasia appears radiographically diffuse with imperceptible borders and a radiolucent to radiodense "ground glass" or "cotton wool" trabecular pattern. The radiographic appearance coordinates with the underlying microscopic changes that consist initially of replacement of bone by fibrous tissue followed by the progressive deposition of calcified tissue within this matrix (Fig. 23–6). Histologically, the lesions develop in stages that are characterized by greater or lesser evidence of stromal activity.

The degree of stromal activity seems to correlate with the age of the patient. Lesions in younger individuals generally show hypercellularity and have more lush-appearing cells and greater numbers of mitotic figures compared with the lesions in older children. Initially, cellular fibrous connective tissue is the prevailing element. Within this foundation, the fibroblastic cells appear stellate, spindly, and morphologically "busy," with rare mitotic figures observed. Between the stromal cells, highly irregular osteoid, woven bone spicules, and trabeculae arise metaplastically by what appears to be a featherlike condensation of the fibrous connective tissue stroma rather than by conventional osteoblastic activity.

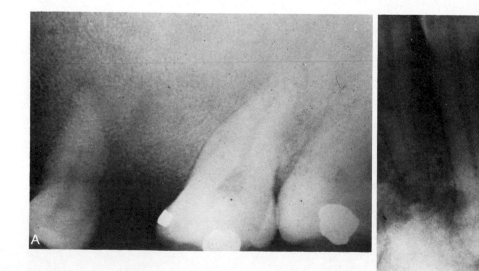

Figure 23–6. *A,* Fibrous dysplasia of the maxilla, with the appearance of ground glass. *B,* Fibrous dysplasia of the mandible, with the appearance of cotton wool.

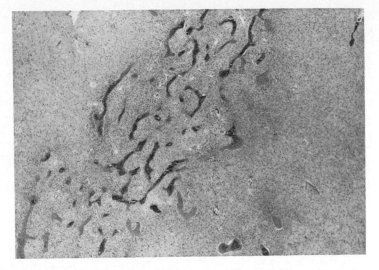

Figure 23–7. Fibrous dysplasia. Delicate spicules of bone and osteoid arising in a featherlike manner within fibrous stroma. Note the tendency for the calcified tissues to remain separate from one another (Hematoxylin and eosin, × 80).

Nevertheless, these abnormal trabeculae contain normal osteocytes in lacunae and are frequently referred to as *Chinese characters* or *C forms* because of their myriad shapes and sizes. In addition, they tend to remain separated from one another within the stroma. When observed under polarized light, these osseous tissue islands consistently reveal the refraction pattern characteristic of woven (immature) rather than lamellar bone (Fig. 23–7).

As the lesions "mature," the cellularity of the connective tissue matrix becomes less prominent and greater numbers of abnormal bone trabeculae are seen with varying degrees of calcification. Generally, osteoblastic and osteoclastic activity are not evident and the stroma appears more fibrocollagenous than cellular. In some fields, there may be myxoid stromal change with little, if any, evidence of bone deposition, whereas other fields in the same lesion may show a remarkable amount of woven bone formation.

Many microevolutionary changes in lesions of fibrous dysplasia are analogous to what is seen in the lesions of Paget's disease of bone.

Histopathologic evidence suggests that, like fibrous dysplasia, individual lesions of Paget's disease of bone follow a developmental progression that correlates with well-recognized radiographic findings. In Paget's disease, lucency gradually progresses to density and results in the classic "cotton wool" effect. The corresponding early microscopic picture reveals highly vascular areolar connective tissue within which the osseous component may be scanty. Frequently, the new bone trabeculae are delicate and may be indistinguishable from typical reparative bone. As the disease advances, erratic osteoblastic and simultaneous haphazard osteoclastic activity take place; thus, the fibrous tissue is succeeded by mosaic-appearing new bone trabeculae. As contrasted with what is seen in fibrous dysplasia, the cells responsible for both apposition and resorption can be recognized on the surfaces of the mosaic Paget's bone spicules, yet the bone itself is not particularly cellular. In the surrounding stroma, blood vessels are ubiquitous, often dilated, and closely associated with the bony fragments; numerous osteoclastic cells may be scattered throughout the background tissue, not necessarily in direct contact with bone trabeculae.

With time, as in fibrous dysplasia, Paget's disease becomes more quiescent. The degree of cellularity diminishes and bone apposition and resorption seems to stop. In addition, however, unlike fibrous dysplasia, the fibrous marrow generally is replaced by less vascular adipose tissue.

CHONDROGENIC NEOPLASMS

Chondrogenic neoplasms are distinctly rare entities in the bones of the craniofacial complex. The incidence of chondrosarcoma in the jaws is practically negligible compared with that in other skeletal sites.

Considerable controversy exists as to whether true benign cartilaginous neoplasms occur in the maxilla and mandible. The few chondromas reported in the jaws are probably analogous to the enchondromas encountered in long bones and digits, which, it has been suggested, are more likely to be hamartomas than neoplasms. These lesions manifest roentgenographically as well-defined, expansile, cystlike lucencies and arise either as solitary findings or as one of several similar-appearing lesions.

The equivalent jaw lesions are more prevalent in the mandibular ascending ramus and coronoid process and the anterior maxilla, respectively. They grow slowly but are frequently locally invasive. This fact, plus their tendency to recur, has served to raise the level of suspicion with regard to the alleged benignity of chondromas in the jaws, and in fact, many pathologists share concerns that a diagnosis of chondroma merely heralds the inevitable development of chondrosarcoma, its malignant counterpart.

In spite of these implications, the diagnosis chondroma is predicated on the pathologist's understanding of benign histologic features. The lesions consist of readily recognizable hyaline cartilage, and although lacunae may be abundant and appear in closely arranged groups throughout the matrix, the bulk of the chondroid mass is generally not hypercellular. Typically, there is one nucleolus per chondrocyte and virtually all the cells are small and uniform in size. However, even the most innocuous-appearing chondrogenic lesions must be approached with caution, because the microscopic picture alone may be deceiving and not at all indicative of the demonstrated propensity of these lesions to precede the development of chondrosarcoma. Therefore, it is the responsibility of the pathologist to demand as much supportive clinical and radiographic information as possible and to review adequate tissue samples from multiple areas within a lesion in order to establish a final benign diagnosis.

Chondrosarcoma, in contrast, is characterized by atypical cytomorphology. However, the malignant nature of the neoplasm may be obfuscated when only a small specimen is available and the cartilage appears to be well-differentiated. In order to decrease the margin of diagnostic error, tissue blocks must be studied from many areas within the lesion.

In chondrosarcoma, there is no evidence of encapsulation and usually islands, nodules, and sheets of hypercellular cartilage are seen. Interspersed within this tissue, myxochondroid tissue and relatively normal-appearing, well-differentiated cartilage may be present. Nuclei have strikingly abnormal forms and appear large, irregular, and darkly staining. Frequently, several nuclei occupy a single lacuna and these, in turn, appear confluent with one another in the hyaline matrix. Despite the distinctly grotesque cell forms, evidence of mitotic activity is either scant or absent (Figs. 23–8 and 23–9).

In myxomatous foci, the cells are usually stellate, pleomorphic, and variably hyperchromatic. There may be evidence of osteoid deposition and bone formation, which is reactive rather than malignant in appearance. This, in addition to the tendency for the malignant cartilage to calcify, is responsible for the radiographic evidence of opacification in chondrosarcoma. Prognosis is generally more favorable in lesions that show better cartilaginous differentiation. Other prognostic factors include the location of the mass, its recurrence, and its accessibility for complete removal.

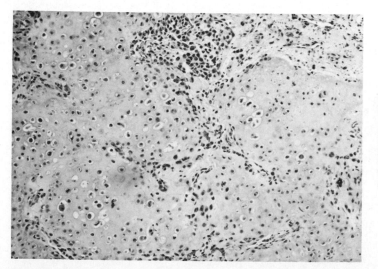

Figure 23–8. Chondrosarcoma. Multilobulated nodules of malignant chondroid characterized by hyperchromatic, pleomorphic chondrocytes in lacunae. In the adjacent fibrous stroma, numerous hyperchromatic, polygonal chondroblasts can be seen (Hematoxylin and eosin, × 250).

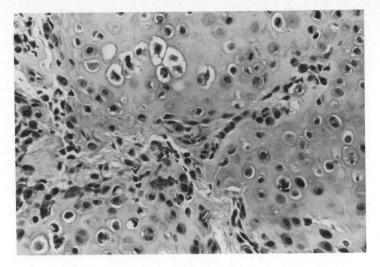

Figure 23–9. Chondrosarcoma. Higher-power view of bizarre chondrocytes. Note the variation in size of the lacunae, their tendency to cluster, and the pleomorphism of chondrocytes (Hematoxylin and eosin, × 450).

The mesenchymal chondrosarcoma is another type of chondrogenic malignancy that has manifested in the jaws, other bones, and extraskeletal locations. Microscopically, it can provide a considerable diagnostic challenge, because the primitive, extremely cellular stroma may be abundant, whereas cartilaginous elements are not as obvious. Thus, inadequate surgical sampling could result in misdiagnosis of a mesenchymal malignancy other than chondrosarcoma.

The cells in mesenchymal chondrosarcoma are generally spindly and hyperchromatic and are often arranged in sheets. Frequently, interstitial cartilaginous islands are seen intimately associated with dense collections of these cells. The cartilage itself is hypercellular with rather primitive-appearing nuclei.

OSTEOID OSTEOMA AND OSTEOBLASTOMA

Osteoid osteoma and osteoblastoma are uncommon lesions with a predilection for the bones of the appendicular skeleton and vertebral column. In spite of their apparent rarity in the bones of the craniofacial complex, the microscopy of osteoid osteoma and osteoblastoma is included in this discussion to alert the diagnostician to their existence, to familiarize the pathologist with their appearance, and to explain the features that distinguish them from osteogenic sarcoma, with which they have been confused.

The lesions affect young patients, and clinical awareness is often prompted by low-grade pain, which occurs at night and is characteristically relieved by aspirin. Although few cases

of either lesion have been reported in the jaw bones, when they do occur, the mandible is the most common site.

Many clinicians regard the osteoid osteoma and osteoblastoma as closely related benign osteoblastic neoplasms separated from one another primarily on the basis of their discrepancies in growth potential, their individual growth patterns, and their ultimate differences in gross clinical dimension. Others are convinced that the osteoid osteoma represents an unusual reparative process rather than a neoplasm because of its slower, more indolent growth pattern and considerably smaller size compared with the osteoblastoma. In addition, the lesion has several characteristic radiographic features, including an unusually round rarefaction (Fig. 23–10) (which may contain central radiodensities) circumscribed by a distinct perilesional radiopacity that suggests reactive cortical sclerosis. The latter is typically absent in the osteoblastoma. Excluding these

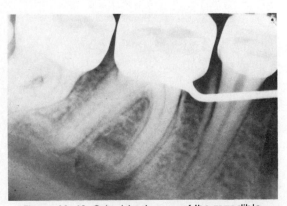

Figure 23–10. Osteoid osteoma of the mandible.

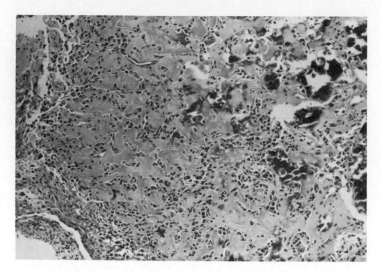

Figure 23–11. Osteoid osteoma. Plump, hyperchromatic osteoblasts are entrapped and incorporated into dense, partly calcified osteoid (Hematoxylin and eosin, × 250).

differences, the two entities exhibit comparatively few disparate clinicopathologic features.

The microscopic similarity of the lesions is sufficiently striking as to justify describing them in tandem. Based on histology alone, it is difficult to distinguish between the two. However, because osteoid osteomas rarely exceed 1 cm in size, microscopic survey on low power may reveal the diagnostic topographical relationship between the relatively contained central nidus of the lesion and its circumferential bed of cortical bone. In other respects, the lesional tissue of osteoid osteoma reveals only subtle features that serve to distinguish it from the osteoblastoma. These features consist principally of quantitative differences in stromal vascularity and the morphology of osteoid trabeculae. Neither is critical in terms of diagnosis or prognosis.

Both osteoid osteomas and osteoblastomas show a loose, richly vascular stroma that contains abundant osteoid and woven bone. The latter may range in appearance from delicate, young bone trabeculae to aggregates and sheets of osteoid with prominent cement lines that show varying degrees of calcification. Often, multinucleated giant cells are present surrounding vessels and in association with hemorrhage. They are also present in their capacity as osteoclasts and may be actively engaged in bone resorption.

Osteoblasts are ubiquitous. They proliferate densely throughout the stroma and appear to pile up in multiple layers or in pyramidal fashion on the surfaces of bone spicules and osteoid. Frequently, they are seen entrapped and incorporated into irregularities in the intercellular osteoid matrix (Fig. 23–11). In more

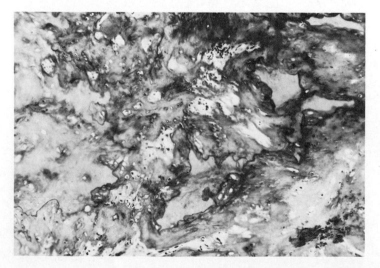

Figure 23–12. Central nidus of osteoid osteoma. This view of dense osteoid reveals bizarre, haphazard appositional lines. Several osteocytes can be seen (Hematoxylin and eosin, × 250).

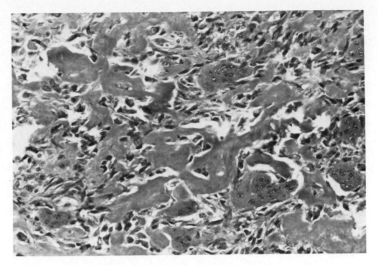

Figure 23–13. Osteoblastoma. Large hyperchromatic polygonal osteoblasts associated with osteoid. Note the multinucleated osteoclastic giant cell (Hematoxylin and eosin, ×450).

highly mineralized foci (that is, the central portions of the lesions) (Fig. 23–12), this may be an impressive finding.

The morphology of the osteoblasts merits further description. They appear active, plump, and hyperchromatic. To the uninitiated microscopist or the hasty pathologist who gives the specimen only cursory, superficial review, these features may be regarded as ominous and conceivably may be misinterpreted as indicative of malignancy. However, on careful examination, nuclear and cellular pleomorphism and atypism are conspiciously absent. Recognition of this latter feature becomes of even more critical differential diagnostic significance as the lesions evolve and more and more osteoid is deposited in the markedly cellular stroma. It may be the deciding factor by which the pathologist avoids confusing this osteoid

with the malignant osteoid of osteogenic sarcoma (Figs. 23–13 and 23–14).

Other important criteria that aid in the histologic differentiation of these benign conditions from osteogenic sarcoma include the absence of necrotic foci; lack of chondroid, chondromyxoid, or evidence of endochondral ossification; and, in the osteoid osteoma in particular, the presence of sclerotic bone at the periphery.

CEMENTOBLASTOMA

Cementoblastoma or true cementoma, a benign neoplasm, bears a striking microscopic resemblance to osteoid osteoma and osteoblastoma. Typically, patients are in the same age group as those affected by the latter lesions. Clinically, pain may be a presenting

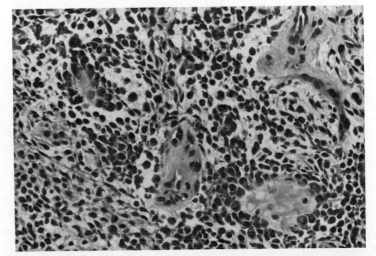

Figure 23–14. Osteoblastoma. Delicate spicules and spherules of osteoid laid down by abundant osteoblasts with hyperchromatic nuclei. Note the tendency for the blastic cells to "pile up" in pyramid formation (Hematoxylin and eosin, × 500).

symptom, either on a continuous or intermittent basis. Rarely, the mandibular cortex is expanded, resulting in subtle facial asymmetry. The most significant feature that distinguishes the cementoblastoma from the benign osteoblastic neoplasms is the roentgenographic evidence of a radiopaque mass, usually contiguous with the root of a tooth, circumscribed by a radiolucency reminiscent of periodontal ligament space. The teeth most often affected are mandibular molars and premolars. In most cases, the lesions are submitted for microscopic analysis adherent to the root of the affected extracted tooth.

On low-power histologic survey, cementoblastomas are apparently neoplastic extensions of the cementum rather than separate lesions that are composed of osseous tissue that originate in the adjacent bone. This is the only histologic feature that distinguishes between the benign cementoblastoma and the benign osteoblastic neoplasms. Whorls, clumps, and dense sheets of cementum or osteocementum are the most outstanding microscopic features of cementoblastoma; these mineralized tissues are accompanied by abundant, obviously active plump, stellate, and densely packed blastic-appearing cells. In most areas, these cells are incorporated into the neoplastic cementum sheets and resemble hypertrophic osteocytes within large lacunae.

AMELOBLASTOMA

Odontogenic tumors occur relatively infrequently and are, with very few exceptions, benign. Microscopically, they consist of either odontogenic epithelial or mesenchymal tissue or mixtures of the two. Each neoplasm is fascinating in that its histomorphology reflects the normal reciprocal inductive influences exerted by the odontogenic epithelium and its surrounding mesenchyme during the process of odontogenesis and, in effect, appears to recapitulate a stage of tooth development. The inductive effects shown in these neoplastic tissues form the basis of their classification by the World Health Organization.

The most commonly seen odontogenic tumors are the odontomas, which in actuality are not neoplasms but hamartomas composed of aberrantly arranged but mature dental tissues. Such composition reflects the full spectrum of epitheliomesenchymal inductive effects, which result in completed tooth development.

In contrast, ameloblastomas are true neo-

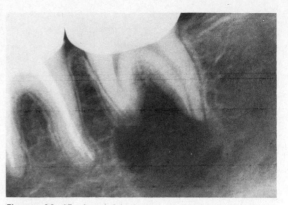

Figure 23–15. Ameloblastoma of the mandible, appearing as a cystic area of radiolucency.

plasms composed exclusively of odontogenic epithelium, which resembles the primitive enamel organ and shows virtually no evidence of induction. The neoplasm fails to show a propensity to metastasize and thus is considered benign. However, ameloblastomas are capable of extensive local invasion of intraosseous and contiguous soft tissue and may recur, often repeatedly, if inadequately excised. In many instances, the degree to which treatment is successful is dictated by the neoplasm's location and surgical accessibility. It is interesting that despite striking microscopic and clinical similarities to ameloblastomas, basal cell carcinomas of the skin are, in contradistinction, regarded as low-grade malignancies. Radiographically ameloblastomas appear as cystic or multicystic radiolucencies (Figs. 23–15 and 23–16).

Histologically, ameloblastomas tend to exhibit various patterns, but the prototypic follicular or simple form is most commonly seen.

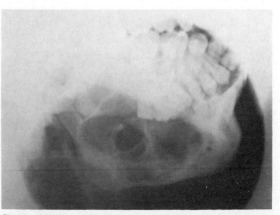

Figure 23–16. Ameloblastoma, appearing as a multicystic radiolucency.

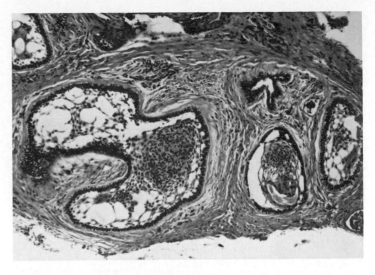

Figure 23–17. Ameloblastoma, follicular type. Columnar ameloblastic cells palisaded around the central delicate stellate reticulum. The latter reveals a tendency toward squamous (acanthomatous) change (Hematoxylin and eosin, × 250).

The follicles consist of neoplastic epithelial islands arranged like the enamel organ, with peripherally palisading columnar cells reminiscent of inner enamel epithelium or ameloblasts, which envelop loose, delicate stellate reticulum-like cells centrally. There is no mitotic activity, and the cells are generally uniform in appearance. The neoplastic follicles are not encapsulated and proliferate in a fibrous tissue stroma that tends to vary in its degree of collagenization. Usually, several histologic variations on the follicular "theme" can be seen within the same lesion (Figs. 23–17 and 23–18).

Cystic ameloblastoma occurs when the stellate reticulum undergoes microdegeneration, leaving a cystlike cavity bounded by columnar cells. It is not unusual to find that several of these cysts have coalesced to form large, cavernous, fluid-filled spaces that may be evident radiographically as well as grossly.

Other possible alterations in the stellate reticulum include a change to squamous appearance with keratin pearl formation (acanthomatous ameloblastoma) and substitution of the loosely arranged stellate cells by large round cells with distinct cell borders, small basophilic nuclei, and granular eosinophilic cytoplasm (granular cell ameloblastoma). Regardless of the morphology of the internal cells, the columnar cells remain at the periphery of the follicles in their palisaded configuration.

Another micropresentation of ameloblastoma is the plexiform type, in which the neoplastic epithelium is architecturally arranged in a network or broad sheet of interconnected complexes of stellate reticulum and ameloblastic cells, rather than in individual islands (see

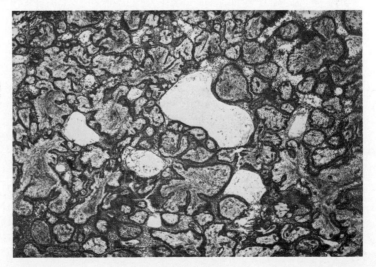

Figure 23–18. Ameloblastoma, plexiform type. Network of interconnecting ameloblastic and stellate reticulum–type cell complexes, with intervening dense fibrous stroma. In several foci, the stellate reticulum has undergone cystic degeneration (Hematoxylin and eosin, × 125).

Fig. 23–18). The fundamental ameloblastoma pattern is recognizable despite the usually extensive epithelial anastomoses. As in the follicular type of ameloblastoma, the stellate reticulum in plexiform ameloblastoma may also show cystic degeneration or metaplasia to acanthomatous or granular cell forms. Any or all of these possible variations may be seen in a single lesion; apparently none of them have any bearing on the prognosis or management of the neoplasm.

Ameloblastoma may be seen manifesting in the lining of a dentigerous cyst. In these instances, the tumor begins as a budding of the lining epithelial basal cells toward the fibrous capsule. As it develops, the ameloblastoma may proliferate extensively through the cyst wall as well as into the lumen. Any of the previously described histologic patterns can be seen. If the neoplasm is confined to the cyst wall and has not invaded the surrounding bone, it is amenable to conservative cyst enucleation and curettage, which should result in a favorable prognosis.

OSTEOGENIC SARCOMA

Osteogenic sarcoma, a primary malignancy of the bone, manifests relatively infrequently in the jaws. When it does occur, the mandible is the most frequent site. Males are affected more often than females, which is consistent with the overall sex predilection for this tumor. Patients who have jaw tumors are generally older than those who have osteogenic sarcomas in other locations.

Symptoms of this malignancy vary. There may be numerous signs that mimic odontogenic infection or periodontal disease, including radiographic widening of the periodontal ligament space and loosening of teeth. Typical clinical findings consist of a rapidly enlarging mass that is usually accompanied or preceded by pain, which becomes progressively severe. Another ominous sign is paresthesia or numbness of the lower lip and other similarly innervated structures. Radiographs classically reveal a ragged, ill-defined lucency with evidence of cortical destruction. Scattered throughout the rarefaction, radiopaque flecks may be noted (Fig. 23–19). The so-called "sunray" configuration, which has popularly been accepted as a characteristic diagnostic sign of this malignancy, is not, in actuality, a consistent finding and is usually absent in early lesions. It may be seen in other malignancies and should not

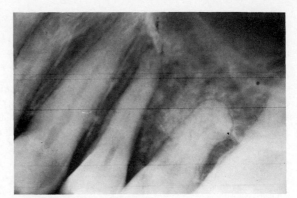

Figure 23–19. Osteogenic sarcoma of the maxilla, appearing as a radiodense area. Note widened periodontal ligament space and indistinct lamina dura around first premolar.

be considered pathognomonic of osteogenic sarcoma.

Generally speaking, the clinical and radiographic features may be strongly suggestive of sarcoma, but none are unequivocal for osteogenic sarcoma specifically. Therefore, final diagnosis is dependent upon microscopic evidence of malignant osteoid and bone formation. However, these factors may not be present or obvious in all fields of the specimen, and it is impossible to make a definitive diagnosis of osteogenic sarcoma when only a small tissue specimen is available in which neither bone nor osteoid is recognized.

The microscopic patterns of osteogenic sarcoma are diverse. This accounts for the considerable variety that may be seen in comparing material from several patients, from multiple metastases in the same patient and even areas remote from one another within an individual tumor. Essentially, the stroma is sarcomatous, consisting of hyperchromatic, spindly and stellate pleomorphic cells engaged in the formation of osteoid and bone. Mitoses may be plentiful and bizarre. Cells that occupy the osteoid and mineralized spicules show marked atypia in contrast to what is seen in the benign osteogenic neoplasms. Multinucleated giant cells of the osteoclastic variety are common and appreciably distinct from bizarre tumor giant cells in their morphology. They are also present in a reactive phagocytic capacity and may be associated with necrotic and hemorrhagic material (Figs. 23–20 and 23–21).

It is not unusual to find malignant cartilage focally in the stroma, either isolated from or intermingled with osteoid elements; or cartilage may be an impressive finding, accounting

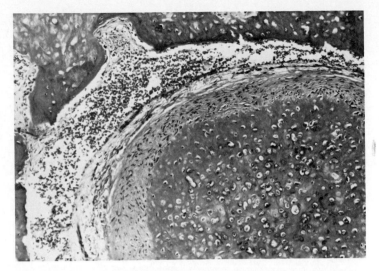

Figure 23–20. Osteogenic sarcoma. Large, bizarre lacunae that contain pleomorphic osteocytes (Hematoxylin and eosin, × 125).

for the major solid or calcified component of the neoplasm. Often, fields in a single specimen are completely devoid of recognizable osteoid or bone. Instead, hypercellular fibrous connective tissue with anaplastic fibroblasts or more primitive-appearing mesenchymal connective tissue showing hyperchromatic stellate nuclei predominates. It is not unusual for the malignancy to harbor any or all three of these mesenchymal derivatives; thus, some researchers have applied the adjectives osteoblastic, chondroblastic, and fibroblastic to further describe the histopathologic picture. Similarly, the tumors that have many tortuous, dilated vascular channels, alternating with heavy bone and osteoid deposition, frequently are referred to as "telangiectatic." It has been found that these appellations have little, if any, bearing

on the prognosis of osteogenic sarcomas of the jaw. Overall, the site of occurrence seems to be a more reliable prognostic indicator, and tumors that manifest in the jaws have a more favorable prognosis than those that arise in long bones.

Transformation to osteogenic sarcoma (or rarely chondrosarcoma or fibrosarcoma) may take place in the stroma of Paget's disease of bone (Fig. 23–22) and the picture is similar to that seen in osteogenic sarcoma that arises in bone not affected by Paget's disease. Spindly, pleomorphic bizarre cells, frequently with many mitotic figures, tumor giant cells, and benign osteoclastic multinucleated giant cells may all be present. Osteoblastic activity is associated with malignant bone formation. The malignant osteoid and bone differs from neigh-

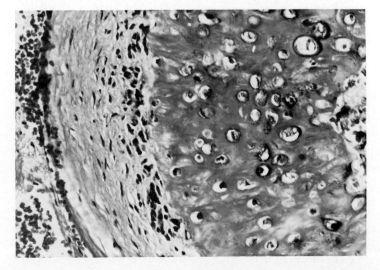

Figure 23–21. Higher-power view of osteogenic sarcoma. Note the clumps of hyperchromatic malignant osteoblasts within the dense fibrous connective tissue peripheral to the malignant bone (Hematoxylin and eosin, × 450).

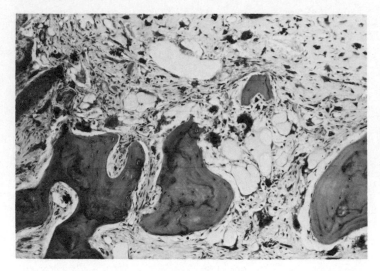

Figure 23–22. Osteogenic sarcoma manifesting in Paget's disease. Spicules of mosaic-appearing Paget's bone are separated by delicate, highly vascular intervening stroma that contain many pleomorphic, hyperchromatic bizarre cells incorporated into malignant osteoid (at top of illustration) (Hematoxylin and eosin, × 250).

boring nonsarcomatous Paget's bone, because it does not have the typical mosaic appositional pattern. This difference is retained and readily apparent throughout the specimen.

HISTIOCYTOSIS X

Histiocytosis X is the designation applied to a group of clinical conditions that result from proliferation and infiltration of organs by histiocytic cells. To date, neither an infectious nor other etiologic source has been implicated as a precipitating factor for the disorder. Classically, three clinical forms have been discussed. In descending order of severity these are:

1. Letterer-Siwe disease, which manifests in very young children as an acute, fulminating, ultimately fatal systemic disease.

2. Hand-Schüller-Christian disease (multifocal eosinophilic granuloma), which may also involve many sites but typically follows a more chronic course, affecting older children or adults. It is the form classically associated with the clinical triad of exophthalmus, diabetes insipidus, and lytic bone lesions.

3. Eosinophilic granuloma, which is by far the mildest form, characterized primarily by unifocal, often isolated osseous or soft-tissue lesions resulting from histiocytic infiltration.

In clinical practice, however, it is rare for histiocytosis X to present in a form which even remotely adheres to such strict categorical boundaries. Thus, it has been postulated that each classical presentation merely represents a different expression of a single disease complex, and furthermore, that the degree and extent of organ involvement may be a function of the immune integrity of the patient.

Some researchers have proposed that the acute, diffuse disease be regarded as a malignant type of histiocytosis, categorically separate from uni- or multifocal forms of eosinophilic granuloma. Moreover, it has been suggested that the latter forms represent a single, essentially benign disease that modulates in its severity with respect to the degree of visceral involvement and morbidity shown. Unfortunately, little meaningful information about the nature of any one of the clinical divisions is gained by comparing the histomorphology of their respective lesions, because each appears remarkably similar to the others.

In the jaws, eosinophilic granuloma manifests as an osteolytic defect that is sometimes accompanied by pain and swelling. Radiographically, it may mimic periapical periodontitis in terms of its location, but distinct from

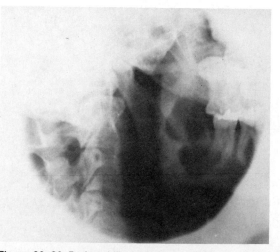

Figure 23–23. Eosinophilic granuloma of the mandible.

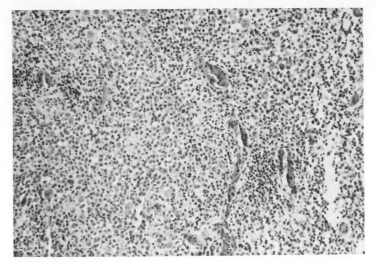

Figure 23–24. Eosinophilic granuloma. Most of the cells are abnormal histiocytes. Bone fragments and scattered neutrophils are present (Hematoxylin and eosin, × 125).

the inflammatory condition, the lesion may progress to destroy the bone cortex and eventually infiltrate overlying mucosa (Fig. 23–23). On the other hand, eosinophilic granuloma may originate in and remain confined to the oral mucous membrane.

Microscopically, the lesions consist of sheets of atypical epithelioid-appearing histiocytes. Usually, they are tightly packed together, making it difficult to discern cytoplasmic boundaries. The nuclei are generally vesicular and mature rather than pleomorphic. Although mitotic figures may be seen, they are not an outstanding feature. The degree of infiltration by eosinophils varies. In some lesions, there may be very few of these cells focally aggregated or scattered sparsely throughout the histiocytic background. In other lesions, eosinophils may be ubiquitous in all fields. Chronic inflammatory infiltrates that consist of lympho-

cytes, plasma cells, and phagocytic cells are typically superimposed on the background of histiocytic proliferation. Foci of necrosis and fibrosis commonly interrupt the collections of histiocytes so that they appear to be aggregated in epithelioid cell "clumps" rather than in sheets (Figs. 23–24 and 23–25).

PRIMARY LYMPHOMA OF BONE

In rare instances, lymphoma may manifest as a solitary primary tumor of bone. It is established as such if it is a unifocal lesion that is microscopically consistent with a diagnosis of lymphoma, if extensive lymphoma work-up fails to disclose distant metastatic or multifocal disease, and if, after six months following local radiation therapy, there continues to be no evidence of disseminated lymphoma other than regional lymph node involvement.

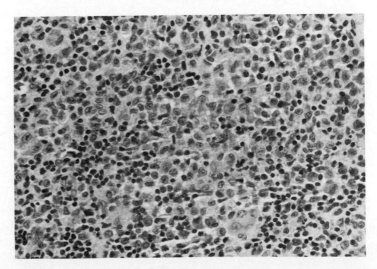

Figure 23–25. Higher-power view of eosinophilic granuloma. Some multinucleated histiocytes as well as a few eosinophilic neutrophils can be seen (Hematoxylin and eosin, × 250).

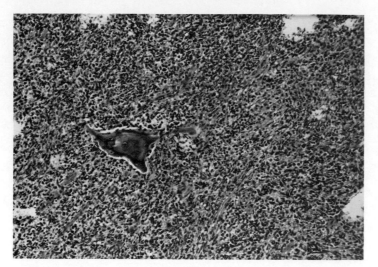

Figure 23–26. Malignant lymphoma that manifested as a periapical lesion. A dense sheet of bizarre mononuclear cells invading the bone. Residual bone spicule is present (Hematoxylin and eosin, × 125).

The incidence of primary lymphoma of bone is highest in older adults. Despite the impressive size that some lesions attain, patients often appear surprisingly healthy otherwise. In the jaws as in other bony sites of primary extranodal lymphoma, the most common presenting symptom is nonspecific boring pain, sometimes long-standing, often accompanied by a palpable mass. Paresthesia and tooth mobility may also develop. The radiographic findings indicate a diffuse destructive process that involves the medullary cavity with extension through the cortex and periosteum.

In the past, most primary lymphomas of bone were referred to as "reticulum cell sarcomas." This designation referred to the alleged neoplastic cell of origin in the marrow tissues; however, it did not reflect the remarkably varied histomorphologic spectrum that these lesions actually display. Nevertheless, because the classification of non-Hodgkin's lymphoma continues to be a source of controversy, it is more useful to emphasize the fundamental microscopic features that distinguish a malignant lymphoma of the jaw bones from inflammatory disease (with which it can be confused) rather than attempt to precisely subcategorize each tumor on the basis of its predominant cell type and overall architectural pattern.

The prevailing microscopic feature in osseous lymphoma is the diffuse, uniform distribution of the neoplastic cells that is interrupted only by residual bone spicules or, rarely, by trabeculae of reactive bone. Hemorrhagic and necrotic foci are usually evident on low power view. In areas of stromal fibrosis, the cells may be arranged in nestlike clusters. True nodular

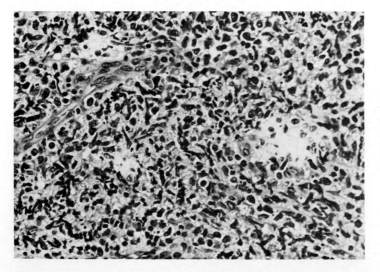

Figure 23–27. Higher-power view of malignant lymphoma. Despite the many artifactually crushed cells, many cells show large hyperchromatic nuclei surrounded by vascular cytoplasm, suggesting a histiocytic origin (Hematoxylin and eosin, × 450).

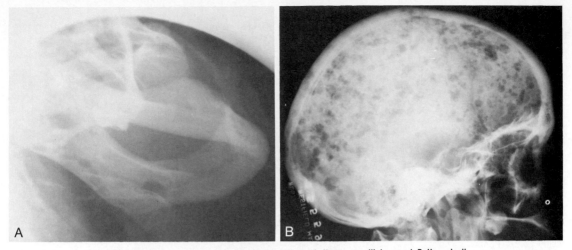

Figure 23-28. Multiple myeloma involving *A*, the mandible and *B*, the skull.

architectural patterns that are prognostically significant and frequently seen in lymphomas manifesting in lymph nodes are virtually never identified in lymphoma of bone (Fig. 23–26).

The classic malignant lymphoma of bone, reticulum cell sarcoma, is composed of cells that resemble histiocytes. They characteristically show abundant cytoplasm surrounded by reticulin fibers that are elicited on appropriate staining with the silver reticulin technique. The nuclei possess prominent nucleoli and are generally ovoid but may show some pleomorphism. Cell boundaries are frequently indistinct (Fig. 23–27).

Most lymphomas of bone consist of a mixed lymphoid cell population that varies chiefly in the degree to which there is prevalence of lymphocytes. Thus, a tumor may be classified as histiocytic, poorly differentiated lymphocytic, mixed histiocytic-lymphocytic, or undifferentiated lymphoma. The malignant cellular infiltrates are dense; cytologic features may be monotonously similar or show marked variation with respect to size, shape, and mitotic activity. Immature cell forms are frequently a striking feature. In contrast to what is seen in malignant lymphomas, inflammatory lesions show proliferation of fibroblasts and vascular elements with mixed infiltrates of mature lymphocytes, plasma cells, and macrophages. The inflammatory stroma is fibrous and highly vascular, and reactive bone formation may be seen throughout.

MULTIPLE MYELOMA

Multiple myeloma is a relatively common malignancy of middle-aged and elderly adults.

It is a plasma cell lymphoma that originates in the bone marrow, (thus, myeloma) and manifests as a widespread, multifocal disease that involves numerous skeletal sites or, rarely, as a solitary osseous lesion. More rare is the extramedullary plasmacytoma that arises chiefly in the lymph nodes or oronasal tonsillar tissue. The latter type may result in disseminated multiple myeloma.

Patients complain of progressive pain, weakness, and weight loss. Jaw involvement may manifest with tooth migration, pain, or sudden increased susceptibility to odontogenic infection. As is seen in other affected bones, the radiographic picture is typically one of medullary destruction and reduction of the width of the cortex with confluent "punched out" osteolytic defects (Fig. 23–28). Because of generalized osseous devastation, both urine and serum calcium are elevated. There is progressive anemia and a predisposition to multiple pathologic fractures. Other findings include Bence Jones urine proteins and dysproteinemia.

The serologic evidence of monoclonal gammopathy in many patients suggests that multiple myeloma may be derived from proliferation of a single clone of immunoglobulin-producing cells that either arises simultaneously in numerous bone marrow sites or is initiated in a single location and subsequently metastasizes.

In multiple myeloma, the bone is replaced by homogeneous infiltrates of plasmacytoid cells arranged in sheets or clusters in a vascular, delicate fibrous stroma. There may be considerable cellular pleomorphism, yet features such as nuclear eccentricity, "clock-face"

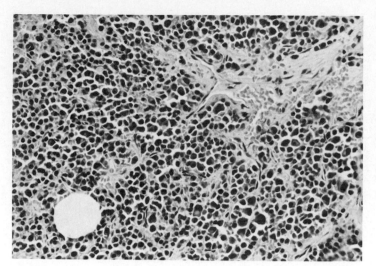

Figure 23-29. Multiple myeloma. Large, bizarre, plasmacytoid cells fill the marrow spaces between the bone trabeculae (hematoxylin and eosin, × 350).

chromatin pattern, and perinuclear haloing, which are characteristic of plasma cells, reveal the fundamental nature of the proliferating cells. Occasionally, there are conglomerates of immature plasma cell forms mingled with less differentiated, often binucleate, large, bizarre tumor cells and recognizable mature plasma cells (Fig. 23–29).

Reticulin stains will usually elicit an intercellular reticulin network. The plasma cell identity is confirmed by red coloration of the cytoplasm on staining with methyl-green pyronine.

Solitary osseous myeloma (plasmacytoma) similarly reveals a microscopic picture of monotonous plasmacytoid cell proliferation. However, the tumor cells tend to be very closely apposed to one another and, despite the presence of occasional mutinucleate cell forms, the mature plasma cell is clearly dominant.

In contrast to what is seen in multiple myeloma, in this form of myeloma clinical and serologic findings are frequently negative for signs of systemic disease. Therefore, it is especially important to appreciate the histologic features that distinguish the solitary intraosseous myeloma from the inflammatory periapical or periodontal granuloma of the jaws, because in the latter, plasma cells are often ubiquitous. In inflammatory lesions, if one looks carefully, one can see a mixture of mature round cell infiltrates on a background of active fibrovascular proliferation. This, combined with adequate clinical and radiographic evidence of a focal inflammatory source,

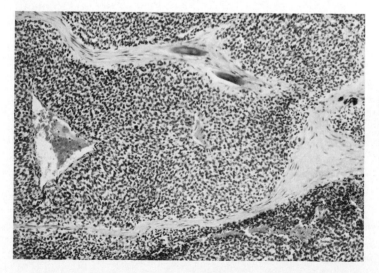

Figure 23-30. Ewing's sarcoma. Highly cellular, densely packed sheets of small cells in perithelial distribution. Note the dense fibrous tissue cords that interrupt the tumor nodules (Hematoxylin and eosin, × 125).

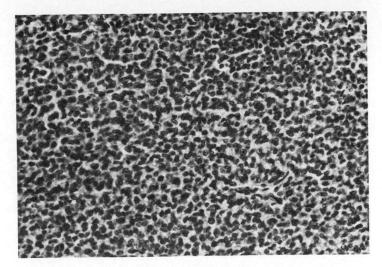

Figure 23–31. Higher-power view of Ewing's sarcoma. Biphasic character of the cells is evident. *Lower right*, cells surround a small blood vessel in pseudorosette formation (Hematoxylin and eosin, × 250).

should provide sufficient differential diagnostic information so that a misdiagnosis of malignant disease can be circumvented.

EWING'S SARCOMA

Ewing's sarcoma is a rare, highly malignant neoplasm with a predilection for people in the first and second decades of life. It is seldom seen in the jaws. Like myeloma, Ewing's sarcoma has been known to arise in extraosseous tissues. However, the tumor is, in essence, a primary malignancy of bone that originates in the marrow. It is composed of primitive-appearing, highly undifferentiated mesenchymal cells, of which the precise cytoderivation remains undetermined despite continuing investigative efforts.

The usual presenting symptoms are a rapidly expanding mass and pain. Mandibular lesions may be heralded by lip or other soft-tissue paresthesia. Regardless of the location of the malignancy, there are no radiographic changes that are pathognomonic of Ewing's sarcoma. The roentgenographic findings include expansion of the medullary cavity and cortical bone with a moth-eaten osteolytic pattern and ill-defined borders. There may be evidence of pathologic fracture or cortical lamellation in an "onion-skin" effect. This is suggestive of a periosteal reaction to dissection of the bone cortex by advancing tumor cells.

Microscopic sections reveal randomly growing clusters and sheets of closely packed cells punctuated by septae of fibrous connective tissue. The cells may be arranged in a perithelial manner around capillaries, primarily adjacent to areas where necrotic and hemorrhagic debris have accumulated. Pseudorosette formation is effected by the aggregation of cells around small foci of necrosis. There is proliferation of basically two cell types that differ in nuclear morphology. In one, the nucleus is somewhat ovoid, large, and pale-staining; in the other, there is characteristically a smaller, more intensely staining round nucleus. It may be difficult to discern the cytoplasmic boundaries of either cell type in areas in which there is dense cell distribution. In more sparsely populated fields, the cells clearly show a tendency to separate from one another (Figs. 23–30 and 23–31).

Results of ultrastructural studies have shown that most Ewing's sarcoma cells contain intracytoplasmic glycogen, which can be seen under the light microscope by a positive reaction to staining with the periodic acid–Schiff (PAS) technique. The PAS-positive material disappears following digestion with diastase. This information is particularly helpful in the microscopic differentiation of Ewing's sarcoma from other small cell malignancies, such as neuroblastoma, embryonal rhabdomyosarcoma, and undifferentiated lymphoma, with which it may be confused.

REFERENCES

1. Akinosi, J. O., Olumide, F., and Ogunbiyi, T. A. J.: Retrosternal parathyroid adenomas manifesting in the form of a giant cell "tumor" of the mandible. Oral Surg., *39*:724, 1975.
2. Azar, H. A., and Potter, M. (eds.): Multiple Myeloma and Related Disorders, Vol. I. New York, Harper and Row Publishers, Inc., 1973.
3. Batsakis, J. G.: Nonodontogenic tumors of the jaws. *In* Tumors of the Head and Neck: Clinical and

Pathological Considerations, 2nd ed. Baltimore, The Williams & Wilkins Co., 1979, pp. 381–419.

4. Campbell, R. L., Kelly, D., and Burkes, E. J.: Primary reticulum-cell sarcomas of the mandible. Review of the literature and report of a case. Oral Surg., *39*:918, 1975.

5. Cataldo, E., and Meyer, I.: Solitary and multiple plasma cell tumors of the jaws and oral cavity. Oral Surg., *22*:628, 1966.

6. Cataldo, E., Goldman, H., and Shklar, G.: Oral Pathology. An Atlas of Microscopic Pathology, 2nd ed., Boston, Oral Pathology Press, 1980.

7. Churg, J., and Gordon, A. J.: Multiple myeloma. Lesions of the extraosseous hematopoietic system. Am. J. Clin. Pathol., *20*:934, 1950.

8. Dehner, L. P.: Tumors of the maxilla and mandible in children. I. Clinicopathologic study of 46 histologically benign lesions. Cancer, *31*:364, 1973.

9. Dehner, L. P.: Tumors of the maxilla and mandible in children. II. A study of 14 primary and secondary malignant tumors. Cancer, *32*:112, 1973.

10. Farman, A. G., Nortje, C. J., and Grotepass, F.: Periosteal benign osteoblastoma of the mandible. Report of a case and review of the literature pertaining to benign osteoblastic neoplasms of the jaws. Br. J. Oral Surg., *14*:12, 1976.

11. Gardner, D. G., and Pecak, A. M. J.: The treatment of ameloblastoma based on pathologic and anatomic principles. Cancer, *46*:2514, 1980.

12. Hamner, J. E., Scofield, H. H., and Cornyn, J.: Benign fibro-osseous jaw lesions of periodontal membrane origin. An analysis of 249 cases. Cancer, *22*:861, 1968.

13. Hirschl, S., and Katz, A.: Giant cell reparative granuloma outside the jaw bone: diagnostic criteria and review of the literature with the first case described in the temporal bone. Human Pathol., *5*:171, 1974.

14. Huvos, A. G.: Bone Tumors: Diagnosis, Treatment, and Prognosis. Philadelphia, W. B. Saunders Company, 1979.

15. Ivins, J. C., and Dahlin, C. D.: Malignant lymphoma (reticulum cell sarcoma) of bone. Mayo Clin. Proc., *38*:375, 1963.

16. Jaffe, H. L.: Giant cell reparative granuloma, traumatic bone cyst and fibrous (fibro-osseous) dysplasia of the jaw bones. Oral Surg., *6*:159, 1953.

17. Lichtenstein, L.: General remarks on the clinical management of bone lesions that may be tumors.

In Bone Tumors, 5th ed. St. Louis, The C. V. Mosby Co., 1977, pp. 1–2.

18. Lieberman, P. H., Jones, C. R., Dargeon, H. W. K., et al.: A reappraisal of eosinophilic granuloma of bone, Hand-Schüller-Christian syndrome and Letterer-Siwe syndrome. Medicine, *48*:375, 1969.

19. Pahor, A. L.: Extramedullary plasmacytoma of the head and neck, parotid, and submandibular salivary glands. J. Laryngol. Otol., *91*:241, 1977.

20. Pindborg, J. J., Kramer, I. R. H., and Torloni, H.: Histological Typing of Odontogenic Tumors, Jaw Cysts, and Allied Lesions. International Histological Classification of Tumors, No. 5. Geneva, World Health Organization, 1971.

21. Pritchard, D. J., Dahlin, D. C., Dauphine, R. T., et al.: Ewing's sarcoma. A clinicopathological and statistical analysis of patients surviving five years or longer. J. Bone and Joint Surg., *57*:10, 1975.

22. Rosen, B. J.: Multiple myeloma. A clinical review. Med. Clin. North Am., *59*:375, 1975.

23. Schajowicz, F.: Ewing's sarcoma and reticulum cell sarcoma of bone: with special reference to the histochemical demonstration of glycogen as an aid to differential diagnosis. J. Bone and Joint Surg., *41*:349, 1959.

24. Schnitzer, B., and Weaver, D. K.: Lymphoreticular disorders. *In* Batsakis, J. G. (ed.): Tumors of the Head and Neck. Clinical and Pathological Considerations, 2nd ed. Baltimore, The Williams & Wilkins Co., 1979, pp. 448–481.

25. Shoji, H., and Miller, T. R.: Primary reticulum cell sarcoma of bone. Significance of clinical features upon the prognosis. Cancer, *28*:1234, 1971.

26. Spjut, H. J., Dorfman, H. D., and Fechner, R. E.: Tumors of bone and cartilage. *In* Atlas of Tumor Pathology, 2nd series, Fascicle 5. Washington, D.C., Armed Forces Institute of Pathology, 1971.

27. Topolnicki, W., and White, R. J.: Primary reticulum cell sarcoma of the skull: response to irradiation. Cancer, *24*:569, 1969.

28. Waldron, C. A.: Fibro-osseous lesions of the jaws. J. Oral Surg., *28*:58, 1979.

29. Waldron, C. A., and Shafer, W. G.: The central giant cell reparative granuloma of the jaws: an analysis of 38 cases. Am. J. Clin. Pathol., *45*:437, 1966.

30. Webb, H. E., Devine, K. N., and Harrison, E. G.: Solitary myeloma of the mandible. Oral Surg., *22*:1, 1966.

24

Surgical treatment of tumors of the jaws

R. BRUCE DONOFF, D.M.D., M.D.

Treatment of any pathologic condition is based on proper diagnosis. This requires biopsy, a complete history of the patient, and clinical, radiographic, and laboratory examination to narrow the choice of diagnosis. For example, the presence of an impacted tooth within a radiolucent lesion markedly reduces the differential diagnosis. Knowledge of the clinical behavior of the lesion permits proper surgical treatment based on sound technique, resulting in total removal of the lesion, minimal morbidity, and uncomplicated healing. A lesion known to be encapsulated, for example, can be removed more simply than one showing infiltration to the adjacent bone.

Most lesions discussed in this chapter are odontogenic in origin and benign. Therefore, discussion of the treatment will be generalized, but description of specific treatment methods will allow the reader to gain an understanding of surgical judgment. Surgical judgment is based on training and experience. This discussion is designed to give the student and clinician an appreciation for the management of tumors of the jaws.

TREATMENT INDICATIONS

1. *Presence of a lesion without symptoms or clinical findings (for example, a radiolucent area around an impacted wisdom tooth)*. Clinically, the dentigerous cyst may grow to reach a very large size. Potential for bone destruction and the ability of the cyst epithelium to undergo ameloblastic and squamous change dictates removal.

2. *Symptoms*. Expansion of the jaws, reported as swelling by the patient, is a common finding. Pain is unusual unless secondary infection or nerve involvement is present. Paresthesia is rare in nonmalignant lesions.

3. *Infection*. Infection often draws attention to an otherwise innocuous lesion. An area of infection without obvious odontogenic pathology demands radiographic views to exclude underlying pathology. An index of suspicion is a must for the astute clinician.

4. *Clinical findings*. Tooth vitality, mobility, or migration should be noted. Root resorption suggests tumor, with ameloblastoma high on the list. Occasionally, other lesions may cause root resorption, but ameloblastoma must be ruled out first.

5. *Pathologic fracture*. This is an uncommon finding, but one which, in the absence of trauma, raises the question of underlying disease.

Contraindications to Surgical Treatment

1. *General condition of the patient.*

2. *Nature of the lesion*. An osteoma has little or no potential for growth. Unless prosthetic considerations warrant treatment, no treatment is indicated.

TYPES OF TREATMENT

The general principle of treatment for these lesions is total removal of pathology with preservation or immediate restoration of jaw continuity. Treatment details are beyond the scope of this presentation, but some specific points will be made. The patient's age, clinical behavior of the tumor, and size of the tumor are the most important factors to be considered in determining surgical therapy.

The following four types of treatment are generally recognized:

1. Curettage—the mechanical removal of tissue with instruments designed to "scoop

263

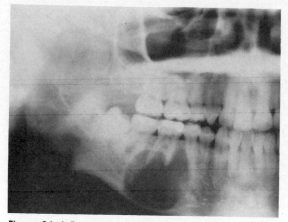

Figure 24–1. Panorex view showing radiolucency of the mandible representing an ossifying fibroma.

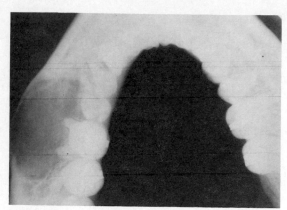

Figure 24–2. Occlusal film view of the same lesion showing buccal expansion.

out" material and "scrape" the remaining bony walls (Figs. 24–1 through 24–3).

2. Enucleation—removal of a lesion as one piece, usually possible because the lesion is encapsulated.

3. Bloc resection—removal of a geometric piece of bone that includes the lesion and surrounding normal bone without interrupting the continuity of the jaw. Removal of a large portion of the mandible while preserving the integrity of the inferior border is an example of bloc resection (Fig. 24–4).

4. Partial resection—removal of bone in continuity, leaving a gap in the bone. Hemimandibulectomy is removal of half the lower jaw with or without disarticulation of the condyle (Figs. 24–5 through 24–9). This procedure may be performed intraorally or extraorally. Hemimaxillectomy is removal of a large sec-

tion of the upper jaw, so that there is continuity established between the oral cavity and the maxillary sinus. This is usually accomplished by a Weber-Fergusson approach.

Enucleation (Figs. 24–10 through 24–17)

Following incision, a mucoperiosteal flap is raised. Frequently, the bone overlying the lesions is paper thin. In the molar ramus area, there is usually a perforation that may be widened for access of rongeurs. If the lesion's wall is attached to the periosteum, it must be separated. With adequate exposure, the lesion can usually be teased from its bony bed. Using the convex side of a curette with gentle counter traction works efficiently. Nerves and vessels are usually pushed aside and are not in the

Text continued on page 270

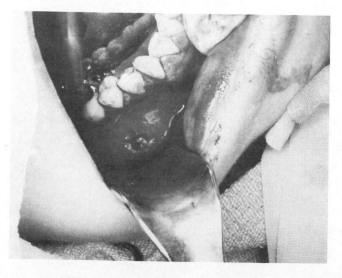

Figure 24–3. Operative view of the lesion, which was treated by curettage. No endodontic treatment of the teeth was performed. The patient is free of disease 8 years postoperatively.

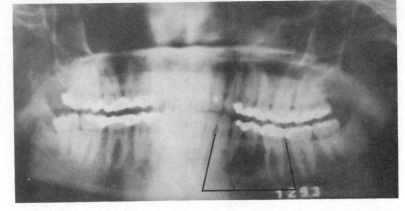

Figure 24–4. Technique of block resection. Panorex view showing radiolucency of the mandible and resorption of tooth roots. Block resection was performed as outlined. The lesion was an ameloblastoma. The patient is free of disease 10 years postoperatively.

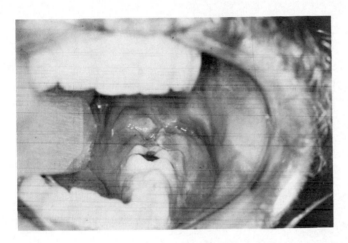

Figure 24–5. Technique of hemimandibulectomy. Intraoral view of an expanding lesion of the left mandible. The patient had paresthesia, and the biopsy findings revealed malignant schwannoma.

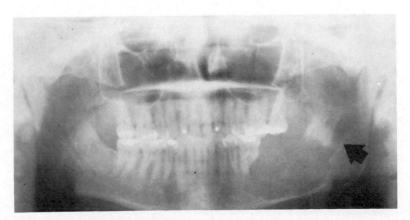

Figure 24–6. Technique of hemimandibulectomy. Panorex view showing large multilocular radiolucency of the left mandible. Note resorption of the first molar root and widening of the mandibular canal.

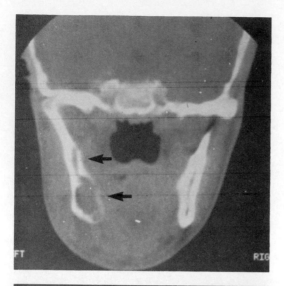

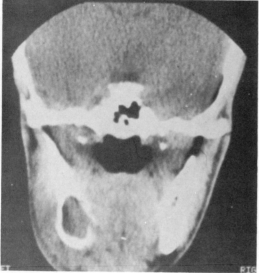

Figure 24–7. Technique of hemimandibulectomy. Coronal views of a computerized tomography (CT) scan showing perforation of the lingual mandible and widening of the mandibular canal.

Figure 24–8. Technique of hemimandibulectomy. Intraoperative view following splitting of the lip and hemimandibulectomy. The stump of condyle was left intact. Suture is tied to the remaining inferior alveolar nerve.

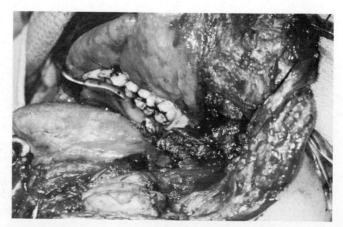

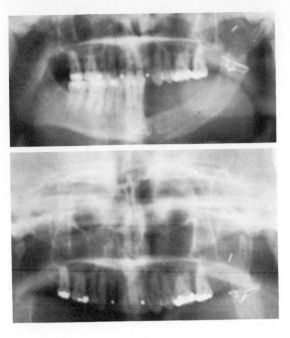

Figure 24–9. Technique of hemimandibulectomy. Panorex view of an immediate iliac bone graft 2 years postoperatively.

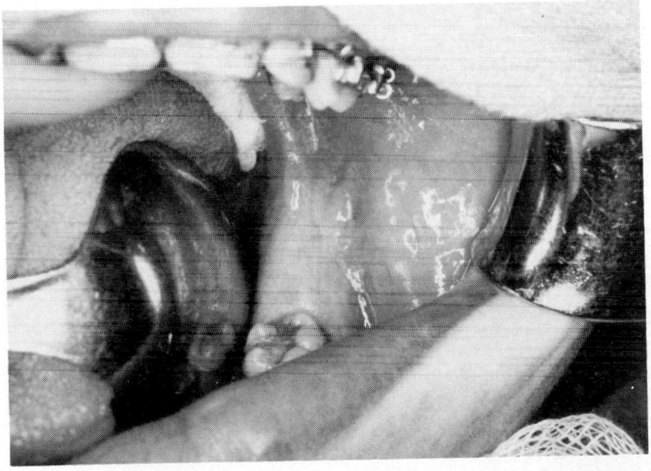

Figure 24–10. Technique of enucleation (for cyst or benign tumor). Clinical examination shows expansion of the mandible laterally.

Figure 24–11. Technique of enucleation (for cyst or benign tumor). Panorex view showing radiolucent lesion with impacted second and third molars.

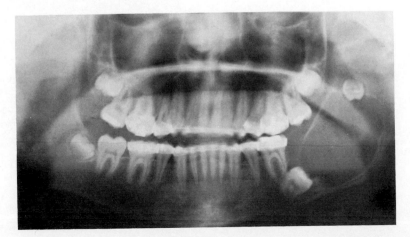

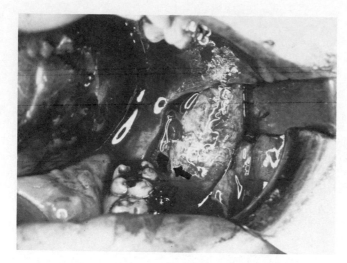

Figure 24–12. Technique of enucleation (for cyst or benign tumor). Intraoperative view showing exposure of the expanded bone with small perforation noted distal to the first molar (arrow).

Figure 24–13. Technique of enucleation (for cyst or benign tumor). Intraoperative view showing exposure of the cyst wall after removal of the lateral bone.

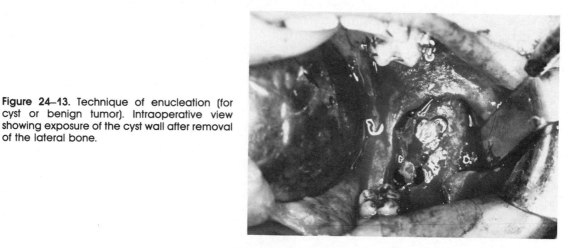

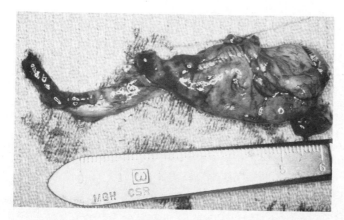

Figure 24–14. Technique of enucleation (for cyst or benign tumor). Pathologic specimen of the collapsed cyst.

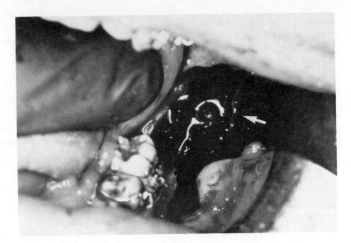

Figure 24–15. Technique of enucleation (for cyst or benign tumor). Intraoperative view of cavity in the bone after cystectomy. The inferior alveolar neurovascular bundle is indicated by the arrow.

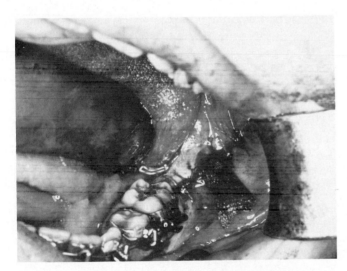

Figure 24–16. Technique of enucleation (for cyst or benign tumor). Intraoperative view showing closure with balsam of Peru–soaked gauze pack.

Figure 24–17. Technique of enucleation (for cyst or benign tumor). Panorex view showing healing and remodeling of the left mandible 1 year postoperatively.

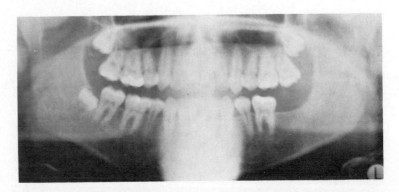

operative field. Because cysts and tumors expand in one direction, usually buccally, lingual bone is intact and indeed thickened in compensatory fashion; thus, fracture is possible, but unusual, with a good surgical technique. This statement is supported by a recent study of a large number of cystectomies. No fractures of mandibles occurred.

The bone edges of the defect should be trimmed and the area should be irrigated and inspected for hemostasis. Teeth in the area of a large cyst or benign tumor do not usually require special treatment. If devitalization is a concern, preoperative endodontics may be performed.

DRESSINGS

The size and location of the lesion determine whether a dressing is needed. Ideally, a dressing should control bleeding, prevent hematoma formation with resultant breakdown of clot and septic drainage, and promote healing. In defects up to 20 mm, no dressing is needed, because the wound will heal by primary intention. This is particularly true in the maxilla, where drainage by gravity reduces the risk of contamination of the suture line. In these instances, proliferation of connective tissue in an organized blood clot is matched by stability of the mucosal wound. In larger cavities, the blood clot does not usually survive. Lysis of the blood clot occurs before it can be invaded by new vessels to form granulation tissue. In mandibular defects, the amount of dead space and the tendency to liquefaction and breakdown of the blood clot with failure of organization can simultaneously be reduced by trimming the bone margins of the defect until it is saucerized. In addition to eliminating part of the dead space, this measure allows the reapproximated flap to collapse into the cavity.

Several types of dressings may be used, including:

1. Gauze. A gauze dressing of ½ to 1 in. plain or iodoform gauze, saturated with balsam of Peru, is used. It is well placed in the cavity and usually removed either partially or totally between the fifth and seventh postoperative days. If considerable bleeding is encountered at surgery, it is advisable to remove the dressing gradually over a period of 10 to 12 days. The defect can be irrigated at the time that the dressing is removed and can be redressed once or twice a week until healing occurs.

2. Gelfoam. Gelfoam has no significant advantage over gauze other than hemostasis.

Because this is a foreign body, the risk of clot breakdown and infection is greater.

3. Bone. Cortical and cancellous bone may be packed into large cavities of bone. Currently, it is thought that such bone prevents lysis of clot as well as stimulating osteogenesis. Although obtaining autogenous marrow from the anterior iliac crest is a simple and benign procedure, its use is questionable in filling a bone cavity that resulted from cystectomy. Commercially available bone is of very limited value. Results of recent trials with osteogenic bone powder and bone stabilizing hydroxyapatite ceramics suggest that these materials may be useful in these situations.

POSTOPERATIVE COMPLICATIONS

Proper treatment should include explaining the more common complications to the patient. Such complications include:

1. Edema. Edema is a normal complication following surgery. It is usually most noticeable on the second day and subsides if there is no secondary infection. Cold compresses are beneficial during the initial 8 to 10 hours.

2. Infection. Any acute infection in these wounds must be controlled before surgical intervention. Antibiotics, good surgical technique, and aseptic procedures minimize the risk of infection.

3. Hematoma. Hemostasis in the cavity must be checked by irrigation, pressure, and dressings. Persistent hematoma that is accessible should be aspirated and drained. Liquefaction of the clot leads to soft-tissue breakdown and possible sepsis.

4. Paresthesia. If the nerve can be seen during the procedure, it is usually in the inferior portion of cavity. Sensory nerve dysfunction is usually transient because the injury is a neuropraxia.

5. Hemorrhage. Primary hemorrhage is controlled at surgery. Secondary bleeding is usually due to large vessel rebleed or trauma to newly proliferated capillary bed when dressings are removed. Treatment by pressure is usually successful.

6. Oronasal or oroantral fistulas. These are often the result of poor technique. Adhesion between lesion and antral or nasal mucosa must be separated. Prevention of undue pressure on the area of intraoral closure is very important. Excessive sneezing, use of straws, smoking, and so on should be avoided.

7. Fracture. It is most unusual for fracture to occur, as discussed previously.

The decision to explore a tumor by the intraoral or extraoral route is based on several considerations. The most important factor is the adequacy of access. Thus, severe mucosal involvement necessitating excision of soft tissue intraorally makes intraoral resection the logical method. Most surgeons prefer to perform immediate bone grafting via the extraoral route, thereby reducing the potential for oral contamination of the bone graft.

Although successful bone grafting can be carried out intraorally, an extraoral approach is surgically "cleaner." In cases in which there are teeth in the jaw that is to be resected, extractions may be performed prior to resection, permitting adequate time for healing of the extraction wounds. The mucosa may then be spared during the extraoral resection. This approach is possible when treating benign lesions, but malignant lesions require a less conservative approach.

SPECIFIC TUMORS

Ameloblastoma

Despite reports of metastasis, this odontogenic tumor must still be considered benign, albeit invasive. Lack of encapsulation usually makes curettage a poor treatment for any but the smallest lesion. Saucerization of surrounding bone is sound practice in these situations. Bloc resection may permit total tumor removal in certain cases, based primarily on the size of the lesion. Resection is indicated for large lesions and for certain recurrent lesions. Some sacrifice of normal bone is indicated. Variants of ameloblastoma with connective tissue components, such as ameloblastic fibroma, are less aggressive and may be treated more conservatively.

Central Giant Cell Reparative Granuloma (CGRG) (Giant Cell Tumor)

This lesion is most prevalent in young patients and has a tendency to grow more rapidly than most odontogenic lesions. Most likely this is a different lesion than the true giant cell tumor of long bones, but several cases have appeared that show alarmingly aggressive clinical behavior. If malignant lesions such as Ewing's sarcoma or osteogenic sarcoma can be ruled out, treatment should be based on size. Treatment by curettage may be sufficient, and judiciously aggressive removal without needless sacrifice of normal bone structure is indicated for large lesions.

Myxoma

Myxoma is another example of a lesion that may destroy cortical bone and grow to a very large size. Excision of the entire lesion is necessary; thus, a more aggressive treatment choice is indicated.

Fibro-osseous Lesions

The two most common examples worthy of discussion are the ossifying fibroma and fibrous dysplasia. The former may be treated by local excision, best carried out by enucleation. The gritty material of the lesions can be scraped out, leaving a normal bony architecture. Fibrous dysplatic lesions usually require treatment because of deformity or functional impairment. Although there are reports of irradiated fibrous dysplasia that undergo sarcomatous change, the biopsy or contouring surgery does not result in more aggressive growth.

Vascular Tumors

The diagnosis of hemangioma or arteriovenous (A-V) malformation is of the utmost importance in preventing a surgical catastrophe. Preoperative angiography is useful for diagnosis and treatment. Blockage of feeding primary vessels to such tumors by tissue fragments or gelfoam can markedly reduce blood flow to the lesion and permit more simple and less morbid surgical treatment. Identification of major vessels permits control of these vessels during surgery. True A-V malformations have been treated by irradiation.

Histiocytosis

The lesions of eosinophilic granuloma are best treated by a combination of surgical curettage and irradiation. The reader is referred to several recent discussions of this topic in the literature. Chemotherapy also seems to play a role in the management of such lesions.

INDICATIONS FOR SURGERY OF MALIGNANT TUMORS OF BONE

Only in rare cases of primary malignant lesions of bone is radical soft-tissue surgery indicated. Indications for such surgery include fibrosarcoma, osteosarcoma, and chondrosarcoma. Radical neck dissection is an operation for actual or potential lymph node involvement. Thus, malignant lesions such as osteosarcoma may be treated by combined resection of the primary lesions and radical neck dissection. Certainly, treatment of squamous cell carcinoma may include radical neck dissection for nodal involvement. Therapy for malignant tumors of the jaws may also involve a combination of surgery and appropriate chemotherapy. None of the benign lesions included in this discussion undergo lymph node metastases. Despite the benign nature of these entities, recurrences may plague the most meticulous surgeon. The ameloblastoma and giant cell tumor (granuloma) are characterized by recurrence.

Because metastases are of no importance even with recurrent benign lesions, lesions that require resections that leave discontinuities may be bone grafted in immediate fashion. Rib or iliac bone grafts are used most often. They provide an important service for the patient, both psychologically and functionally. Recurrence in grafts has been reported but is very rare. Alloplastic materials may also be used to reconstruct the mandible in particular. These trays are filled with cancellous bone to induce osteogenesis. Because large resections may sacrifice the interior alveolar nerve, microsurgical methods provide a nerve graft to restore sensation.

In summary, knowledge of the lesion that is being treated is of paramount importance. Entire maxillas has been resected in children who have adenoameloblastomas—a very unfortunate occurrence. Current methods of clinical and radiographic assessment include CT scanning to determine perforation of bone and soft-tissue involvement. The type, size, and location of the lesion are the most important determinants of the correct extent of surgical treatment.

REFERENCES

1. Adamo, A. K., and Szal, R. L.: Timing, results, and complications of mandibular reconstructive surgery: report of 32 cases. J. Oral Surg., 37:755, 1979.
2. Chuong, R., Donoff, R. B., and Guralnick, W.: The odontogenic keratocyst. J. Oral Maxillofac. Surg., 40:747, 1982.
3. Guralnick, W., and Schwartz, H. D.: Myxoma of the mandible: resection and immediate reconstruction. Br. J. Oral Surg., 11:217, 1974.
4. Mehlisch, D. R., Dahlin, D. C., and Masson, J. K.: Ameloblastoma: a clinico-pathologic report. J. Oral Surg., 30:9, 1972.
5. Voorsmit, R. A. C. A., Stoelinga, P. J. W., and Van Haelst, U. J. G. M.: The management of keratocysts. J. Maxillofac. Surg., 9:228, 1981.
6. Zhao-ju, Z., et al.: Clinical application of angiography of oral and maxillofacial hemangiomas. Oral Surg., 55:437, 1983.

25

Tumors metastatic to the mouth and jaws

GERALD SHKLAR, D.D.S., M.S.

Malignant tumors metastatic to the jaws are encountered occasionally and usually represent one manifestation of a widespread involvement of the skeletal system. Clausen and Poulsen[4] reviewed 92 cases of carcinoma metastatic to the jaws, as recorded in the medical literature between 1884 and 1961. An analysis of the 92 cases, together with an additional 5 cases that were seen by themselves, revealed that the major sites of the primary lesions were breast (30 cases), lung (17 cases), and kidney (15 cases). Thyroid, colon and rectum, and prostate were represented by 6 cases of each and stomach by 5 cases. There were also 5 cases of melanoma. Lesions from testes, bladder, liver, ovary, and uterine cervix were also recorded. The mandible was involved four times as often as the maxilla, and simultaneous involvement of both jaws was extremely unusual (only 2 cases). Major symptoms included swelling, pain, anesthesia, and loosening of teeth. Other reviews of the medical literature were carried out by Castigliano and Rominger[3] (176 cases) and by Richard and associates.[7] Their statistics were comparable to those of Clausen and Poulsen, but their criteria for acceptable documentation of cases were not as rigid.

Few investigators have been able to study a large series of carefully documented oral metastatic lesions. Cash, Royer, and Dahlin[2] reported on 20 cases seen at the Mayo Clinic between 1911 and 1957. These included 5 hypernephromas, 2 breast adenocarcinomas, 2 sigmoid adenocarcinomas, 2 carcinomas of the face, 5 carcinomas of the lip, and single cases of adenocarcinomas of the colon, prostate, and rectum. All lesions except one were in the mandible rather than the maxilla, and the radiographic pattern of the lesions was extremely variable.

Meyer and Shklar,[6] in 1965, reported on 25 cases of tumors that were metastatic to the mouth and jaws that they saw within a 12-year period. These tumors included 5 breast adenocarcinomas, 3 hypernephromas, 3 rectal adenocarcinomas, 2 prostatic adenocarcinomas, and single cases of adenocarcinoma of the stomach, submandibular gland, parotid gland, and ovary (Figs. 25–1 through 25–4). Single cases of other metastatic tumors were also described in this series, including carcinoma of the lower lip, melanoma of the scalp, and osteosarcoma of the femur. Only 2 cases of metastases to oral soft tissues were seen, indicating the rarity of such lesions. Symptoms were similar to those previously reported: pain and swelling of membranes of the affected jaw and mobility of the teeth. Pain was found to be the most striking feature of the lesions, and it affected the bone, teeth, and even the soft tissues.

Therapy in these 25 cases included surgery, radiation, chemotherapy, and hormonal therapy. It was unsuccessful in all cases, because the jaw involvement represented only one focus of the overall metastatic spread. The rarity of metastatic lesions of the mouth and jaws is indicated by the fact that Meyer and Shklar's experience of primary malignant oral tumors within the same 12-year period included more than 2400 cases. These figures suggest that tumors metastatic to the mouth and jaws represent approximately 1 percent of all oral malignancies. Because the jaws are usually not examined radiographically in patients who have generalized tumor metastasis unless symptoms are present, it is possible that the percentage of mandibular involvement in tumor metastasis could be higher. Abrams, Spiro, and Goldstein[1] found skeletal metastases in 27 percent of 1000 autopsied cases of carcinoma, with breast carcinoma, lung carci-

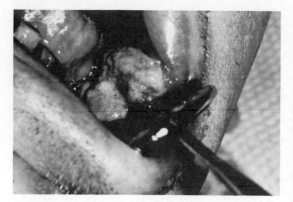

Figure 25–1. Metastatic lesion in the oral cavity from an adenocarcinoma of the stomach.

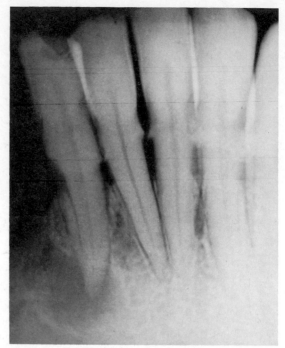

Figure 25–3. Radiolucent lesion in the mandible at the apex of a tooth. Biopsy of the lesion and follow-up investigation revealed an adenocarcinoma of the prostate.

noma, and renal tumors being the lesions most likely to spread to bone.

In Geschichter and Copeland's classic study of bone tumors,[5] the original sites for 334 metastatic lesions were found to be primarily lung (134 cases), breast (100 cases), kidney (22 cases), and gastrointestinal tract (11 cases). Only 3 cases of the 334 metastatic lesions involved the jaws, indicating the relative rarity of jaw metastases.

Tumor metastasis to oral soft tissue is an extremely rare phenomenon. Zegarelli and associates[8] recently reviewed 12 cases of tumors metastatic to the tongue that were seen at Roswell Park Memorial Institute between 1955 and 1971. There were 5 melanomas, 2 breast tumors, 2 lung tumors, and single examples of neoplasms from the colon, esophagus, and breast. In 9 of the 12 cases, there was widespread metastasis and the tongue lesion represented one facet of the overall involvement.

From the various studies that have been carried out, several points can be made concerning malignant tumors metastatic to the mouth and jaws.

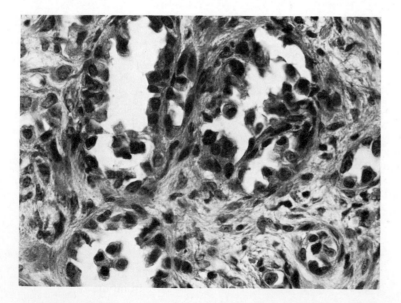

Figure 25–2. High-power view of a biopsy of the oral lesion showing pleomorphic cells forming glandular patterns (× 350).

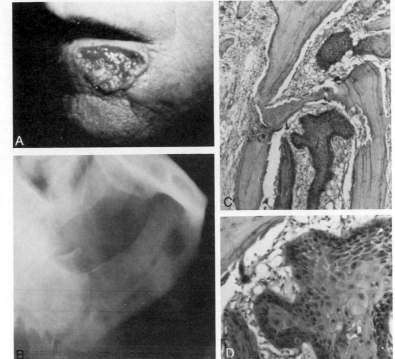

Figure 25–4. Carcinoma of the face metastatic to the mandible. *A*, Primary lesion, on the skin below the lips. *B*, Radiolucencies in the mandible, found to be metastatic epidermoid carcinoma *(C* and *D)*. The metastases can be seen spreading within the bone marrow and stimulate resorption of the adjacent bone.

1. Tumors metastatic to the oral soft tissue are extremely rare (0.1 percent, of the overall spectrum of oral malignancy).

2. Tumors metastatic to the jaws are rare (1 per cent of oral malignant tumors) but must be considered in the differential diagnosis of any radiolucent lesion of the mandible that produces painful symptoms. Biopsy will determine the presence of a primary bone tumor or a possible metastatic lesion.

3. The presence of the metastatic jaw lesion may be the first manifestation of a metastatic malignancy. The primary site is then located by evaluation of the histologic pattern of the jaw lesion and appropriate laboratory and clinical studies relative to the organ system suggested by the jaw biopsy.

4. Diagnosis of a tumor metastatic to the mouth or jaws is primarily of academic interest, because the prognosis for these patients is poor. In our experience, no patient has survived 5 years. On the other hand, many patients who have primary malignancies of the jaws survive with current therapeutic modalities.

5. Because the common tumors that metastasize to the jaws are adenocarcinomas (breast, prostate, and gastrointestinal tract) or hypernephromas, a history of such past involvement may alert a clinician to early asymptomatic but radiographically evident jaw lesions. However, it is doubtful whether early diagnosis would improve prognosis, because other metastatic lesions usually develop prior to jaw involvement in all the common tumors that metastasize to bone. Advances in chemotherapy may eventually lead to significant cure rates for metastatic malignancies with bone involvement.

REFERENCES

1. Abrams, H. L., Spiro, R., and Goldstein, N.: Metastases in carcinoma; analysis of 1000 autopsied cases. Cancer, *3*:74, 1950.
2. Cash, C. D., Royer, R. W., and Dahlin, D. C.: Metastatic tumors of the jaws. Oral Surg., *14*:897, 1961.
3. Castigliano, S. G., and Rominger, C. J.: Metastatic malignancy of the jaws. Am. J. Surg., *87*:496, 1954.
4. Clausen, F., and Poulsen, H.: Metastatic carcinoma to the jaws. Acta Pathol. Microbiol. Immunol. Scand., *57*:361, 1963.
5. Geschichter, C. F., and Copeland, M. M.: Tumors of Bone. New York. Am. J. Cancer, 1936.
6. Meyer, I., and Shklar, G.: Malignant tumors metastatic to mouth and jaws. Oral Surg., *20*:350, 1965.
7. Richard, A., Cernea, P., Henrion, P., et al.: Les epitheliomas metastatiques de la mandible. Rev. Stomatol. Chir. Maxillofac., *57*:652, 1956.
8. Zegarelli, D. J., Tsukada, Y., Pickren, J. W., et al.: Metastatic tumors to the tongue. Report of twelve cases. Oral Surg., *35*:202, 1973.

26

Unusual malignant oral neoplasms

GERALD SHKLAR, D.D.S., M.S.

Primary malignant tumors of oral mucosa, other than epidermoid carcinoma and adenocarcinoma, are extremely rare. In a review of more than 3500 oral malignancies seen in a 25-year period, only 33 cases involved lesions other than carcinoma.[18] These 33 unusual malignant oral mucosal tumors represented less then 0.1 percent of all oral cancers in our continuing investigations and consisted of the following tumors:

Malignant melanoma	4
Malignant lymphoma	11
Fibrosarcoma	7
Rhabdomyosarcoma	1
Liposarcoma	1
Neurofibrosarcoma	3
Angiosarcoma	3
Kaposi's sarcoma	2
Carcinosarcoma	1

The clinical features of these lesions are rarely sufficiently distinctive for clinical diagnosis; they are usually interpreted initially as epidermoid carcinoma or adenocarcinoma. Biopsy then reveals the histologic features of an unusual malignant oral lesion, and the specific microscopic diagnosis is made. Malignant tumors of bone may also extend from the jaws into the oral tissues and may appear clinically as lesions of the oral cavity. Radiographs usually reveal the true derivation of these tumors (see Chapter 23). Metastatic lesions from distant primary sites, such as the prostate, kidney, and breast, may also appear as tumors of oral mucosa, but these are rare. Metastases from distant sites often involve the mandible or maxilla as part of a generalized skeletal involvement. Localized metastasis to the jaws is rare, but cases have been reported (see Chapter 24). Because melanomas, lymphomas, and sarcomas are rarely seen in the mouth, there is little information about their prognosis and appropriate therapeutic modalities.

MALIGNANT MELANOMA

Malignant melanoma is a commonly found malignancy of the skin but an extremely rare tumor of oral mucosa.[2, 6, 8] Chaudry and associates[5] recently reviewed 105 cases from the literature. Benign melanotic tumors (nevi) are also rarely found on oral mucosa, yet they are one of the most frequently observed lesions of the skin. It has generally been believed that malignant melanomas arose from benign nevi, particularly those with junctional activity. This concept has given way to the approach that melanomas usually manifest as "new" lesions from melanoblasts of the skin or mucosa and not from transformation of nevi by continuous irritation of the benign lesions.

Melanoma of the mouth appears as a painless brown or brown-black lesion. It may appear as a pedunculated tumor mass or as a relatively nonraised, large macular lesion. The margins of an oral melanoma tend to be erythematous. Melanoma may be of the amelanotic variety and may appear as a pink or red tumor mass. As the tumor expands, the surface becomes ulcerated in areas and hemorrhage may be noted (Fig. 26–1). Oral melanomas tend to grow rapidly and to be relatively pleomorphic histologically, with numerous mitoses, bizarre mitoses, and abnormal cell forms.

Metastasis occurs early in oral malignant melanoma, involving regional lymph nodes and often spreading to distant organs as blood-borne metastases.

Prognosis tends to be grave, as with melanoma of the skin; however, some cases have been successfully treated by surgical excision.[14]

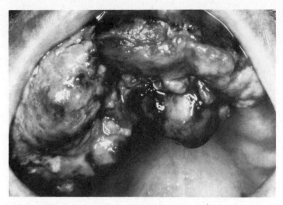

Figure 26–1. Extensive pigmented malignant melanoma of the palate.

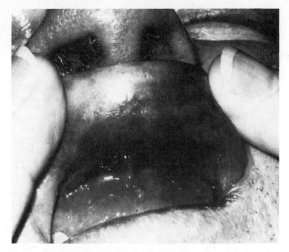

Figure 26–2. Malignant lymphoma involving the lip and maxillary gingiva.

MALIGNANT LYMPHOMA

Various forms of malignant lymphoma occur in the oral cavity. Because terminology is constantly changing, the general term *malignant lymphoma* is appropriate for these tumors. They commonly originate as primary tumors of lymph nodes but in rare instances may appear as primary tumors of the skin or oral mucosa. The older terminology of lymphosarcoma, reticulum cell sarcoma, Hodgkin's disease, and so on, is giving way to the B-cell and T-cell lymphoma terminology of Lukes and Collins,[12] which seems to have somewhat better predictive value for successful chemotherapy. However, criteria other than immunologic markers may be developed as more information becomes available. Hodgkin's disease tends to be considered a separate entity, and the term *non-Hodgkin's lymphoma* is used for the major group.

Mycosis fungoides is a form of malignant lymphoma that starts as a relatively benign condition of the skin and gradually involves lymph nodes in its late stages.[15] The initial lesions that appear on the skin are composed of dysplastic or neoplastic T-lymphocytes and appear as infiltrated red plaques or tumor masses. The lips may be affected as part of an involvement of the facial skin (see Chapter 25) or as a localized lesion. Diagnosis is usually made on the basis of clinical appearance and biopsy. If there is no evidence of internal involvement, therapy may be localized, using topical application of alkylating agents such as nitrosourea or nitrogen mustard,[23] topical corticosteroids, or radiotherapy. If internal involvement is suspected, systemic chemotherapy is used.

Malignant lymphoma of the oral cavity may appear as a rapidly growing tumor mass with areas of surface necrosis and ulceration. Common sites are the palate, gingiva, and dorsal surface of the tongue. The lesion tends to be red in color and of a relatively soft consistency. There is less peripheral induration than in epidermoid carcinoma, but there may be extensive surface necrosis. In some cases, there may be extensive involvement of the gingiva, lip, or palate, with bright red color but with relatively minimal tissue enlargement (Figs. 26–2 and 26–3). There may also be lymph node involvement together with oral involve-

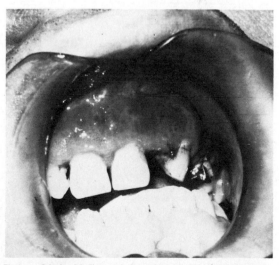

Figure 26–3. Malignant lymphoma of the maxillary gingiva showing notable erythema and erosive areas. Gingival bleeding can also be seen. Mandibular gingiva is unaffected.

ment, and if a positive diagnosis is made by oral biopsy (Fig. 26–4), the patient must be examined carefully for more extensive involvement.[9, 11, 17]

At the present time, prognosis is reasonably good, with remission in more than 40 percent of the cases, following chemotherapy.

Drug combinations that are currently used include cyclophosphamide, vincristine, and prednisone (CVP); Cytoxan, Oncovin, prednisone, and procarbazine (C-MOPP); and bleomycin, Adriamycin, Cytoxan, Oncovin, and prednisone (BACOP).

HODGKIN'S DISEASE

Although Hodgkin's disease represents an unusual form of lymphoma of lymph nodes and other lymphatic tissues, the skin and oral mucosa may develop lesions as part of a generalized involvement. In Hodgkin's disease, oral lesions are extremely rare and manifest as firm, raised nodular masses beneath the mucosa. The lesions tend to be red in color and are biopsied to rule out neoplastic disease. In the absence of notable lymph node involvement or a history of Hodgkin's disease, the oral lesions are suggestive of carcinoma. Biopsy of oral lesions of Hodgkin's disease usually reveals the characteristic microscopic features of lymphoid tissue, with large binucleate Reed-Sternberg cells as well as other multinucleate on mononuclear giant cells. Mitoses are usually evident. In addition to lymphocytes, eosinophil leukocytes, plasma cells, and histiocytes can also be seen.

Early classification of Hodgkin's disease into paragranuloma, granuloma, and sarcoma have given way to more descriptive microscopic terms, such as lymphocytic in the early stage; nodular, sclerotic, fibrotic, or mixed in the next stage; and reticular, lymphocyte depletion or Reed-Sternberg cell increase in the sarcoma or late stage. Prognosis becomes less favorable in the third stage of the disease.

Anatomic staging of the disease is used in planning therapy, with stage I representing one or two contiguous lesions on the same side of the diaphragm, stage II representing two or more noncontiguous sites on the same side of the diaphragm, stage III involving bilateral lesions of lymphoid tissue, and stage IV involving extralymphatic sites.

Etiology is unknown, but a viral agent is strongly suspected, based on epidemiologic studies and immunologic investigations.

Therapy involves both radiation and chemotherapeutic approaches. Megavoltage radiation results in a high cure rate for stage I and stage II disease. Stage III disease is treated by a combination of radiation and chemotherapy. Stage IV disease is treated primarily with combination chemotherapy, and radiation is limited to decreasing the size of the tumor masses in areas of bulk disease. Surgery has also been advocated for the removal of bulk disease. The type of combination chemotherapy currently being used is C-MOPP, which results in an excellent overall response (90 percent of all cases) and complete remission in 75 to 80 percent of all cases. Another combination chemotherapy protocol currently being used is ABVD (Adriamycin, bleomycin, vinblastine, and the nitrosourea drug DTIC).

Overall prognosis for patients who have Hodgkin's disease is very good, with 5-year

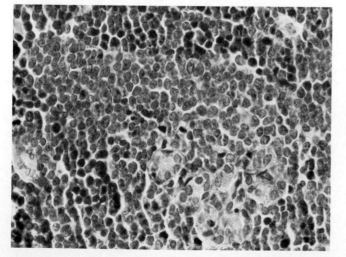

Figure 26–4. Microscopic view of biopsy of gingival lymphoma showing sheets of abnormal lymphocytes with scattered mitotic figures (× 200).

survival rates of over 85 percent for patients with stages I, II, and III disease and 5-year survival rates of over 70 percent for patients with stage IV disease. Prognosis is less favorable with lymphocyte-depletion giant cell histology and in patients who have generalized involvement that is suggested by severe weight loss, elevated temperature, and night sweats. Relapses of disease may occur following initial therapeutic success, and they indicate a poorer overall prognosis.

BURKITT'S LYMPHOMA

Burkitt[4] first described an unusual form of lymphoma in African children, which affects primarily the mouth and jaws but also may involve other sites. The tumors are unusual in that they tend to respond extremely well to antimetabolite drugs such as cyclophosphamide, and they reveal a relatively unique microscopic picture, often described as a "starry sky." The "stars" are individual histiocytes scattered among a dense field of pleomorphic, deeply staining lymphocytes. The histologic pattern is not as unique as was previously believed. Occasional cases of non-Hodgkin's lymphoma throughout the world have the so-called Burkitt's lymphoma microscopic pattern. However, the diagnosis of Burkitt's lymphoma should be based on the clinical manifestations and response to chemotherapy in addition to the histologic features (see Chapter 27). A viral etiology has been postulated that is based on the original epidemiologic studies of Burkitt and the recent findings of antibodies to Epstein-Barr virus in affected children.

The oral tumors originate in the marrow spaces of the alveolar bone of the jaws and rapidly extend beyond the periosteum to develop into large, firm, fungating tissue masses that proliferate within oral mucosa. Ulceration of the tumor surface is commonly seen. Gross distortion of the jaws and oral structures occurs as the tumors reach large size (Fig. 26–5).

FIBROSARCOMA

Fibrosarcoma is occasionally seen as a tumor of the jaws. It is extremely rare as a tumor of oral mucosa. Lesions can occur on the lip, tongue, gingiva, palatal mucosa, or buccal mucosa. The tumor grows slowly but gradually develops into a firm, nodular mass that is bound to adjacent and underlying tissues (Fig. 26–6). The surface may become ulcerated as the tumor increases in size and extends into

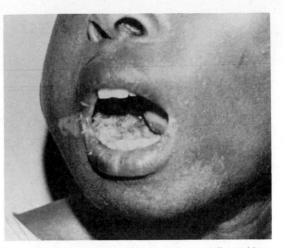

Figure 26–5. Burkitt's lymphoma of the mouth and jaws in a young African patient.

the oral cavity, where it becomes traumatized. Initially, it may be interpreted as a carcinoma, and diagnosis is made from biopsy. Prognosis is usually good. Metastasis to regional lymph nodes is not uncommon, and surgical removal is often curative. Oral fibrosarcomas occasionally develop following extensive injury or radiation therapy.

NEUROFIBROSARCOMA

Neurofibrosarcoma or neurogenic fibrosarcoma is a rare tumor of the mouth and tends to occur in the posterior regions of the oral cavity.[7, 19] Appearing as a firm tumor mass, it may be interpreted clinically as a carcinoma. Biopsy reveals the true nature of the lesion. The microscopic picture often resembles a schwannoma, with large numbers of abnormally shaped hyperchromatic nuclei. Mitoses are present but not usually in large numbers.

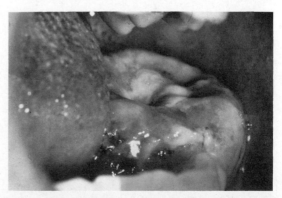

Figure 26–6. Proliferating fibrosarcoma of the mandibular gingiva.

The finely fibrillar structure of the connective tissue stromal element and the occasional pallisading of nuclei are often diagnostic. Therapy usually involves surgical removal. Prognosis is good if the tumor has not spread to regional lymph nodes.

RHABDOMYOSARCOMA

Rhabdomyosarcoma is an extremely rare oral tumor that is usually found in the tongue. Stout,[21] in 1946, reviewed a series of 116 cases of rhabdomyosarcoma and found that 10 cases had occurred in the tongue. Other studies have found a lower incidence of lingual or oral rhabdomyosarcoma.

The lesion develops as a painless mass in the body of the tongue and gradually proliferates, so that the dorsal lingual surface is raised. Metastases to regional lymph nodes are more common in rhabdomyosarcoma than in fibrosarcoma. The microscopic picture is relatively characteristic, and diagnosis is made following biopsy. Numerous large hyperchromatic cells with spindling cytoplasm are seen, and careful examination of the cells reveals cross striations within the cytoplasm of the tumor cells, confirming their skeletal muscle tissue origin. Numerous mitoses are usually observed. Therapy involves surgery, and prognosis is always guarded.

LEIOMYOSARCOMA

Leiomyosarcoma has been reported to be found in the oral cavity.[3] It probably originates from the smooth muscle of larger blood vessels. Leiomyosarcoma is difficult to distinguish both clinically and microscopically from fibro-

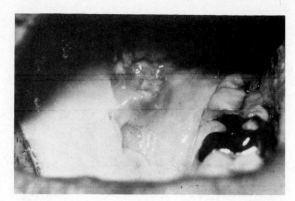

Figure 26–7. Angiosarcoma arising in buccal mucosa. The (dark) lesion represents surface necrosis.

sarcoma. Special stains may reveal the unusual derivation of the tumor.

LIPOSARCOMA

Liposarcoma rarely occurs in the oral regions.[1] It appears as a firm, proliferating tissue mass, and biopsy reveals the true nature of the tumor. Microscopically, there are relatively large numbers of hyperchromatic, pleomorphic cells surrounding numerous spaces that represent fatty material. The cells are often multinucleated, and occasional mitoses may be observed.

ANGIOSARCOMA

Angiosarcoma is a rare malignancy of the mouth. It occurs as a moderately firm, red lesion, usually with a bleeding, ulcerated surface (Fig. 26–7).[20] Biopsy reveals large numbers of bizarre, hyperchromatic cells that tend

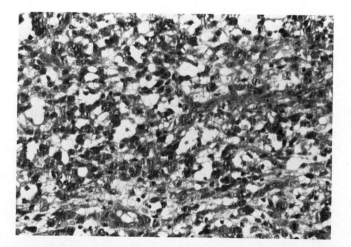

Figure 26–8. Microscopic view of angiosarcoma showing numerous cells with pleomorphic, hyperchromatic nuclei. The endothelial cells are forming small vascular spaces ($\times$ 250).

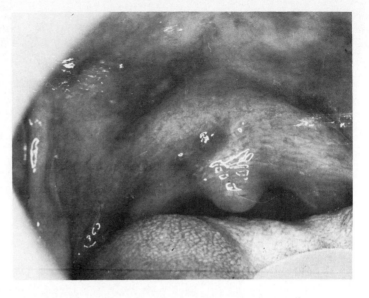

Figure 26–9. Oral lesions of Kaposi's sarcoma. Numerous small, raised, red foci can be seen.

to form small blood vessels. Mitoses are common (Fig. 26–8).

Prognosis tends to be poor. Angiosarcoma grows rapidly, and spread to regional lymph nodes is an early manifestation. Widespread metastases are also common. Therapy usually involves surgical removal of the tumor and affected cervical lymph nodes. Some cases of angiosarcoma may respond to chemotherapy.

KAPOSI'S SARCOMA

Kaposi's sarcoma (idiopathic multiple hemorrhagic sarcoma) is an unusual malignancy of endothelial cells, primarily involving the skin and oral mucosa and arising in multiple sites. The lesions of Kaposi's sarcoma on the skin manifest as small red-purple macules or raised, indurated pigmented plaques (see Chapter 28). Oral lesions appear as multiple red macular configurations of variable size and shape (Fig. 26–9). Some lesions may be ulcerated, with raised indurated margins.[20] Lesions may also occur in the gastrointestinal tract and in lymph nodes. Histopathology is relatively characteristic and consists of numerous dilated engorged blood vessels and nests and sheets of pleomorphic endothelial cells that form small vascular spaces. Mitoses are seen but are not prominent. There may also be a proliferation of fibrous connective tissue. In early lesions of Kaposi's sarcoma, the microscopic picture may resemble a nonspecific granulomatous inflammation with lymphocytic infiltration. Diagnosis is made on the basis of clinical and microscopic features. Prognosis is somewhat better than

that for angiosarcoma. The tumors are relatively radiosensitive, and radiation therapy is widely used. Surgical excision may be performed for isolated, individual lesions.[13]

CARCINOSARCOMA

Carcinosarcoma is probably the most rare of all oral tumors and represents the "collision" of a fibrosarcoma and adenocarcinoma that develop in close proximity to one another. It may also represent a malignant-mixed tumor of minor salivary gland origin with both epithelial and connective tissue components undergoing simultaneous malignant transformation. At the present time, there is no reliable information concerning prognosis, because so few carcinosarcomas have been recorded.

REFERENCES

1. Baden, E., and Newman, R.: Liposarcoma of the oropharyngeal region. Oral Surg., *44*:889, 1977.
2. Baldridge, O. L., and Waldron, C. A.: Malignant melanomas of the mouth. Oral Surg., 7:1108, 1954.
3. Brandjord, R. M., Reaume, C. E., and Wesley, R. K.: Leiomyosarcoma of the floor of the mouth. J. Oral Surg., *35*:590, 1977.
4. Burkitt D., and O'Connor, G. T.: Malignant lymphoma in African children. 1. A clinical syndrome. Cancer, *14*:259, 1961.
5. Chaudry, A. P., Hampel, A., and Gorlin, R. J.: Primary malignant melanoma of the oral cavity; a review of 105 cases. Cancer, *11*:923, 1980.
6. Chaudry, A. P., Burke, R. J., and Gorlin, R. J.: Malignant melanoma of the oral cavity. Oral Surg., *13*:584, 1960.
7. DeVore, D. T., and Waldron, C. A.: Malignant

peripheral nerve tumors of the oral cavity. Oral Surg., *14*:56, 1959.

8. Greene, G. W., Haynes, J. W., Dozier, M., et al.: Primary malignant melanoma of the oral mucosa. Oral Surg., *6*:1435, 1953.

9. Greer, J. L., Crine, J. D., and Tilson, H. B.: Malignant lymphomas of the oral soft tissues. J. Oral Surg., *36*:971, 1978.

10. Kaposi, M.: Idiopathisches multiples Pigmentsarkom der Haut. Arch. Dermatol. Syph., *4*:265, 1872.

11. Lehrer, S.: The presentation of malignant lymphoma in the oral cavity and pharynx. Oral Surg., *41*:441, 1976.

12. Lukes, R. J., and Collins, R. D.: Lukes-Collins classification and its significance. Cancer Treat. Rep., *61*:971, 1977.

13. McCarthy, W. D., and Pack, G. T.: Malignant blood vessel tumors; a report of 56 cases of angiosarcoma and Kaposi's sarcoma. Surg. Gynecol. Obstet., *91*:465, 1950.

14. Nathanson, N., Cataldo, E., and Shklar, G.: Primary malignant melanoma of the oral cavity treated by surgery. J. Oral Surg., *23*:463, 1965.

15. Reed, R. J.: Mycosis fungoides. Cancer, *27*:322, 1977.

16. Safai, B., and Good, R. A.: Kaposi's sarcoma; a review and recent developments. Clin. Bull., *10*:62, 1980.

17. Schuler, S., McDonald, J. S., Strull, N. J., et al.: Soft tissue reticulum-cell sarcoma of the oral cavity. Oral Surg., *45*:984, 1978.

18. Shklar, G.: Unpublished data.

19. Shklar, G., and Meyer, I.: Neurogenic tumors of the mouth and jaws. Oral Surg., *16*:1075, 1963.

20. Shklar, G., and Meyer, I.: Vascular tumors of the mouth and jaws. Oral Surg., *19*:335, 1965.

21. Stout, A. P.: Rhabdomyosarcoma of skeletal muscles. Ann. Surg., *123*:447, 1946.

22. Yoshimura, Y.: Two cases of plasmacytoma in the oral cavity. Int. J. Oral Surg., *5*:82, 1976.

23. Zackheim, H. S., and Epstein, E. H.: Treatment of mycosis fungoides with topical nitrosourea compounds. Arch. Dermatol., *111*:1564, 1975.

27

Burkitt's lymphoma of the mouth and jaws

ADEYEMI MOSADOMI, D.M.D., M.S.

Burkitt's lymphoma is a malignant neoplasm of the hematopoietic system. It is presumed to be a monoclonal outgrowth of immature B-lymphocytes that probably manifest from small transformed follicular center cells. The newer, at times tedious, classification schemes proposed for non-Hodgkin's lymphoma have not spared Burkitt's lymphoma from being referred to by confusing names. Underlying all these nomenclature schemes is an attempt to rationalize the morphological classification of Rappaport and the functional classification of Lukes and Collins. Consequently, Burkitt's lymphoma has been described by the following terms:

1. Diffuse lymphoma—Burkitt's type (Rappaport).
2. Lymphoblastic malignant lymphoma of high-grade malignancy—Burkitt's type (Kiel).[10]
3. B cell (follicular center cell)—small noncleaved variety (Lukes and Collins).[15, 16]
4. Diffuse lymphosarcoma—Burkitt's tumor (World Health Organization).[24]

The predominant and characteristic cells of the lesion are undifferentiated lymphoreticular or primitive stem cells that show moderate nuclear and cytoplasmic variations. These variations are interpreted either as biologic variations within the same cell type or as absence of cytologic or cytochemical evidence of differentiation toward either lymphocytes or histiocytes.[20] The neoplastic cells are generally uniform, with a diameter ranging from 10 to 25 microns and contain round or oval nuclei with coarsely clumped chromatin and well-defined parachromatin. There may be between one and four prominent nucleoli. Mitotic figures are frequently seen with variable degrees of abnormality. The cytoplasm has a strong affinity for pyronine and contains many small vacuoles that are best seen with Wright's stain on imprint slide preparations. Benign macrophages are interspersed among these tumor cells to impart the so-called "starry-sky" or "water-pot" appearance seen histologically. This feature, which may be very impressive in many cases of Burkitt's lymphoma, is no longer regarded as pathognomonic of Burkitt's lymphoma, because the same "starry-sky" appearance has been described in infectious mononucleosis, viral (cat scratch) lymphadenitis, and other juvenile and adult lymphomas.

HISTORICAL BACKGROUND

In 1958, Denis Burkitt, then a British surgeon practicing surgery in Uganda, gave the first definitive description of the lesion that is now known as Burkitt's lymphoma.[3]

A detailed description of most of the features of the disease as a clinical syndrome was published in 1961 by Burkitt and O'Connor.[6] Soon after, as similar cases were being reported all over Africa in the wake of Burkitt's travels throughout tropical Africa, a peculiar geographic distribution of the tumor became evident. It was then suggested that the geographic and climatic determinants of this newly described lymphoma indicated that an etiologic agent carried by the wet-tropics group of mosquitoes may be responsible for the disease.[4, 18] Those who searched for the etiologic agent were rewarded in 1964 by the publication of Epstein, Achong, and Barr[11] in which they described virus particles in cultured lymphoblasts from Burkitt's lymphoma. Once the Epstein-Barr virus (as the virus was later to be designated) was recognized, there was intense activity to determine the clinicopathologic relationship of the tumor and the virus. For several years, the lymphoma was thought to

Table 27–1. COMPARISON OF JAW LESIONS IN AFRICAN BURKITT'S LYMPHOMA AND AMERICAN BURKITT'S LYMPHOMA

Burkitt's Lymphoma—Africa	Burkitt's Lymphoma—America
1. Age-dependent incidence (peak incidence 5–7 yrs; age range 1–15 yrs).	1. Nonage dependent incidence (mean incidence 16 yrs; age range 2–36 yrs).
2. Jaw most frequent tumor site (60% of cases).	2. Jaw infrequent tumor site (18% of cases).
3. Males affected more frequently than females (nonjaw, M/F = 1:1; jaw, M/F = 3:1).	3. Increased female frequency (nonjaw, M/F = 3:1; jaw, M/F = 1.5:1).
4. Epstein-Barr virus deoxyribonucleic acid (EBV-DNA) associated with 95% of tumors.	4. EBV-DNA associated with 10–20% of tumors.

5. *Clinical Presentation*
Toothache rare.
Circumoral paresthesia, "chin numbness" rare.
Loose displaced teeth common.
Maxilla most frequently affected.
Multiple jaw quadrant involvement common (80% of cases).
Massive facial tumor common.
Proptosis common.
Jaw disease essentially limited to children (younger than 15 yrs).
	5. *Clinical Presentation*
	Toothache present in all cases.
	Circumoral paresthesia common.
	Loose displaced teeth rare in adults, but noted in children.
	Mandible most frequently affected.
	Single jaw quadrant involvement most common (14/18 cases).
	Little or no extraoral mass typical for adult, even when bony destruction is extensive.
	Proptosis rare.
	Difference in clinical presentation in children (0–15 yrs) with jaw lesions vs. adults (older than 16 yrs).
	    Children
	        Toothache.
	        Extraoral mass less pronounced than in African children.
	        Loose teeth.
	        Extensive bone loss on radiograph.
	        Developing teeth attacked.
	        Intraoral exophytic mass.
	    Adults
	        Toothache.
	        Paresthesia.
	        Minimal or no extraoral mass.
	        Localized intraoral mass frequently exophytic only after tooth extraction.
	        Early radiographic findings often minimal, resembling tooth infection.

(From Sariban, E., Donahue, A., and Magrath, I.: Jaw involvement in American Burkitt's lymphoma (AMBL). Proc. 13th Int. Congress Against Cancer, Seattle, Washington, 1982.

be specific to the African regions that appeared to be susceptible. However, it soon became apparent that a lymphoma that was morphologically similar to and indistinguishable from Burkitt's lymphoma existed in children in North America, Europe, the Middle East, and Australia. However, there are dissimilarities in clinical presentations (Table 27–1).

ETIOLOGY AND EPIDEMIOLOGY

Cases of Burkitt's lymphoma were found in different parts of Africa in a characteristic manner that suggested the etiologic agents' dependence upon temperature, altitude, and rainfall. Extensive field work in East and Central Africa, as well as numerous "turnover safaris" by ardent researchers, finally delimited Burkitt's lymphoma belt to geographic areas in which the average daily temperature was 60° F or higher, annual rainfall was 20 in. or more, height above sea level was less than 5000 ft, and latitudes approximately 15° north or south of the equator.[23] In 1964 when Epstein, Achong, and Barr[11] described a herpes-like virus in electron micrographs of cultured lymphoblasts in a Burkitt's lymphoma cell line, several findings about the Epstein-Barr virus (EBV) emerged:[13]

1. Patients with Burkitt's lymphoma were found to have a high antibody titer to EBV-determined antigens.

2. Between 80 and 90 percent of the tumors contain multiple copies of the EBV-DNA genome.

3. Since 1968, EBV has been shown to be the cause of infectious mononucleosis.

4. In the African region, more than 80 percent of children younger than 5 years of age are infected with EBV without evidence of clinical disease.

5. EBV selectively infects B-lymphocytes that contain a specific surface receptor that transforms them into a continuous cell line in vitro.

6. EBV produces a malignant lymphoma in marmosets and has also been implicated in nasopharyngeal carcinoma.

7. High EBV antibodies were found in Ugandan children who subsequently developed Burkitt's lymphoma.

These data are consistent with an etiologic association of EBV and Burkitt's lymphoma, although it has been found that only 15 to 20 percent of the cases in nonendemic areas show association with the virus. Klein proposed that malignancy occurs when a B cell clone, perhaps by virtue of some advantageous chromosomal aberration, "escapes" immuno regulatory surveillance of suppressor T-lymphocytes, which control B-cell proliferation.[13] It has also been proposed alternatively that EBV may be an innocent "passenger" resident in a B cell that undergoes transformation by other causes unrelated to the EBV. Other etiologic cofactors have been suggested. The geographic coincidence of Burkitt's lymphoma belt and the hyperendemic or holoendemic malaria areas prompted Burkitt and O'Connor to postulate immune stimulation (or hyperstimulation) by chronic malaria as an etiologic cofactor.[6, 12]

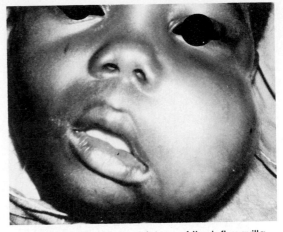

Figure 27–1. Burkitt's lymphoma of the left maxilla.

Growth is predominantly extranodal, multifocal, and widely disseminated, with involvement of one or more of the following sites:[21, 25]

1. Abdominal or pelvic viscera or both.

2. Retroperitoneal soft tissues (bilateral ovarian masses common).

3. Facial bones or long bones or both, particularly jaw bones (Figs. 27–1 through 27–4).

4. Thyroid gland.

5. Salivary glands.

6. Central nervous system.

The mediastinum, spleen, thymus, and peripheral nodes are rarely involved.[6]

Burkitt's lymphoma involves multiple quadrants of the jaws. Involvement of bones other than the jaw is considerably less frequent, occurring singly or as multiple tumors (Table 27–2).[6, 21, 25]

The tumor cells do not significantly manifest

GENERAL CLINICAL FEATURES AND GROSS PATHOLOGY

Burkitt's lymphoma is predominantly a tumor of childhood, although occasionally it occurs in any age group, especially in nonendemic areas. Burkitt's lymphoma accounted for 70 percent of the 230 malignant diseases in children 1 to 14 years of age seen in Ibadan, Nigeria, by Edington and coworkers.[10a] The results of various studies in endemic areas indicate an age-dependent peak incidence between the ages of 5 and 7 years in a range of 1 to 15 years. The frequency of jaw tumors in African cases is definitely related to age, with the incidence rate falling progressively after 8 years of age.

This type of tumor is solid, has a rapid onset, and also is rapidly fatal if untreated.

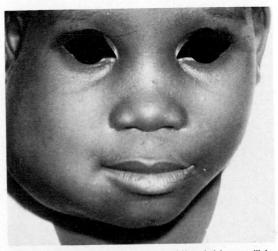

Figure 27–2. Burkitt's lymphoma of the right mandible.

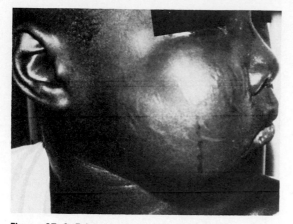

Figure 27–3. Extensive involvement of the right maxilla in Burkitt's lymphoma.

Table 27–2. MAIN PRESENTING CLINICAL FEATURES OF 557 HISTOLOGICALLY PROVEN CASES OF BURKITT'S LYMPHOMA IN UGANDA 1950–1965 (372 male, 183 female, 2 unrecorded)

Clinical Features	Percentage of Patients
Jaw tumours	55
Single jaw tumours	26.5
Multiple jaw tumours	21.5
All 4 quadrants	7.5
Abdominal swelling	25
Ovarian tumour	38 females
Testicular tumour	3.8 males
Paraplegia	6.8
Other Bones	6.7
Femur	3.2
Tibia	1.2
Humerus	0.7
Others	2
Thyroid	9.2
Superficial lymph nodes	5.2
Breast	1.6
Others	1.6

(From Burkitt, D. P., and Wright, D. H.: Burkitt's Lymphoma. Edinburgh, E and S Livingstone, 1970.)

in the peripheral blood, and they do not diffusely infiltrate or replace bone marrow.[6]

Paraplegia may be the presenting clinical feature of patients with Burkitt's lymphoma. The paraplegia is due to compression of the cord by extradural tumor mass or to infiltration by intrathecal deposits. Extension of the tumor mass from the maxilla or periorbital region may also involve the cranial nerves.[25]

Some uncommon features of clinical presentations of Burkitt's lymphoma were described, including anemia, malaise, and fever of unknown origin; arthritis with swelling of and effusion into the joints and an increase in uric acid concentration; cardiac arrhythmia, especially in terminal cases; and gastrointestinal malabsorption.

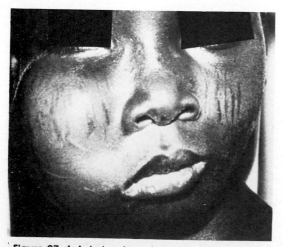

Figure 27–4. Anterior view of patient in Figure 27–3.

GENERAL HISTOPATHOLOGY

Histologic sections usually reveal a monotonous sea of undifferentiated lymphoreticular cells with little variation in size and shape (Fig. 27–5). The cohesiveness of the tumor cells varies considerably, even on the same section, and largely depends upon fixation. Cells located at the periphery of the section, where fixation can be presumed to be prompt, tend to have rounded, oval, or slightly indented nuclei and to have a finely granular nuclear chromatin with inconspicuous nucleoli. Cells in the center of the section, where fixation may be presumably delayed, show vesicular nuclei with slightly more prominent nucleoli. The tumor cell nuclei are, however, generally very uniform in size and similar to the nuclei of scattered macrophages.

The cytoplasm is best visualized in the periphery, where the cells are better separated from one another. The narrow rim of cytoplasm under hematoxylin and eosin stain, results in an amphophilic staining similar to that seen in plasma cells. Cytoplasmic vacuoles that are not readily seen under low and medium powers are best visualized under oil immersion.

Scattered among the tumor cells are large, clear, or vacuolated macrophages (Fig. 27–6). These macrophages (tissue histiocytes) are

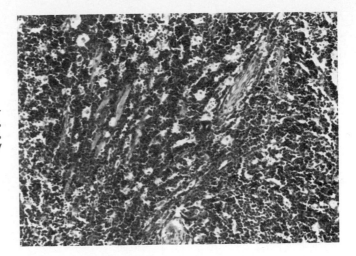

Figure 27–5. Microscopic view of Burkitt's lymphoma in the maxilla. In this low-power view, there is a very dense mass of lymphocytes, with a scattering of clear spaces (starry sky pattern).

often laden with whole or parts of neoplastic cells, pyknotic nuclei, and cell debris from various inflammatory cells. These cellular cytoplasmic inclusions impart the celebrated "starry-sky" or "water-pot" histologic pattern seen in sections of Burkitt's lymphoma. The "starry-sky" pattern becomes less obvious in sections in which fixation has been delayed. For years, this "starry-sky" pattern was thought to be pathognomonic for Burkitt's lymphoma, but it is now an accepted fact that other lymphoproliferative or lymphoreticular diseases may show the same pattern. The reticulin content in Burkitt's lymphoma is scanty and confined mainly to the blood vessels within the tumor or the residual non-neoplastic tissue.

CYTOLOGY

Imprint cytology is especially suited to the study of lymphoreticular diseases, particularly when used along with usual histologic preparations. Imprints are made essentially as they are with smear preparations, by gently touching the freshly cut surface of a tumor tissue onto clean glass slides. The average size of a Burkitt's lymphoma cell in an imprint preparation is 10 to 12 microns and approximately the same degree of immaturity is shown. Cells tend to be slightly larger in marrow smears than in imprint preparations. Large macrophages are often present in the imprint preparation and are usually laden with pyknotic cells and cellular debris. Smears of body fluids reveal equally useful cellular details for imprints.

CYTOCHEMISTRY AND HISTOCHEMISTRY

Burkitt's tumor cells show marked cytoplasmic pyroninophilia that can be abolished by prior digestion with fibonuclease, indicating

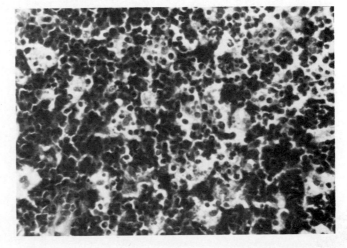

Figure 27–6. Higher-power view showing the clear spaces that contain macrophages with lightly staining cytoplasm.

that RNA is being shown. The acridine orange staining method may also be used to show the high RNA content of Burkitt's lymphoma cells. In this method, the cytoplasm of Burkitt's lymphoma cells gives a brilliant orange-red fluorescence that is uniformly intense throughout the specimen.[25] Most cells of a majority of Burkitt's lymphomas are negative when stained with periodic acid Schiff (PAS), although occasional cells may contain coarse PAS positive cytoplasmic granules. Neutral fat stain may be used to show lipid granules in frozen sections of Burkitt's lymphoma. These granules, dissolved away during fixation for hematoxylin and eosin stain preparation, correspond with the vacuoles that prominently feature in imprint preparations. The demonstration of abundant cytoplasmic lipid droplets may aid in the diagnosis of Burkitt's lymphoma, although this feature should not be regarded as diagnostic enzyme histochemistry; it does not show the presence of alkaline phosphatase or nonspecific esterase in Burkitt's lymphoma cells. Results of very sensitive tests, however, show weak presence of acid phosphatase in the tumor cells and a larger amount in the scattered macrophages (see Tables 27–1 and 27–2).

ULTRASTRUCTURE

Monomorphism of the dominant cells is very striking at low magnifications. The cells are round or oval with a relatively high nucleocytoplasmic ratio. The nucleus is round or oval with generally shallow indentations. Projections of the nuclear membrane, although nonspecific, may appear as satellites or as invaginations of the nucleus. Chromatin is abundant. Nucleoli are large, with visible nucleolonemas. The cytoplasm is moderate, variable in amount, and relatively dense. Polyribosomes are plentiful and ergastoplasmic lamellae are rare, whereas the few mitochondria are large and polarized. Large inclusions consistent with lipid vacuoles are found in some cells. Evidence from ultrastructural studies tends to confirm the lack of differentiation of these neoplastic cells from lymphocytes or histiocytes.

DENTAL ASPECTS OF BURKITT'S LYMPHOMA

As mentioned previously, in geographic regions in which Burkitt's tumor is endemic, the jaws are involved in approximately half the cases. In areas in which the tumor is rare, the jaws are involved in at least 15 percent of the cases. Of the 557 histologically proven cases of Burkitt's lymphoma in Uganda from 1950 to 1965, 55.5 percent involved the jaws: single jaw involvement, 26.5 percent; multiple jaw involvement, 21.5 percent; and all quadrants, 7.5 percent.

Clinical Features

Loosening of Teeth

One of the earliest signs of jaw involvement in Burkitt's lymphoma is loosening of the teeth. In the absence of local causes, loosening of the teeth should be investigated when the patient is at the age when this lymphoma most commonly occurs in the endemic areas (Fig. 27–7).

Premature Eruption

The tumor mass initially destroys the compact bone of the dental sockets and infiltrates the periodontal membrane. As the tumor increases in size, the teeth are pushed out of their sockets. When permanent teeth are involved, premature eruption results. There may be little or no change in the contour of the jaw, and pain may be minimal.

Displacement of Teeth

The expansion of the jaw that occurs with increased growth of lymphoma in the jaws

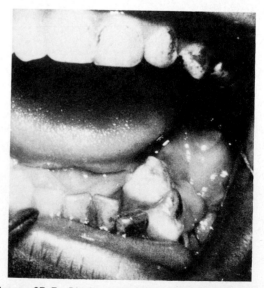

Figure 27–7. Displacement and mobility of teeth caused by proliferating Burkitt's lymphoma of the mandible.

causes gross displacement and distortion of the teeth. In spite of gross displacement, exfoliation occurs very late in the disease. The displacement of teeth, resulting in derangement of the arch and impairment of dental occlusion, causes the so-called "dental anarchy" (see Fig. 27–7).

Expansion of the Alveolus

A simultaneous buccal and palatal bulging of the maxilla in a child who lives in an endemic region is almost diagnostic of Burkitt's lymphoma, in the absence of other known causes. Lingual expansion is also common in the mandible. Rapid growth causes the tumor to burst through the bone, erupt through the periosteum, and reach the tissues of the face, where it obliterates all facial grooves, resulting in a tense, shiny skin (see Fig. 27–3).

Peripheral Nerves

Characteristically, the mandibular and maxillary nerves are not affected, even in very advanced cases.[2] Anesthesia of the lips and oral mucosa or paralysis of the muscles of mastication have not been recorded for Burkitt's lymphoma, in marked contrast to the frequency with which these features are recorded in other forms of malignant lymphoma involving the jaws.

Radiologic Features

The tumor appears to begin as small osteolytic foci in the posterior aspect of the jaw that coalesce to form larger foci that eventually cause loosening and avulsion of the teeth. One of the earliest signs of this process is the loss of or break in the lamina dura around the teeth. Involvement of the dental pulp is also common, causing an enlargement of the radiographic shadow of the crypt of a developing tooth. This enlargement may even precede the loss of lamina dura.[2] The results of radiologic examination of the jaws invariably show the disease to be more widespread than the clinical presentation would suggest. In Table 27–3 a comparison of the distribution of Burkitt's lymphoma on clinical and radiologic examination in 80 patients in Uganda is shown.[2] The usefulness of extraoral and intraoral radiographs (when the latter is possible) as an adjunct to diagnosis cannot be overemphasized, especially in the endemic regions.

Table 27–3. DISTRIBUTION OF BURKITT'S LYMPHOMA IN THE JAWS ON CLINICAL AND RADIOLOGIC EXAMINATION OF 80 PATIENTS IN UGANDA

| | Examination | |
	Clinical	Radiologic
Right maxilla	16	7
Left maxilla	7	2
Bilateral maxilla	2	3
Right mandible	9	2
Left mandible	6	3
Bilateral mandible	0	10
Incisor area of mandible	2	0
Ipsilateral maxilla and mandible	11	13
Three quadrants	6	8
Four quadrants	19	32
No obvious jaw involvement	2	0
Total	80	80

Radiographs taken later, as the disease progresses, show complete disappearance of the lamina dura, gross displacement of the remaining teeth or buds, and coalescence of the small osteolytic foci to form large radiolucent areas. Adatia has reported occasional cases of pathologic fracture of the mandible as well as reactive subperiosteal osteoplasia in patients whose tumor is confined by the periosteum.[2] In the maxilla, as the tumor advances, antral shadows are blurred, and the details of the facial skeleton become difficult to identify.

Histopathology

As the tumor grows, the marrow is replaced by tumor tissue and the lamina dura is destroyed. Osteoclasts are evident as the bone is being destroyed. Invasion of the pulp is a characteristic feature of Burkitt's lymphoma, and there is hardly any other lesion of the jaws in patients who are in the age group that exhibits this pulp involvement.[14] Adatia has reported alteration in the shape of the root tip, irregular dentin formation, and a high resistance of odontogenic epithelium to destruction of the developing tooth in Burkitt's lymphoma.[2]

Postchemotherapy Effects

The dramatic response shown by patients who receive chemotherapy for Burkitt's lymphoma is paralleled by the return of displaced teeth to their normal positions.[2] Alveolar bone recovery and diminution of radiolucent areas take place. Antral opacity, if present, clears quickly. Within 3 weeks, radiographs show reconstruction of the lamina dura, reformation of the dental crypts, further root development, and appearance of teeth at appropriate ages.[2] Examination of autopsy material in which regression of the tumor in the jaw was achieved showed that the formation of new bone begins at the periphery and advances inward, filling the defect at the center.

MANAGEMENT

Successful management is preceded by clinical staging of the tumor. The commonly used staging classification is as follows:

A. Single extra-abdominal site.

B. Multiple extra-abdominal sites.

C. Intra-abdominal tumor.

D. Intra-abdominal tumor with involvement of multiple extra-abdominal sites, or abdominal mass with sites of tumor other than facial or marrow involvement.

AR. Stage C but with more than 90 percent of the tumor surgically resected.

For other than jaw lesions, the rigorous diagnostic procedures that are used include gallium 67 scintigraphy, computerized axial tomography (CAT) scanning, ultrasound localization, determination of the serum lactate dehydrogenase level, examination of cerebrospinal fluid for malignant cells, and iliac crest aspiration.

The treatment of choice is chemotherapy, usually administered systemically. Radiotherapy has little or no use. Because it has been shown that the prognosis is directly proportional to the volume of the tumor, surgery, consisting of resection of the bowels, ovaries, kidney, or any other affected organ, may be carried out before or in conjunction with chemotherapy. The phenomenal chemotherapeutic drug sensitivity of Burkitt's lymphoma may be related to the fact that, from kinetic studies, Burkitt's lymphoma has been found to be one of the fastest growing tumors in humans (Figs. 27–8 and 27–9). Many drugs are effective in the treatment of Burkitt's lymphoma, and combination therapy is usually used. Cyclophosphamide was found to give excellent results in the original studies of Burkitt and Wright.[7]

Several factors concerning the prognosis and treatment of Burkitt's lymphoma have emerged.

1. Prognosis depends upon whether the patient survives during the period of treatment

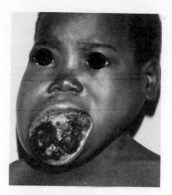

Figure 27–8. Extensive intraoral proliferation of Burkitt's lymphoma of the right mandible.

and whether there is complete regression of all tumors. This means there must be prompt diagnosis, careful medical and surgical (for large abdominal masses) management, and aggressive chemotherapy.

2. Chemotherapy must be of adequate quantity. Whereas a single dose of a selected drug may be sufficient for small tumors, multifocal tumors invariably require multiple and combination doses.

3. Patients who are at greater risk of having frequent relapses in the central nervous system are those with bone marrow involvement, head, neck, or paraspinal tumors. Such cases require aggressive intrathecal chemotherapy with a drug that crosses the blood-brain barrier.

4. Burkitt's lymphoma has an unusual relapse pattern. If a relapse occurs within 3 months following therapy, it is suggestive of a regrowth at the original tumor site that is resistant to the initial treatment. Such cases have a high incidence of central nervous system (CNS) involvement, and the prognosis is poor. When relapse occurs after 3 months, it is

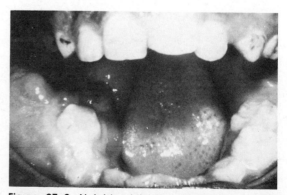

Figure 27–9. Notable shrinkage of the tumor mass during chemotherapy.

suggestive of tumors in new sites with infrequent CNS involvement. Patients with the latter type of relapse respond well to reinduction chemotherapy, with prolonged second remissions.

In any case, initial management must include high doses of cyclophosphamide. There is evidence that combination chemotherapy with vincristine, methotrexate, or cytarabine lowers the relapse rate. Prognosis in Burkitt's lymphoma is directly related to the tumor size on initial presentation and to the age of the patient. Younger patients survive longer than older patients. A correct management approach must include prompt histologic diagnosis, aggressive and adequate initial chemotherapy, vigilant clinical management in the period surrounding treatment (for example, during tumorlysis syndrome), careful follow-up of remission, and prompt treatment of relapse, particularly if CNS is involved.

DIFFERENTIAL DIAGNOSIS

The list of diseases that mimic Burkitt's lymphoma could logically be divided into those that pertain more to the jaw and facial bones and those that pertain to the viscera and other sites. The jaw conditions include odontogenic tumors (for example, ameloblastoma, ameloblastic fibroma, and adenomatoid odontogenic tumor), dental cysts (dentigerous cysts and keratocysts), cancrum oris (gangrenous stomatitis or noma), and fibro-osseous and related lesions (fibrous dysplasia, cherubism, myxoma, and ossifying fibroma). The clinical characteristics of these disease categories are such that they create little or no difficulty in ruling them out in arriving at a clinical impression of Burkitt's lymphoma.

The list of diseases in the viscera and at other sites includes neuroblastoma; abdominal distention due to tuberculous adenitis, peritonitis, or Hodgkin's disease; Wilms' tumor (nephroblastoma); ovarian tumors; bone lesions such as osteogenic sarcoma, reticulum cell sarcoma, osteomyelitis, and hemoglobinopathies; and paraplegia due to tuberculosis of the spine.

BURKITT'S LYMPHOMA-TYPE LESIONS SEEN OUTSIDE AFRICA

Following the observation that Burkitt's lymphoma-type lesions in North American and European children were histologically indistinguishable from the classical Burkitt's lymphoma of children in Africa, considerable discussion was initiated as to why the predilection for the jaw has such a high incidence among children in Africa (about 60 percent). As yet, no answers have been offered. What has emerged, however, is a clinicopathologic picture that clearly delineates Burkitt's lymphoma seen in Africa from that seen in North America. Several reports have detailed and delineated the "African Burkitt's Lymphoma," AFBL, from the American Burkitt's Lymphoma, AMBL.[9]

SUMMARY

From the vast amount of data now available concerning Burkitt's lymphoma, it is clear that this disease entity cannot be regarded as an exclusively African disease, because it has been proved that it occurs throughout the world. This awareness does not preclude delimiting geographic zones in which the disease is endemic from those in which only sporadic cases occur. What Denis Burkitt started as a "nosogeographic adventure" has evolved into a complex and fascinating study of lymphoproliferative disorders. A growing awareness of the immunologic parameters of subtypes of lymphomas and leukemias has resulted in a deeper appreciation of differences in the course of diseases related to immunologic subtypes. The extreme sensitivity of Burkitt's lymphoma to alkylating cell-cycle specific agents underscores the fact that this lymphoma is the fastest growing neoplasm in man.[26] When more information is known about normal B-cell regulation and blocking factors, immunotherapy may also find a role in the management of the lymphomas.

REFERENCES

1. Achong, B. G., and Epstein, M. A.: Fine structure of the Burkitt tumor. J. Nat. Cancer Inst., *36*:877, 1966.
2. Adatia, A. K.: Dental tissues and Burkitt's tumor. Oral Surg., *25*:221, 1968.
3. Burkitt, D. P.: A sarcoma involving the jaws in African children. Br. J. Surg., *46*:218, 1958.
4. Burkitt, D. P.: Lymphomas of African children. Br. J. Cancer, *16*:379, 1962.
5. Burkitt, D. P.: Etiology of Burkitt's lymphoma: an alternative hypothesis to a vectored virus. J. Nat. Cancer Inst., *42*:19, 1969.
6. Burkitt, D. P., and O'Connor, G. T.: Malignant lymphoma in African children. 1. A clinical syndrome. Cancer, *14*:259, 1961.
7. Burkitt, D. P., and Wright, D. H.: Burkitt's Lymphoma. Edinburgh, E and S Livingstone, 1970.
8. Byrne, G. E.: Rappaport classification of non-Hodg-

kin's lymphoma: histologic features and clinical significance. Cancer Treat. Rep., *61*:935, 1977.

9. Dorfman, R. F.: Diagnosis of Burkitt's tumor in the United States. Cancer, *21*:563, 1968.

10. Dorfman, R. F.: Pathology of the non-Hodgkin's lymphomas: new classifications. Cancer Treat. Rep., *61*:945, 1977.

10a. Edington, G. M., and MacLean, C. M. U.: Incidence of Burkitt's tumour in Ibadan, Western Nigeria. Brit. Med. J. *1*:264, 1964.

11. Epstein, M. A., Achong, B. G., and Barr, Y. M.: Virus particles in cultured lymphoblasts from Burkitt's lymphoma. Lancet, *1*:702, 1964.

12. Kafuko, G. W., and Burkitt, D. P.: Burkitt's lymphoma and malaria. Int. J. Cancer, *6*:1, 1970.

13. Klein, G.: The Epstein-Barr virus and neoplasia. N. Engl. J. Med., *293*:1353, 1975.

14. Lehner, T.: The jaws and teeth in Burkitt's tumour (African lymphoma). J. Pathol. Bact., *88*:581, 1964.

15. Lukes, R. J., and Collins, R. D.: Immunologic characterization of human malignant lymphomas. Cancer, *34*:1488, 1974.

16. Lukes, R. J., and Collins, R. D.: New approaches to the classification of the lymphomata. Brit. J. Cancer, *31*:1, 1975.

17. Lukes, R. J., and Collins, R. D.: Lukes-Collins classification and its significance. Cancer Treat. Rep., *61*:971, 1977.

18. MacMahon, B.: Epidemiologic aspects of acute leukemia and Burkitt's tumor. Cancer, *21*:558, 1968.

19. Nathwani, B. N.: A critical analysis of the classification of non-Hodgkin's lymphomas. Cancer, *44*:347, 1979.

20. Nathwani, B. N., et al.: Non-Hodgkin's lymphomas. A clinicopathologic study comparing two classifications. Cancer, *41*:303, 1978.

21. Nkrumah, F. K., and Perkins, I. V.: Burkitt's lymphoma. A clinical study of 110 patients. Cancer, *37*:671, 1976.

22. Pagano, J. S., Huang, C. H., and Levine, P.: Absence of Epstein-Barr viral DNA in American Burkitt's lymphoma. N. Engl. J. Med., *289*:1395, 1973.

23. Williams, E. H., Spit, P., and Pike, N. C.: Further evidence of space-time clustering of Burkitt's lymphoma patients in the West Nile District of Uganda. Brit. J. Cancer, *23*:235, 1969.

24. World Health Organization: Histopathological definition of Burkitt's tumour. WHO Bull., *40*:601, 1969.

25. Wright, D. H.: Burkitt's tumour; a postmortem study of 50 cases. Brit. J. Surg., *51*:245, 1964.

26. Ziegler, J. L., Cohen, M. H., and Gerber, P.: Burkitt's tumor. Ann. Intern. Med. *70*:817, 1969.

28

Cancer of the face

PHILIP L. McCARTHY, M.D.

Of all the new malignant tumors that will be diagnosed in any year, more than half will originate in the skin.[13] Fortunately, the cure rate is high; however, there will be considerable morbidity and extensive utilization of medical personnel and facilities, both in time and cost, to care for these patients. One variety of skin cancer, namely malignant melanoma, is associated with a significant mortality rate.

ETIOLOGY

As with most cases of malignant disease, there is no generally accepted cause. However, there are factors involved in the development of skin cancer that can be better documented and are more accepted than for cancer of most other organ systems.[12]

Skin Type. People who have light complexions, especially those with red hair, freckles, and blue eyes, are at highest risk of skin cancer. This is particularly true for those of Celtic origin. The incidence decreases with darker skinned people and is extremely rare in blacks.

Sun Exposure. In every study concerning skin cancer, the amount of sun exposure is directly related to incidence. Because the skin of the face is constantly exposed, it is logical to expect that skin cancer is most commonly encountered in this area.

Other Factors. There are other situations that may influence the development of skin cancer, such as exposure to ionizing radiation, chemical carcinogens, and genetic errors in metabolism, as with xeroderma pigmentosum.

Immunologic Factors. It has been well established that the host's immune response plays a significant role in the development of malignant tumors.[6] When the patient is immunocompromised either by a naturally occurring disease such as lymphoma or artificially by the administration of immunosuppressive drugs, the incidence of malignant tumors increases. The increased incidence and aggressive behavior of malignant tumors, which may be rapidly invasive and are prone to recurrence after appropriate therapy, are worthy of note.

CLASSIFICATION OF SKIN CANCER

Epithelial origin
  Basal cell carcinoma
  Epidermoid (squamous cell) carcinoma
    Bowen's disease
Connective tissue origin
  Fibrosarcoma
  Neurofibrosarcoma
  Liposarcoma
  Leiomyosarcoma
Vascular tissue origin
  Kaposi's hemorrhagic sarcoma
Melanoma
  Lentigo maligna
  Superficial spreading
  Nodular
Lymphoma
  Mycosis fungoides
  Hodgkin's
Metastatic lesions
Special lesions
  Keratoacanthoma
  Cutaneous horn

CLINICAL TYPES

Basal Cell Carcinoma

This is by far the most common malignant tumor of the face. Although it is destructive and in rare instances may be fatal, it rarely produces metastatic lesions. The term *epithelioma* is preferred by many clinicians to differentiate this type of locally malignant tumor from more potentially serious carcinomas with significant metastatic capabilities.

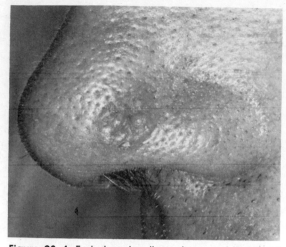

Figure 28–1. Early basal cell carcinoma of the tip of the nose.

Varieties

The classical basal cell carcinoma originates as a small insignificant papule (Figs. 28–1 and 28–2). As it enlarges, with varying rapidity, certain clinical features become apparent. The papule is a grayish semitranslucent lesion, softer to the touch than most tumors, and generally laced with telangiectatic vessels. A central depression eventually develops (Fig. 28–3), and ulceration is a common feature. The term *rodent ulcer* has been used over the years to describe the destructive nature of the lesion. As the tumor progresses further, extension is characterized by necrosis, deep ulceration, hemorrhage, crusting, and secondary infection (Fig. 28–4).

Less obvious varieties of basal cell carcinoma include the superficial type, which can appear as an eczematous patch, with scaling and crusting as the main features (Figs. 28–5 and 28–6). It may mimic benign lesions such

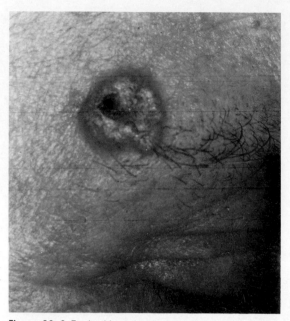

Figure 28–3. Typical basal cell carcinoma, with crusting in the center.

as psoriasis and eczema, but with close scrutiny, an elevated border can be detected.

The malignant tumor of the face that may be the most difficult to diagnose and manage is the morphea variety of basal cell carcinoma, which may appear as an indurated area of the skin with rather indefinite borders (Fig. 28–7). Extensive periods of time may elapse before a correct diagnosis is established, which may further complicate successful management.

Finally, there are several varieties of adnexal basal cell carcinomas as well as cystic varieties that may have lesions that are atypical.[8] A

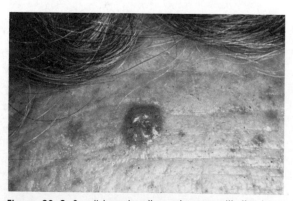

Figure 28–2. Small basal cell carcinoma, with the beginning of central depression.

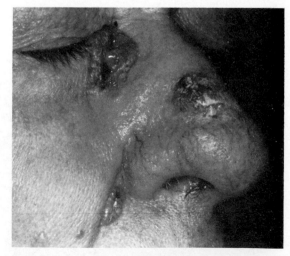

Figure 28–4. Multiple advanced basal cell carcinomas, with significant ulceration and necrosis.

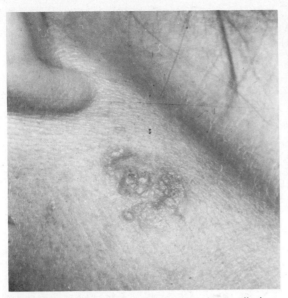

Figure 28–5. Superficial basal cell carcinoma that resembles an eczematous patch.

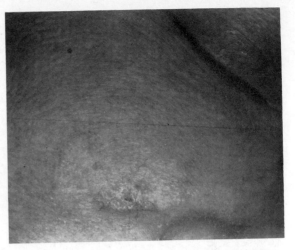

Figure 28–7. Morphea variety of basal cell carcinoma.

biopsy must be performed before a definite diagnosis can be established.

Basal Cell Nevus Syndrome

This rare and fascinating syndrome is manifested by the development of multiple basal cell carcinomas, usually at an early age.[5] Genetic studies reveal an autosomal dominant pattern with good penetration and variable expression.

In addition to basal cell carcinomas, a variety of other findings are noted, including palmar and planter pits, keratinous cysts of the jaws, rib abnormalities, shortening of the fourth metacarpal bones, frontoparietal bosses, and a broad nasal root. Several other less common conditions have been associated with this syndrome. The multiplicity of the lesions results in a significant challenge to the therapist to successfully manage the cutaneous malignancies in a manner best suited for each individual patient.

Epidermoid Carcinoma

This variety of malignant tumor is the second most commonly encountered malignant lesion on the skin of the face. Although it generally arises from pre-existing actinic keratosis, an epidermoid carcinoma may develop in otherwise normal-appearing skin. Although it may be confused with basal cell carcinoma, it tends to be firmer to the touch, and develops a more verrucous or hyperkeratotic surface (Figs. 28–8 and 28–9). Obvious surrounding cutaneous

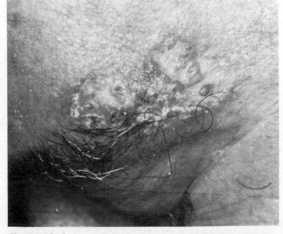

Figure 28–6. Superficial basal cell carcinoma, with psoriasiform features.

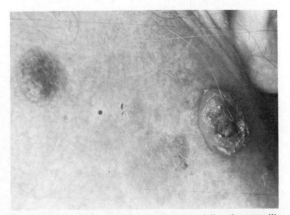

Figure 28–8. Epidermoid carcinoma of the face, with two adjacent benign keratoses.

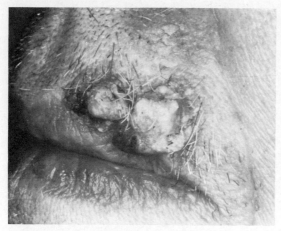

Figure 28–9. Epidermoid carcinoma of the upper lip, with heaped-up keratinous surface.

changes from excessive sun exposure are frequently present.

Bowen's Disease (epidermoid carcinoma-in-situ)

The lesions of this condition closely resemble superficial basal cell carcinomas except that they lack the slightly elevated pearly border. In most instances, they are diagnosed as a papulosquamous eruption such as nummular eczema or psoriasis (Fig. 28–10). They are easily managed in their superficial stage, but over a period of time, they may show the characteristics of an invasive epidermoid carcinoma.

Connective Tissue Tumors

There are a wide variety of malignant tumors that are manifested from the subcutaneous tissue of the face. Most of them are unusual. It is beyond the scope of this chapter to list and discuss them in detail.

Vascular Tissue Tumors

Kaposi's hemorrhagic sarcoma is a unique tumor that is characterized by multiple reddish-violaceous plaques and nodules (Fig. 28–11). Most of the lesions originate as part of a multicentric phenomenon, although there may be metastatic spread. Facial lesions are not common.

Melanoma

Malignant melanoma is a tumor composed of malignant melanocytes. It may develop de

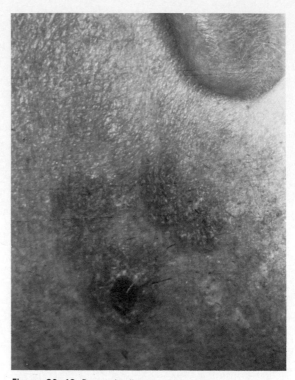

Figure 28–10. Bowen's disease. The crusted area is the site of biopsy.

novo or may be preceded by a benign nevus.

In order to properly classify malignant melanomas, it is necessary to examine them histologically and to determine the depth of the invasion.

Level I—Tumor cells are limited to the epidermis (melanoma in situ).

Level II—Tumor cells invade the papillary dermis but do not fill it.

Level III—Tumor cells fill the papillary dermis but do not invade the reticular dermis.

Level IV—Tumor cells invade the reticular dermis.

Level V—Tumor cells invade the subcutaneous fat.

Lentigo Maligna (Hutchinson's freckle; malignant melanoma-in-situ)

The typical lentigo maligna lesion is characterized by macular areas of brown pigmentation with irregular borders (Figs. 28–12 and 28–13). The color tends to be mottled rather than diffuse. The most common site is the malar region, and most patients are females in their fifth to eighth decades. The melanoma may remain macular and relatively harmless for years, but usually it eventually becomes invasive and thus should be dealt with definitively in its early development.

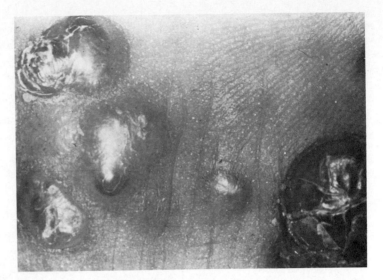

Figure 28–11. Kaposi's sarcoma, with typical nodules.

Superficial Spreading Melanoma

This form of melanoma is usually characterized by a lesion of varying clinical criteria. The general rule is that it has a variegated appearance with an irregular border and a spectrum of colors, including light brown interspersed with white areas, darker brown, and frequently erythematous patches (Figs. 28–14 and 28–15). Histologically, the depth usually ranges from Level II to III.

Nodular Melanoma

This form of malignant melanoma usually arises de novo as a distinct nodule with fairly regular margins and varying degrees of elevation that range from a plaque to a dome-shaped lesion (Figs. 28–16 and 28–17). Nodular melanoma is usually a serious form of the disease, because it indicates an early deep invasion, quite often to Level IV or V.

Lymphomas

These malignant tumors originate from the extramedullary portion of the lymphoreticular system.[2] They may be of multicentric origin or may spread by metastasis. There also may be a leukemic phase. Included are the monomorphous lymphocytic and histiocytic types as well as the polymorphous type, which includes Hodgkin's disease and mycosis fungoides.

The skin lesions vary considerably from insignificant, slightly indurated areas of discoloration (Figs. 28–18 and 28–19) to large nodules (Fig. 28–20). The color ranges from a light erythema to a brownish-violaceous hue. Ulceration may result in poorly differentiated tumors (Fig. 28–21).

THERAPY

Skin cancer may be treated by a variety of successful modalities.[7, 9] The most common

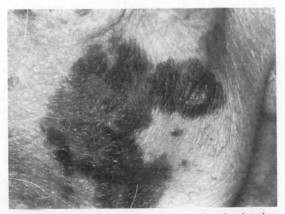

Figure 28–12. Lentigo maligna, with extensive involvement, in an elderly female.

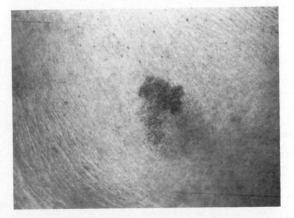

Figure 28–13. Early lesion of lentigo maligna in a middle-aged male.

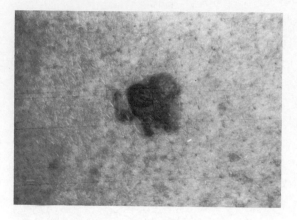

Figure 28–14. Typical early superficial spreading melanoma.

Figure 28–15. More advanced superficial spreading melanoma, with typical irregular configuration.

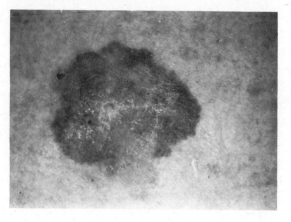

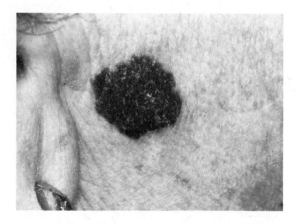

Figure 28–16. Nodular malignant melanoma of the preauricular area.

Figure 28–17. Small, nodular dome-shaped malignant melanoma that has reached level IV.

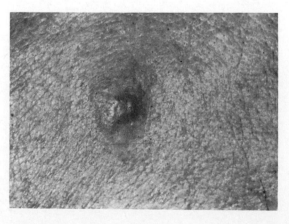

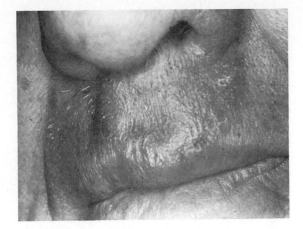

Figure 28–18. Superficial plaque of mycosis fungoides.

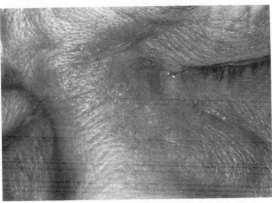

Figure 28–19. Early lesion of mycosis fungoides that could be confused with seborrheic dermatitis.

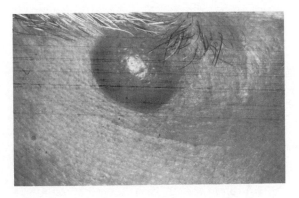

Figure 28–20. Prominent nodule of lymphoma.

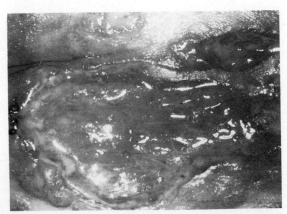

Figure 28–21. Advanced lesions of reticulum cell (histiocytic) sarcoma.

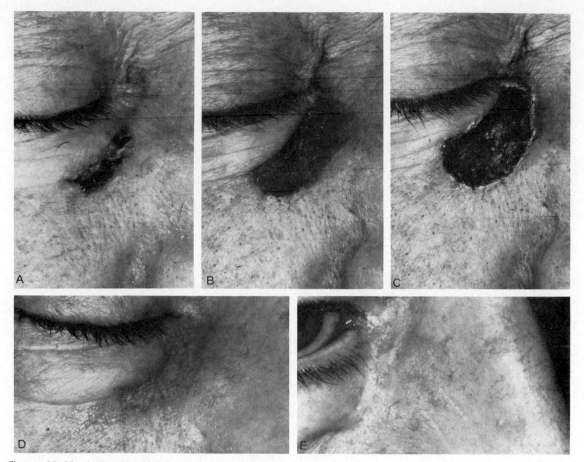

Figure 28–22. *A*, Basal cell carcinoma of the cheek pretreatment. *B*, Post-curettage. *C*, Post-curettage and coagulation. *D*, Six weeks post-treatment. *E*, Three months post-treatment.

basal cell and epidermoid varieties are excised or destroyed by radiation therapy, cryosurgery, or electrocoagulation and curettage (Fig. 28–22). The cure rate approximates 96 to 97 percent by all four methods. There are several sites that require special attention, namely the nasolabial fold, the eyelids, and the ear near the opening of the external auditory canal. In these sites, x-ray therapy is usually the treatment of choice.

Malignant tumors of connective tissue origin are usually best treated by excision or radiation therapy.

Melanomas generally are treated by wide excision and may be followed with regional lymph node resection if the tumor has reached Level IV or V. These tumors are usually radioresistant except for the lentigo maligna type, which can frequently be eradicated by radiation therapy.

Lymphomas of the skin are usually part of a generalized process and are treated by a team of oncologists who utilize both radiation therapy and chemotherapy.

Mohs Chemosurgery

This method of managing malignant cutaneous tumors is generally reserved for those that have recurred after conventional therapy or for primary tumors that are extensive or deeply invasive or that involve critical areas.[11] The essential feature of this method is microscopic examination of each section of the tumor, at all margins and depths, as it is removed until all areas are tumor free. It may be performed in the originally described method using zinc chloride paste or by modifying the procedure using a fresh tissue technique. By either method, the cure rate is generally about 97 to 99 percent despite the difficult challenge of the tumor.

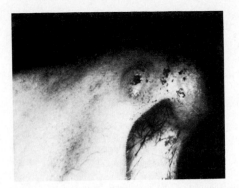

Figure 28–23. Metastatic lesion at the tip of the nose caused by primary lung cancer.

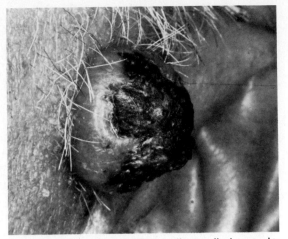

Figure 28–25. Typical keratoacanthoma that grew to the present size in 6 weeks.

Metastatic Lesions

Although the skin is the largest organ of the body, metastases from underlying malignant tumors are not common. Although cutaneous lesions have been reported from most sites of origin, the more likely primary sites include the breast, lung, prostate, kidney, and bowel.[4]

The lesions are difficult to diagnose clinically and frequently appear as small subcutaneous papules (Figs. 28–23 and 28–24). Histologically, the cell of origin may be recognized, but occasionally the pathologist may have difficulty in determining the type of tumor, particularly in very anaplastic varieties.

Special Lesions

Keratoacanthoma[1]

These rapidly developing tumors are a constant concern, because they closely mimic ep-

idermoid carcinomas, both clinically and histologically. The typical lesion develops in a few weeks and is characterized by a fleshy, firm nodule with bulging sides and a prominent central hyperkeratotic crater (Figs. 28–25 and 28–26). If untreated, they generally regress spontaneously and eventually disappear, leaving some scarring. In critical areas, such as the face, one is rarely content with a clinical diagnosis, and the keratoacanthoma is removed. The histologic structure is important, and a mere biopsy is usually inadequate for a definitive diagnosis. It is commonly believed that keratoacanthomas are of viral origin, which may account for their clinical behavior. Simple excision should be curative, but occasionally they may recur; radiation therapy is effective in these instances.

Cutaneous Horn

These rather spectacular lesions probably represent an actinic keratosis that produces an exaggerated hyperkeratotic response. The horn portion may grow to several centimeters and may assume various configurations (Fig. 28–27). Typically, there is an elevated indurated base (Fig. 28–28), which, on histologic examination, may be interpreted as a well-differentiated epidermoid carcinoma. Cutaneous horns probably never metastasize, and they may be cured with a simple excision (Fig. 28–29).

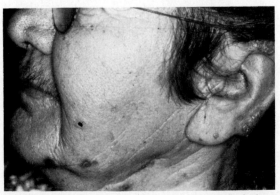

Figure 28–24. Several small papular metastatic lesions caused by renal carcinoma.

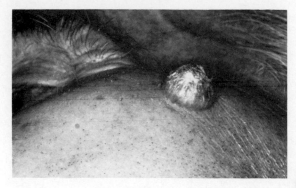

Figure 28–26. Keratoacanthoma that developed in 4 weeks.

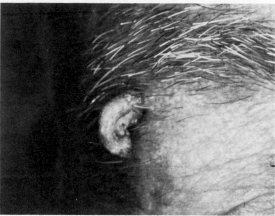

Figure 28–27. Cutaneous horn showing characteristic configuration of keratinous portion.

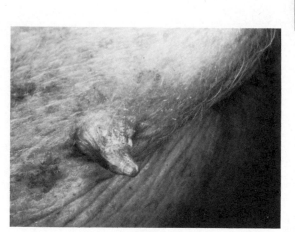

Figure 28–28. Cutaneous horn with a prominent base, which was an early epidermoid carcinoma.

Figure 28–29. Cutaneous horn at the margin of the lower lip.

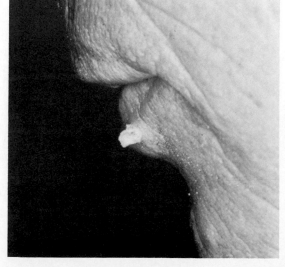

REFERENCES

1. Baer, R. L., and Kopf, A. W.: Keratoacanthoma. *In* Yearbook of Dermatology, 1962–1963 Series, Chicago, Year Book Medical Publishers, Inc., 1963.
2. Berard, C. W., Gallo, R. C., Jaffe, E. S., et al.: Current concepts of leukemia and lymphoma: etiology, pathogenesis, and therapy. Ann. Intern. Med., *85*:351, 1976.
3. Bluefarb, S. M.: Kaposi's Sarcoma. Springfield, Illinois, Charles C Thomas, Publisher, 1957.
4. Brownstein, M. H., and Helwig, E. B.: Patterns of cutaneous metastasis. Arch. Dermatol., *105*:862, 1972.
5. Clendenning, W. E., Block, J. B., and Radde, I. C.: Basal cell nevus syndrome. Arch. Dermatol., *90*:38, 1964.
6. Fisher, B.: The present status of tumor immunology. Adv. Surg., *5*:189, 1971.
7. Freeman, R., Knox, J., and Heaton, C.: The treatment of skin cancer. A statistical study of 1341 skin tumors comparing results obtained with irradiation, surgery, and curettage followed by electrodesiccation. Cancer, *17*:535, 1964.
8. Hashimoto, K., and Lever, W. F.: Appendage Tumors of the Skin. Springfield, Illinois, Charles C Thomas, Publisher, 1968.
9. McLean, D. I., Haynes, H. A., McCarthy, P. L., et al.: Cryotherapy of basal cell carcinoma by a simple method of standardized freeze-thaw cycles. J. Dermatol. Surg. Oncol., *4*:175, 1978.
10. Mihm, M. C., Jr., Clark, W. H., and Fro, L.: The clinical diagnosis, classification, and histogenic concepts of the early stages of cutaneous malignant melanoma. N. Engl. J. Med., *284*:1078, 1971.
11. Mohs, F. E.: Chemosurgery for skin cancer: fixed tissue and fresh tissue techniques. Arch. Dermatol., *112*:211, 1976.
12. Schottenfield, D. (ed.): Cancer Epidemiology and Prevention: Current Concepts. Springfield, Illinois, Charles C Thomas, Publisher, 1975.
13. Third National Cancer Survey, Incidence Data. Biometry Branch, National Cancer Institute, Bethesda, Maryland, DHEW, Publication No. (NIH) 75–787, 1975.

29

Oral lesions in leukemia

GERALD SHKLAR, D.D.S., M.S.

Leukemia represents a malignant neoplastic proliferation of poorly differentiated cells in the various blood-forming organs. The normal hematopoietic cells gradually become replaced by the abnormal leukemic cells, and the resultant disease state is not only leukemia but also anemia, thrombocytopenia, and neutropenia. As the neoplastic condition progresses, many organs and tissues may become infiltrated with leukemic cells, producing a complex array of signs and symptoms. The oral cavity is often involved in leukemia, and the changes may represent a true infiltration of leukemic cells into oral tissues such as the gingiva, but more commonly, they reflect oral pathogenesis resulting from the thrombocytopenia, neutropenia, or anemia. The problems one usually faces in leukemia are hemorrhage, ulceration, and generally decreased resistance to oral bacterial and mycotic infection. Oral disease in leukemic patients is often exaggerated or complicated by the chemotherapeutic protocols used to treat the leukemia. The chemotherapeutic agents are antimetabolites and immunosuppressants.

CLASSIFICATION OF LEUKEMIA

Classification of leukemia into acute and chronic forms and into cell types is important for treatment planning and for overall prognosis. Acute leukemia is the most common form in children, whereas chronic leukemia is the usual form in adults. Differentiation by cell types involves cell morphology and immunologic markers. Cellular morphology may indicate the degree of differentiation of the cells, and this in turn may assist in prognosis. In the future, further classification may be possible using chemical markers, enzyme activity, or cell surface characteristics. A typical classification of the leukemias is primarily morphologic,[1] with the acute leukemias subdivided into several groups (Table 29–1).

The etiology of leukemia is unknown. Viruses are suspected, because there are models of both murine and simian leukemia in which viral agents have been identified as etiologic agents.

Leukemia is most commonly found during childhood and is the major cancer killer in both males and females younger than 15 years. It is also the major cancer killer in males between the ages of 15 and 34 years and is second to breast cancer as a cancer killer in females between the ages of 15 and 35 years.

SIGNS AND SYMPTOMS

In acute leukemia, there is usually several weeks of nonspecific symptoms such as malaise, fatigue, and anorexia. Low-grade fever may also be present. Bone pain and vague muscle pain may also be present. As anemia develops, there may be pallor and further debilitation. As the thrombocytopenia develops, there may be evidence of a hemorrhagic disorder such as bleeding gingiva, petechial hemorrhages of the skin and mucosa, and larger ecchymoses of the skin, resulting from minor trauma or pressure (Figs. 29–1 through 29–3). In acute lymphocytic leukemia of childhood, there will be adenopathy and hepatosplenomegaly in a significant number of patients. With the clinical impression of leukemia, diagnosis is made by hematologic studies. White cell count usually ranges from 5000 to 30,000 cells per cubic millimeter. Peripheral blood smear is usually suggestive of a diagnosis of leukemia, and the cellular morphology may indicate the cell type. Bone marrow aspiration and smear is usually diagnostic. Normal mar-

Table 29–1. CLASSIFICATION OF THE LEUKEMIAS

Acute Lymphocytic (Lymphoblastic) (ALL)

L1   Small cells predominate but may vary, with some cells up to twice the diameter of the small lymphocytes. Nuclei are generally round and regular with occasional clefts. Nucleoli are often not visible. Cytoplasm is scanty. The cell population is homogeneous.

L2   Cells are heterogeneous in size and have the features of both L1 and L3. Nuclei often show clefts. Nucleoli are often present.

L3   There is a homogeneous population of large cells (3 to 4 times the diameter of small lymphocytes). Nuclei are round to oval with prominent nucleoli. Cytoplasm is abundant and deeply basophilic.

Chronic Lymphocytic (CLL)

Cells constitute a homogeneous population of small mature lymphocytes, often associated with lymphocytic, well-differentiated lymphoma.

Acute Myelocytic (Myeloblastic) (AML)

M1   Myeloblastic leukemia without maturation—Cells are dominantly blasts without Auer rods or granules.

M2   Myeloblastic leukemia with maturation—Many blasts are evident, but there is some maturation to promyelocytes or beyond.

M3   Hypergranular promyelocytic leukemia—It is mainly composed of promyelocytes, with the cytoplasm packed with peroxidase-positive granules. There are many Auer rods.

M4   Myelomonocytic leukemia—Both myeloid and monocytic differentiation are evident. Myeloid element resembles M2.

M5   Monocytic leukemia—Both "monoblasts" and monocytes are present, the former having large round nuclei with lacy chromatin and prominent nucleoli. Diagnosis must be confirmed by fluoride-inhibited esterase reaction.

M6   Erythroleukemia—Erythropoietic elements constitute more than 50% of the cells in marrow and have bizarre multilobate nuclei. They may also be present in circulating blood in addition to an admixture of myeloblasts and promyelocytes.

Chronic Myelocytic (CML)

The cells are neutrophils, with scattered myelocytes and promyelocytes.

Acute Monocytic

(included as M4, myelomonocytic leukemia)

Chronic Monocytic

This type of leukemia is very uncommon. It is composed of mostly mature monocytes, with scattered blasts. Some cells are peroxidase positive.

Special Rare Types

Histiocytic leukemia—This may occur in histiocytic lymphoma.

Hairy-cell leukemia associated with leukemic reticuloendotheliosis—It is of uncertain cell type; it may be a B cell or possibly a histiocyte.

Leukemia associated with Sézary syndrome—This type is thought to be of T-cell origin.

Stem cell leukemia—Cells are so immature that they are unidentifiable.

From Robbins, S. L., and Cotran, R. Z.: The Pathologic Basis of Disease. Philadelphia, W. B. Saunders Company, 2nd ed., 1979.

row elements are decreased and replaced by a population of undifferentiated leukemic cells. These cells may resemble myeloblasts or lymphoblasts, and definitive diagnosis is made. Other laboratory studies may be necessary to rule out other hematologic disturbances such as infectious mononucleosis.[13]

Symptoms are less notable in chronic leukemias. One may have vague feelings of fatigue and malaise. Adenopathy or splenomegaly is minimal or absent. Diagnosis of chronic leukemia is often made on the basis of routine hematologic studies in a patient who has various vague complaints and recurrent infections and low-grade fever.

THERAPY

Long-term remission for acute lymphocytic leukemia is now possible with chemotherapy, and complete cure is becoming a reality—that is, a 5-year remission following cessation of chemotherapy.

Therapy involves remission induction by prednisone, vincristine, and L-asparaginase.[3, 4, 10, 15] The central nervous system is treated prophylactically with irradiation and intrathecal methotrexate to prevent relapse. It was found that the central nervous system harbored leukemic cells that did not respond to systemic chemotherapy and would subse-

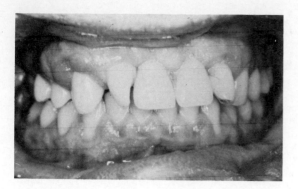

Figure 29–1. Gingival enlargement in a patient who has acute monocytic leukemia.

Figure 29–2. High-power microscopic view of gingival biopsy showing abnormally shaped monocytes and a mitotic figure.

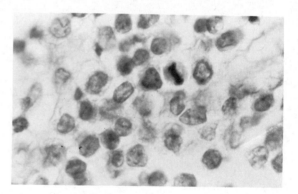

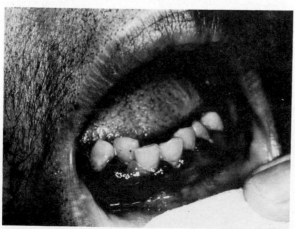

Figure 29–3. Gingival enlargement and hemorrhage in a patient who has acute monocytic leukemia.

quently re-establish disease in the body. Maintenance with drugs such as methotrexate and 6-mercaptopurine prolongs the initial remission. Relapse still occurs in a high proportion of children (almost 50 percent), and this inevitably has a fatal outcome. In acute myelocytic leukemia, the prognosis is less promising than in acute lymphocytic leukemia.

Various alkylating agents are used in the treatment of chronic leukemia.

ORAL MANIFESTATIONS

The oral lesions of leukemia result from three possible underlying pathologic entities: leukemic infiltration of tissues, neutropenia, and granulocytopenia. The classically described lesions are gingival enlargement, gingival bleeding, nonhealing ulcers, and increased susceptibility to oral infection.[2, 6-8, 14]

Gingival Enlargement. Hyperplasia or gingival enlargement usually results from an exaggerated or conditioned inflammatory response to local irritation, rather than from an actual infiltration of leukemic cells. Normally, the marginal gingivae are reasonably well protected against the irritation of dental plaque, a mass of bacteria that tenaciously clings to the tooth surface. There tends to be a mild to moderate gingivitis, with erythema of the gingival margin. If tartar develops on the tooth surface near the gingival margin or in the gingival crevice, the inflammation tends to be more severe. The tartar or calculus is calcified and is both a mechanical and bacterial irritant. Poor oral hygiene also results in food debris on the tooth surface, in addition to plaque and tartar. In leukemia, particularly acute monocytic or acute myelocytic leukemia, the gingival inflammatory response is exaggerated by the underlying leukemic state. The gingivae become enlarged and edematous, with increased vascularity and dense infiltrations of chronic inflammatory cells. In many cases, there may also be dense infiltrations of abnormal white cells, with mitoses and notable pleomorphism. In the conditioned gingivitis of leukemia, a significant improvement in gingival health may be gained by better oral hygiene, removal of irritating deposits on the teeth, and the use of such antibacterial mouthwashes as hydrogen peroxide. In the true leukemic infiltration of the gingiva, significant improvement results mainly from control of the leukemia itself by chemotherapy. Usually, even the leukemic infiltration is combined with the conditioned inflammatory response, and local gingival therapy does result in some improvement.

In leukemic infiltration of the gingiva, the leukemic cells appear as a dense sheet of immature or abnormally shaped leukocytes within the corium of the gingiva and separated from the overlying epithelium by a zone relatively free of leukemic cells. Scattered mitoses are usually noted. The abnormal leukocytes and the mitoses are suggestive of the possibility or even probability of leukemia. However, hematologic studies are necessary for definitive diagnosis.

Superimposed upon the gingival enlargement, there may be ulceration and necrosis of the marginal gingiva, with evidence of fusospirochetal infection (acute necrotizing ulceromembranous gingivitis). There may also be gingival bleeding, particularly in response to slight trauma, abrasion, or even pressure. Gingival hemorrhage usually indicates an associated underlying thrombocytopenia. The abnormality of normal coagulation mechanisms may also result in subepithelial hemorrhages in the skin as well as in the oral mucosa. These may be small petechiae or larger ecchymoses.

In chronic leukemia, the gingival pathology is less severe than in acute leukemia, and associated problems also tend to be less severe.

Ulcers. In acute leukemia, ulcers of the oral mucosa are often seen and result from an associated leukopenia. Absence of protective leukocytes in response to some irritation or trauma, such as hard crusts of food, of the oral mucosa results in tissue breakdown and ulceration. The oral bacterial-mycotic flora then further exaggerates the nonhealing ulcer. With careful cleansing of the ulcer and the use of hydrogen peroxide mouthwash, eventual healing will occur.

REFERENCES

1. Bennett, J. M., Catovsky, D., Daniel, M. T., et al.: Proposals for the classification of the acute leukemias. Brit. J. Haematol., 33:451, 1976.
2. Curtis, A. B.: Childhood leukemias; initial oral manifestations. J. Am. Dent. Assoc., 83:159, 1971.
3. Frei, E., III, and Sallan, S. E.: Acute lymphoblastic leukemia: treatment. Cancer, 42:828, 1978.
4. Holland, J. F.: Therapeutic considerations in acute lymphocytic leukemia. Am. J. Pathol., 90:521, 1978.
5. Hustic, H. O., and Aur, R. J.: Extramedullary leukemia. Clin. Haematol., 7:313, 1978.
6. Lynch, M. A., and Ship, I. I.: Initial oral manifestations of leukemia. J. Am. Dent. Assoc., 75:932, 1967.
7. McCarthy, P. L., and Shklar, G.: Diseases of the Oral

Mucosa, 2nd ed. Philadelphia, Lea and Febiger, 1980, pp. 408–412.

8. Michaud, M., Bachner, R. L., Bixler, D., et al.: Oral manifestations of acute leukemia in children. J. Am. Dent. Assoc., *95*:1145, 1977.

9. Moloney, W. C.: Natural history of chronic granulocytic leukemia. Clin. Haematol., *6*:41, 1977.

10. Pinkel, D.: Treatment of acute lymphocytic leukemia. Cancer, *43*:1128, 1979.

11. Silverberg, E.: Cancer statistics, 1982. CA, *32*:15, 1982.

12. Simone, J. V., Aur, R. J., Hustu, H. O., et al.: Combined modality therapy of acute lymphocytic leukemia. Cancer, *35*:25, 1975.

13. Smithson, W. A., Li, C. Y., Pierre, R. V., et al.: Acute lymphoblastic leukemia in children: immunologic, cytochemical, morphologic, and cytogenetic studies in relation to pretreatment risk factors. Med. Pediat. Oncol., *7*:83, 1979.

14. White, G. E.: Oral manifestations of leukemia in children. Oral Surg., *29*:420, 1970.

15. Wintrobe, M. M., et al.: Clinical Hematology, 7th ed. Philadelphia, Lea and Febiger, 1974.

30

Psychological impact of oral cancer

GERALD SHKLAR, D.D.S., M.S.

The mouth and facial architecture represent a highly significant part of the body in terms of its psychological background and its importance in the overall emotional development of the individual. The mouth relates both directly and symbolically to our basic instinctive drives. The physiologic requirements for food and water and the enjoyment of nourishment when availability and leisure permit are among the oldest pursuits of humans. To this may be added an aesthetic and cultural element in the way the food is prepared and eaten, as well as the social act in which people join one another in eating and drinking. The role of the oral tissues in sexual development is one of the fundamental concepts in current psychological and psychoanalytic theory, and the function of the mouth, lips, and tongue in sexual activity requires no elaborate description. The role of the mouth and facial structures in communication must also be emphasized, whether in communicating information, casual pleasantries, or the deeper emotions of love, hatred, hostility, or aggressiveness. The mouth may enunciate the words, but the entire orofacial architecture assists in presenting the appropriate expressions and gestures that enhance the meaning of the words and their emotional impact. The oral tissues are also of extreme importance to musicians, such as singers and performers on wind instruments.

Obviously, a dysfunction or impending dysfunction, or even a threat of dysfunction of the oral tissues will have a very significant impact upon the patient's emotional state. Furthermore, unlike other cancer sites, the mouth and face must be constantly exposed to view, and even small defects in function and appearance are obvious not only to the patient but also to all observers, and particularly to those who are close to the patient, such as family, friends, business associates, academic associates, clients, and students. The fear of facial deformity or loss of normal function is a very real and rational fear and must be handled with compassion by the clinician. The patient may have many questions, and these should be answered with patience and gentleness, so that he or she will feel that the clinician is a friend offering kind advice rather than an enemy merely bringing catastrophic news and then brusquely dismissing the patient's pleas for information and understanding. Ignorance generally breeds fear, and the patient should be given as much information as possible, consistent with a positive approach to therapy and prognosis.

The psychological impact of cancer in such tissues as the breast, stomach, and rectum has been adequately reviewed. The loss of a limb and its psychological problems have been considered in some detail. However, the problems related to the mouth and face have received considerably less attention but are constantly confronting clinicians who deal with the diagnosis and treatment of oral cancer and the rehabilitation of the patient following successful therapy, which may result in dysfunction and disfigurement.

In the classic studies of Sutherland, the cancer patient is seen as a person who is under a particular and severe form of stress that threatens to disrupt important patterns of adaptation that have evolved. A pattern of adaptation is defined by Sutherland as "a system of beliefs and behaviour designed in order to bring the individual's physical and emotional needs into harmony with demands of the environment". . . "Whenever a pattern of adaptation is threatened or disrupted, a considerable amount of anxiety is generated, as the individual may believe himself unable to meet environmental demands or fulfill his own emotional needs. He loses self-esteem and believes himself vulnerable to loss of esteem from others or to explicit condemnation or isolation."[8]

The anxiety created by cancer of the mouth is severe. The patient immediately worries about damage to the oral structures by surgery or radiation. The very thought of extensive treatment to this region with its enormous psychological potential is unnerving. Removal of the rectum, with its psychological relations to toilet training and cleanliness, often produces profound feelings of worthlessness in patients. Removal of the breast obviously may relate to feelings of sexual inadequacy and rejection. Likewise, any mutilation or dysfunction of the mouth may lead to the fear of rejection, both sexually and socially.

The impact of cancer in the so-called normal individual generally depends upon how the overall experience challenges the patient's patterns of adaptation. By overall experience, we are referring to the initial assimilation of the diagnosis, consideration of treatment, traumatic experience of the treatment, results of the treatment and their acceptance, rehabilitative phase, and lastly, the return to previous activity or professional life. If the challenge is severe or is perceived to be severe by the patient, his or her emotional status may suffer. If therapy is successful and deformity is absent or minimal, the patient may respond extremely well and anxiety may be minimal. Obviously, a patient who has a neurotic personality will respond in a more unpredictable manner, and one who has a borderline psychopathic personality may have a bizarre response that requires psychiatric intervention.

The major role of the dentist or physician is to attempt to minimize the patient's anxiety. The dentist plays an extremely important role in the overall management of oral cancer. He or she is often the person who makes the original diagnosis or arranges for the diagnostic procedures. The dentist also maintains contact with the patient following therapy. This continuity of care offers the generalist practitioner the opportunity to serve as a friendly and sympathetic figure, a role with an importance that cannot be overemphasized in treating a cancer patient.

Anxiety in normal patients can always be reduced by listening carefully to their questions and apprehensions and answering them as completely and positively as possible. There is now enough known about oral cancer therapy and its prognosis to offer reassurance that there is a good chance for successful treatment together with an excellent aesthetic result. Radiation therapy has become much more effective in recent years, and gross, mutilating surgery is rarely used today. In fact, various combinations of surgery and radiation are successfully used for superior aesthetic and functional results. Even chemotherapy may play a role in reducing tumor bulk so that less surgery may be required.

However, in most cases, the effects of oral cancer still result in some distortion in an important part of the body that is constantly exposed to careful scrutiny. Inevitably, the patient must learn to accept the result, and this is always easier if the patient's family and friends can accept the result. A supportive family always facilitates the patient's social rehabilitation. A hostile marital partner will delay the patient's rehabilitation and may produce emotional problems beyond those anticipated. Basically, the patient's psychological well-being will relate directly to the ease with which he or she can re-establish former life patterns or patterns of adaptation. There is evidence that patients who have strong emotional control may have a better overall prognosis.[7]

In psychiatric terms, following cancer therapy, patients may display a variety of clinical reactions, such as dependency, anxiety, depression, hypochondriasis, and obsessive-compulsive and paranoid reactions. These reactions may not be sufficiently severe to require psychotherapy, and some are to be realistically anticipated. Excessive dependency upon various professionals may be prolonged until the patient feels that he can cope with his environment. He may continue to seek specialists who he believes may be able to improve his appearance. Anxiety is common and may persist. The patient knows that cancer may recur and that it may eventually destroy him. This type of anxiety will continue at some level and may determine many of the plans that the patient makes for the future.

Depression may occur together with anxiety or as a separate clinical entity. It is invariably a "reactive depression" and may persist if the patient's basic adaptation pattern has been altered. Hypochondriasis is a more severe type of clinical behavior pattern. The patient may be convinced that the cancer or treatment or both has ruined him as a person and that he will always be defective and inferior. He may become unfriendly and suspicious of others. He may become unproductive and may change his type of work, because he feels that his body is no longer capable of carrying out its previous function. Paranoid reactions may accompany some of these other behavior patterns. They are often bizarre and based on delusions of the cancer being caused in some way by the patient. Strong feelings of guilt may be directed at others, or there may be self-directed rage.

Obsessive-compulsive reactions are not uncommon in patients who have oral cancer. The feeling that the mouth is damaged and unclean may cause patients to brush their teeth excessively and to constantly use mouthwashes with strong flavors to remove the perception of a foul taste or odor.

Sexual problems may also arise from the emotional trauma of oral cancer. The patient may avoid sexual contact, feeling that he has been damaged sexually. Impotence may occur in male patients. Hostility may develop if the patient feels that his partner is avoiding sexual intimacy because of his perceived oral abnormality.

At some point, the perceptive oral cancer clinician may believe that psychiatric consultation will be of value. The psychiatrist must determine whether the patient's symptoms indicate a true affective disorder such as depression or whether the symptoms are primarily caused by the neoplastic disease and its treatment modalities. The problem becomes particularly complex in the patient who has advanced or recurrent cancer.

Psychiatrists have developed reasonably reliable criteria for diagnosing a disorder such as depression, including the presence of somatic symptoms such as sleep impairment, appetite disturbance, fatigue, and anorexia. Severe mood alterations, irritability, and withdrawal are also suggestive manifestations. In patients who have advanced cancer, it is difficult to determine whether these symptoms represent a primary affective disorder or whether they are secondary to the cancer itself. In fact, true depression has been found to be relatively uncommon, even in patients who have advanced or recurrent cancer.

Plumb and Holland found that 23 percent of the patients who had advanced cancer were moderately or severely depressed.[4] However, although their somatic symptoms resembled those of control psychiatric depressive patients, their psychologically or nonsomatic symptoms were similar to those of control healthy individuals. Sebberfarb and associates found that only 15.1 percent of a group of patients who had recurrent breast cancer and only 4.5 percent of a group of patients who had advanced breast cancer had both somatic and nonsomatic features of depression.[5]

It is apparent that although patients who have cancer may be unhappy and depressed, the depression usually does not represent true psychiatric disease, even in those with advanced cancer. Furthermore, patients who have advanced disease may develop psychiatric changes that resemble depression or psychosis that are caused by the cancer therapy. They may be caused by drug reactions or may be reactions to severely compromised nutritional status.

PSYCHOSOCIAL ISSUES

Although the cancer patient requires a warm and supportive environment in order to minimize emotional problems, friends, relatives, and business associates often tend to shun the patient, resulting in his having a feeling of isolation or abandonment. Some people still believe that cancer may be a contagious disease and that one should avoid contact with cancer patients so that one does not, in some way, become contaminated. It would be convenient to say that this antiquated notion is held only by uneducated lay persons. Unfortunately, even some health professionals share this innate irrational feeling. They will attempt to avoid physical contact with the patient and, if they touch the patient, they will rush to wash their hands afterward.

There is also the social awkwardness of not knowing what to say to a cancer patient, and the resultant silence further gives the patient a feeling of isolation. With oral cancer, the visitor may stare at the patient's face and then uncomfortably react with feelings of guilt and foolish remarks. These reactions increase the patient's anxiety about his appearance and the way it offends or frightens those who look at him.

Education about cancer is obviously needed not only by the patient but also by society at large and often even by health professionals. Unfortunately, society is being educated slowly about oral cancer and even about cancer in general. The oral cancer patient will face problems in his social environment, and it is best to prepare him for these unpleasant possibilities. The patient's close family should be educated together with the patient and become helpful and supportive to him.

ADVANCED DISEASE AND DEATH

Unfortunately, many patients who have oral cancer develop advanced disease and die. Denial mechanisms may keep the patient functional up to a point. However, at some point, the patient must face the hopelessness of cure and the inevitability of death. Psychiatric consultation may be helpful in suggesting antidepressant drugs, if necessary. Patients may wish to talk about death, and the physician or dentist should be prepared to listen. Often, the patient tends to withdraw socially and may not wish to carry on a falsely cheerful conversation. A patient's wish to cease further therapy should be respected if the situation is indeed hopeless. He should be given all treatment necessary for palliation—treatment to make him reasonably comfortable—but aggressive and active cancer therapy should be stopped at the point when it merely serves to make the patient more uncomfortable.

REFERENCES

1. Abrams, R. D., and Finesinger, J. E.: Guilt reactions in patients with cancer. Cancer, 6:474, 1953.
2. Goldberg, R. J.: Management of depression in the patient with advanced cancer. J.A.M.A., 246:373, 1981.
3. Peck, A.: Emotional reactions to having cancer. J. Roentgenol. Radium Ther. Nucl. Med., 114:591, 1972.
4. Plumb, M. M., and Holland, J.: Comparative studies of psychologic function in patients with advanced cancer. Psychosom. Med., 39:264, 1977.
5. Sebberfarb, P. M., Mauer, L. H., and Crouthamel, C. S.: Psychosocial aspects of neoplastic disease. I. Functional status of breast cancer patients during different treatment regimens. Am. J. Psychiatry, 13:450, 1980.
6. Shands, H. C., Finesinger, J. E., Cobb, S., et. al.: Psychological mechanisms in patients with cancer. Cancer, 4:1159, 1951.
7. Stavraky, K. M., Buck, C. W., Lott, S. J., et. al.: Psychological factors in the outcome of human cancer. J. Psychosom. Res., 12:251, 1968.
8. Sutherland, A. M.: Psychological impact of cancer and its therapy. Med. Clin. North Am., 40:705, 1956.
9. Sutherland, A. M., and Orback, C. E.: Psychological impact of cancer and cancer surgery. I. Depressive reactions associative with surgery of cancer. Cancer, 6:958, 1953.

Index

Page numbers in *italics* refer to illustrations; page numbers followed by (t) refer to tables.